Skin Health Information for Teens

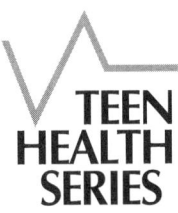

TEEN HEALTH SERIES

First Edition

Skin Health Information for Teens

Health Tips about Dermatological Concerns and Skin Cancer Risks

Including Facts about Acne, Warts, Hives, and Other Conditions and Lifestyle Choices, Such as Tanning, Tattooing, and Piercing, That Affect the Skin, Nails, Scalp, and Hair

◆

Edited by Robert Aquinas McNally

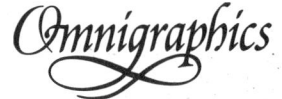

615 Griswold Street • Detroit, MI 48226

Bibliographic Note

Because this page cannot legibly accommodate all the copyright notices, the Bibliographic Note portion of the Preface constitutes an extension of the copyright notice.

Edited by Robert Aquinas McNally

Teen Health Series
Karen Bellenir, *Managing Editor*
David A. Cooke, M.D., *Medical Consultant*
Elizabeth Barbour, *Permissions Associate*
Dawn Matthews, *Verification Assistant*
Laura Pleva Nielsen, *Index Editor*
EdIndex, Services for Publishers, *Indexers*

***

Omnigraphics, Inc.
Matthew P. Barbour, *Senior Vice President*
Kay Gill, *Vice President—Directories*
Kevin Hayes, *Operations Manager*
Leif Gruenberg, *Development Manager*
David P. Bianco, *Marketing Consultant*

***

Peter E. Ruffner, *Publisher*

Frederick G. Ruffner, Jr., *Chairman*

Copyright © 2003 Omnigraphics, Inc.

ISBN 0-7808-0446-5

Library of Congress Cataloging-in-Publication Data

Skin health information for teens : health tips about dermatological concerns and skin cancer risks / edited by Robert Aquinas McNally.--1st ed.
  p. cm. -- (Teen health series)
  "Including facts about acne, warts, hives, and other conditions and lifestyle choices, such as tanning, tattooing, and piercing, that affect the skin, nails, scalp, and hair."
  ISBN 0-7808-0446-5
  1. Teenagers--Health and hygiene. 2. Skin--Care and hygiene. 3. Beauty, Personal. I. McNally, Robert Aquinas. II. Series.
  RA777.S546 2003
  616.5'00835--dc21
                                                              2003053631

Electronic or mechanical reproduction, including photography, recording, or any other information storage and retrieval system for the purpose of resale is strictly prohibited without permission in writing from the publisher.

The information in this publication was compiled from the sources cited and from other sources considered reliable. While every possible effort has been made to ensure reliability, the publisher will not assume liability for damages caused by inaccuracies in the data, and makes no warranty, express or implied, on the accuracy of the information contained herein.

This book is printed on acid-free paper meeting the ANSI Z39.48 Standard. The infinity symbol that appears above indicates that the paper in this book meets that standard.

Printed in the United States

Table of Contents

Preface ix

Part I—Skin Basics

Chapter 1—Skin, Hair, And Nails 3
Chapter 2—Oily Skin, Dry Skin 15
Chapter 3—Flushing And Blushing 19

Part II—Managing The Appearance Of Skin, Nails, And Hair

Chapter 4—Clearing Away Confusion About Cosmetics 25
Chapter 5—Skin Problems From Cosmetics 33
Chapter 6—Brown Spots, Freckles, And Moles 41
Chapter 7—Birthmarks 47
Chapter 8—Stretch Marks 53
Chapter 9—Cellulite: Is There Any Such Thing? 55
Chapter 10—Body Piercing: A Guide For Teens 67
Chapter 11—Tattoos And Permanent Makeup 75
Chapter 12—Making Decisions About Tattooing And
    Body Piercing 81
Chapter 13—Healing Body Piercings 95
Chapter 14—Fingernails: Looking Good, Playing Safe 99
Chapter 15—Head Off Hair-Care Disasters 107
Chapter 16—The Luster In Your Locks 113

Chapter 17—Losing Your Hair 117
Chapter 18—Removing Hair You Don't Want 123

Part III—Acne: Understanding Its Causes And Treatments

Chapter 19—The Skinny On Acne 135
Chapter 20—The Psychological And Social Effects Of Acne 147
Chapter 21—Acne Scarring 151
Chapter 22—Medications That Can Cause Acne 159
Chapter 23—Over-The-Counter Acne Treatments 163
Chapter 24—Prescription Medications For Acne 167
Chapter 25—Accutane®: The Breakthrough Acne Drug 175
Chapter 26—Chemical Peeling For Acne Scars 185

Part IV—Understanding And Preventing Skin Cancer

Chapter 27—Everything You Need To Know About Sun And Skin 191
Chapter 28—Seven Steps To Safer Sunning 199
Chapter 29—Sunscreens And Sun Safety 209
Chapter 30—Indoor Tanning Increases The Risk Of Skin Cancer 221
Chapter 31—Treating Skin Cancer 227
Chapter 32—Moles And Cancer 229
Chapter 33—All About Melanoma 237

Part V—Other Diseases And Conditions That Affect The Skin, Nails, And Scalp

Chapter 34—Eczema 247
Chapter 35—Psoriasis 267
Chapter 36—Cellulitis 275
Chapter 37—Lichen Sclerosis 279
Chapter 38—Vitiligo 285
Chapter 39—Sebaceous Cysts 295
Chapter 40—Warts 297

Chapter 41—Fever Blisters And Cold Sores 301
Chapter 42—Lyme Disease 305
Chapter 43—Cat Scratch Disease 311
Chapter 44—Impetigo 315
Chapter 45—Poison Oak, Ivy, And Sumac 319
Chapter 46—Hives 323
Chapter 47—Swimmer's Itch 327
Chapter 48—Athlete's Foot, Jock Itch, And Ringworm 331
Chapter 49—Nail Disorders And Treatments 335
Chapter 50—Dandruff 343
Chapter 51—Bald Too Soon: Alopecia Areata 347

Part VI—Caring For Injuries To The Skin

Chapter 52—Cuts, Scrapes, And Puncture Wounds 357
Chapter 53—Those Big Scars: Keloids 361
Chapter 54—Taking Care Of Burns 365
Chapter 55—Over-The-Counter Medications For Skin Injuries 369
Chapter 56—Bruises And Contusions 377
Chapter 57—Animal Bites 381
Chapter 58—Insect Bites And Stings 387
Chapter 59—Itching 395

Part VII—Additional Help And Information

Chapter 60—Directory Of Skin-Related Resources 403
Chapter 61—Suggested Reading For Skin-Related Concerns 407

Index 413

Preface

About This Book

Of all the organs of the body, the adolescent years focus most sharply on the skin. Just as young people become uniquely aware of how they look, they are beset by pimples and other skin-related embarrassments. The skin also becomes one of the arenas in which teenagers express their individuality and identity through body piercing, tattooing, and cosmetics. Additionally, adolescent lifestyle choices, such as tanning, greatly influence the health of the skin throughout the rest of life.

Skin Health Information For Teens offers a wealth of information on skin, nails, and hair. The book opens with a section on what the skin is and how it functions. Did you know, for example, that the skin is the body's largest organ? Next the book considers a series of dermatological topics relating to appearance, such as cosmetics, birthmarks, freckles, and moles. Acne is the focus of the third section. Here readers learn what the disease is, how best to treat it with over-the-counter and prescription medications, and what to do about acne scars. Cancer is covered in the fourth section. Readers learn to distinguish the various types of skin cancer and to understand the connection between sun exposure and cancer. The many other kinds of diseases—viral, bacterial, fungal, allergic, and inherited—that affect the skin are discussed next. Injuries to the skin, from cuts to itching, are covered in the following group of chapters. The book concludes with a list of organizations that can provide further information and a list of books for further reading.

How To Use This Book

This book is divided into parts and chapters. Parts focus on broad areas of interest; chapters are devoted to single topics within a part.

Part I: Skin Basics provides fundamental information about what the skin is and about the roles it plays in the body's overall functioning.

Part II: Managing The Appearance Of Skin, Nails And Hair takes on a variety of issues centering on how skin looks and how skin can be altered to change appearance. The chapters in this section address such issues as cosmetics, freckles, moles, birthmarks, cellulite, fingernails, hair loss, and hair removal. It also includes information on the popular practices of tattooing and body piercing.

Part III: Acne addresses this commonplace disease that causes many teenagers grief and anxiety. These chapters look at the underlying disease process, detail its psychological and social effects, describe over-the-counter and prescription treatments, and discuss ways of treating acne scars.

Part IV: Understanding And Preventing Skin Cancer looks at the skin disease most likely to cause major disfigurement and even death. Although skin cancer is relatively uncommon among adolescents, sun exposure in the teenage years sets the stage for skin cancer later in life. In addition, teenagers are at risk for melanoma, the deadliest skin cancer of all. This part's chapters examine the various types of skin cancer, discuss sun safety, and tell teens how to detect skin changes that may indicate cancer.

Part V: Other Diseases That Affect The Skin, Nails, And Scalp examines a long list of viral, bacterial, fungal, allergic, and inherited maladies that may affect the skin and its associated structures. These chapters provide information about eczema, psoriasis, cellulitis, lichen sclerosis, vitiligo, sebaceous cysts, warts, cold sores, Lyme disease, cat scratch disease, impetigo, poison ivy, hives, swimmer's itch, athlete's foot, nail disorders, dandruff, and premature baldness.

Part VI: Caring For Injuries To The Skin discusses the variety of ways the skin can be harmed and the measures one can take in the event of injury. Topics covered include cuts, burns, keloid scars, skin-injury medications, bruises, animal and insect bites, and itching.

Part VII: Additional Help And Information includes a directory of national organizations able to provide skin-related information. Many of these organizations have websites that offer a good beginning point for further research. A chapter of additional reading lists books on topics pertaining to the skin.

Bibliographic Note

This volume contains documents and excerpts from publications issued by the following government agencies: California Department of Health, Centers for Disease Control and Prevention, Environmental Protection Agency, Food and Drug Administration, Federal Trade Commission, National Cancer Institute, National Institute of Arthritis and Musculoskeletal and Skin Diseases, and the Wisconsin Department of Health and Family Services.

In addition, this volume contains copyrighted documents and articles produced by the following organizations: A.D.A.M., Inc.; American Academy of Dermatology; American Academy of Family Physicians; American Academy of Orthopaedic Surgeons; American Academy of Foot and Ankle Surgeons; American Society for Dermatologic Surgery; Center for Young Women's Health, Children's Hospital Boston; Student Health and Wellness Center, Johns Hopkins University; Lyme Disease Foundation; MedicineNet, Inc.; National Alopecia Areata Foundation; Nemours Foundation; New Zealand Dermatological Society; Quackwatch; Skin Cancer Foundation; University Health Services, University of California, Berkeley; Campus Health Pharmacy, University of Arizona; University of Iowa Virtual Hospital; and University of Maryland Medicine.

Full citation information is provided on the first page of each chapter. Every effort has been made to secure all necessary rights to reprint the copyrighted material. If any omissions have been made, please contact Omnigraphics to make corrections for future editions.

Acknowledgements

In addition to the organizations listed above, special thanks are due to verification assistant Dawn Matthews and permission specialist Liz Barbour.

Note From The Editor

This book is part of Omnigraphics' *Teen Health Series*. The series provides basic information about a broad range of medical concerns. It is not intended to serve as a tool for diagnosing illness, in prescribing treatments, or as a substitute for the physician-patient relationship. All persons concerned about medical symptoms or the possibility of disease are encouraged to seek professional care from an appropriate health care provider.

At the request of librarians serving today's young adults, the *Teen Health Series* was developed as a specially focused set of volumes within Omnigraphics' *Health Reference Series*. Each volume deals comprehensively with a topic selected according to the needs and interests of people in middle school and high school. If there is a topic you would like to see addressed in a future volume of the *Teen Health Series*, please write to:

Editor
Teen Health Series
Omnigraphics, Inc.
615 Griswold Street
Detroit, MI 48226

Our Advisory Board

The *Teen Health Series* is reviewed by an Advisory Board comprised of librarians from public, academic, and medical libraries. We would like to thank the following board members for providing guidance to the development of this series:

> Dr. Lynda Baker, Associate Professor of Library and Information Science, Wayne State University, Detroit, MI

> Nancy Bulgarelli, William Beaumont Hospital Library, Royal Oak, MI

Karen Imarisio, Bloomfield Township Public Library, Bloomfield Township, MI

Karen Morgan, Mardigian Library, University of Michigan-Dearborn, Dearborn, MI

Rosemary Orlando, St. Clair Shores Public Library, St. Clair Shores, MI

Medical Consultant

Medical consultation services are provided to the *Teen Health Series* editors by David A. Cooke, M.D. Dr. Cooke is a graduate of Brandeis University, and he received his M.D. degree from the University of Michigan. He completed residency training at the University of Wisconsin Hospital and Clinics. He is board-certified in internal medicine. Dr. Cooke currently works as part of the University of Michigan Health System and practices in Brighton, MI. In his free time, he enjoys writing, science fiction, and spending time with his family.

Part 1
Skin Basics

Chapter 1
Skin, Hair, And Nails

The skin is our largest organ. If the skin of a typical 150-pound adult male were stretched out flat, it would cover about two square yards and weigh about nine pounds!

Our skin protects the network of tissues, muscles, bones, nerves, blood vessels, and everything else inside our bodies. The eyelids have the thinnest skin, and the soles of our feet the thickest.

♣ **It's A Fact!!**

Ask someone to name the body's largest organ, and you'll rarely get the right answer. Most people don't think of the skin as an organ, but it is. And it's the largest single organ in the human body.

Hair is actually a modified type of skin. It grows everywhere on the human body except the palms of the hands, soles of the feet, eyelids, and lips. Hair grows more quickly in summer than in winter and more slowly at night than during the day.

About This Chapter: This information was provided by KidsHealth, one of the largest resources online for medically reviewed information written for parents, kids, and teens. For more articles like this one, visit www.KidsHealth.org or www.TeensHealth.org. © 2001 The Nemours Center for Children's Health Media, a division of the Nemours Foundation. This article is available on the website at http://www.kidshealth.org.

Nails are also a type of modified skin—they're not just for beauty. Our nails protect the sensitive tips of our fingers and toes from everyday wear and tear.

How Are Skin, Hair, And Nails Necessary For Living?

Skin is necessary for our survival. It forms a protective barrier against the outside world that prevents harmful substances and microorganisms (germs like bacteria) from entering the body. It guards delicate body structures and organs against injury and prevents the loss of life-sustaining fluids that bathe body tissues.

Skin also helps to regulate body temperature through perspiration (sweating) and protects us from the damaging ultraviolet (UV) rays of the sun. And without the sensory nerve cells in our skin, we wouldn't be able to distinguish the touch of something sizzling hot or dangerously frozen and other sensations that allow us to protect our bodies from injury.

The hair on our heads keeps us warm by preserving heat. The hair found inside the nose and ears and around the eyes provides protection from dust and other foreign particles. Eyebrows and eyelashes protect us by decreasing the amount of bright light and particles that enter the eyes. The fine hair that covers our bodies provides warmth and additional skin protection. Hair also cushions our bodies—especially our heads—against injury.

Although human nails are not necessary for living, they provide support for the tips of the fingers and toes, protect them from injury, and aid in picking up small objects. Without them, we'd have a hard time scratching an itch or untying a knot! The appearance of someone's nails can be an indicator of general health, and illness often affects nail growth.

Basic Anatomy

Skin

Every square inch of skin contains thousands of cells and hundreds of sweat glands, oil glands, nerve endings, and blood vessels. (See Figure 1.1.)

Skin, Hair, And Nails

Skin is made up of three layers: the epidermis, the dermis, and the subcutaneous (pronounced: sub-kue-tay-nee-us) tissue.

The epidermis is the tough, protective outer skin layer. It is about as thick as a sheet of paper throughout most parts of the body and contains four layers of cells. In these four layers are three special types of cells:

- *Melanocytes* (pronounced: meh-lan-uh-sites), which produce melanin, the pigment that gives skin its color. The more melanin in the skin, the darker the skin color.

- *Keratinocytes* (pronounced: ker-at-ih-no-sites), which produce keratin, the basic component of nails

- *Langerhans cells*, which help protect the body against infection

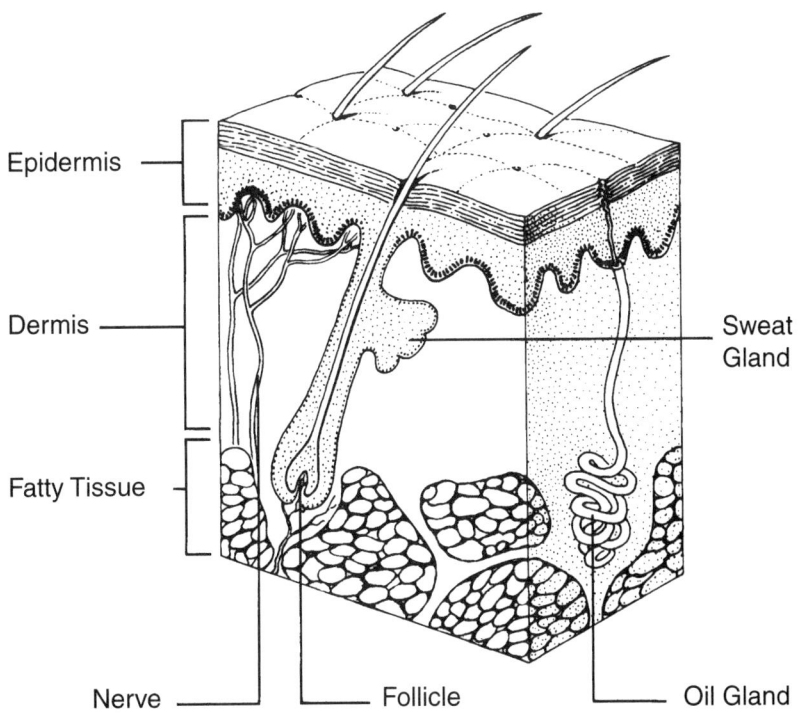

Figure 1.1 *The basic structure of the skin. (Source: National Cancer Institute.)*

The dermis is made up of blood vessels, nerve endings, and connective tissue and connects to the epidermis through tiny projections called papillae (pronounced: puh-pill-ee).

The innermost skin layer, the subcutaneous tissue, is made up of connective tissue, blood vessels, and cells that store fat. Subcutaneous tissue helps protect the body from sudden injury from outside forces, such as falling, and also holds in body heat.

Hair

Human hair consists of the root, a soft, thickened bulb at the base of the hair embedded in the skin, and the shaft, the part we see projecting from the skin's surface. The root ends in the hair bulb, which is lodged in a sac-like pit in the skin called the follicle. Hair grows from the follicle.

At the bottom of the follicle is the papilla (pronounced: puh-pill-uh), where hair growth takes place. The papilla contains an artery that nourishes the root of the hair. As cells are pushed up the follicle, they harden and become the shaft of hair. Each hair has three parts:

- the *medulla*, which is soft and at the center
- the *cortex*, which surrounds the medulla and is the main part of the hair
- the *cuticle*, the hard outer layer that protects the shaft

Nails

Nails are also a type of modified skin. They consist of clear, hardened dead skin cells called keratin.

The epidermis at the base of the nail, under its surface, is called the matrix. The matrix supplies the skin cells that will be transformed into a hardened nail that's continuously growing. At the tip of the matrix is the lunula, the whitish crescent-shaped area that can be seen through the nail at its base. A thin layer of keratin known as the cuticle surrounds the base of the nail and adds protection.

Skin, Hair, And Nails

Normal Physiology

Skin is elastic—it stretches when we bend or smile and repositions itself when we straighten up or return to a relaxed facial expression. This is due to two types of fibers in the dermis: collagen, which is strong and hard to stretch; and elastin, which is elastic and allows skin to move easily.

In older adults, these fibers disappear and skin becomes wrinkled. Because the cells in the epidermis are completely replaced about every 28 days, the skin looks youthful for many years, and cuts and bruises heal quickly.

The dermis layer contains more than 2 million sweat glands. Sweat-producing glands called eccrine glands are found everywhere in the skin, especially in the forehead, palms, and soles of the feet. By producing sweat, these glands help regulate body temperature, and waste products are excreted (removed) through them.

Apocrine glands develop at puberty and are concentrated in the armpits and pubic region. The sweat from the apocrine glands is thick and odorless. When it mixes with bacteria on the skin's surface, this sometimes creates odors. A normal, healthy adult secretes about one pint of sweat each day, but this may be increased by physical activity.

Found mostly on the face and upper body, sebaceous glands lie beneath the walls of the hair follicles. These glands produce an oil called sebum that naturally lubricates the skin and hair. Hair gets its shine from sebum. Sebaceous glands can become overactive during puberty, leading to acne and oily hair that requires frequent shampooing. Later in life, sebaceous glands produce less sebum, often contributing to dry skin and scalp.

Skin gets its color from the melanin produced by epidermal cells called melanocytes. All people have roughly the same amount of melanocytes, but those of dark-skinned people produce more melanin. Exposure to sunlight increases the production of melanin, like when people get suntanned or get freckles.

Hair grows by forming new cells at the base of the root. These cells multiply and push down into the dermis to form a rod of tissue. The cells then move upward as new cells form beneath them. As they move up, they are cut off from their supply of nourishment and start to form a hard protein called keratin (which is also in nails). This process is called keratinization (pronounced: ker-uh-tuh-nuh-zay-shun). As this process occurs, the hair cells die. These dead cells form the shaft of the hair.

The color of a person's hair is determined by how much melanin is in the cortex of each hair and how the melanin is distributed (the same melanin found in the epidermis). Hair also contains a yellow-red pigment; people who have blonde or red hair have only a small amount of melanin in their hair. Hair becomes gray when people age because pigment no longer forms.

Each individual strand of hair grows about one-quarter inch every month and keeps growing in length for up to six years. A hair then falls out and another grows in its place. The length of someone's hair depends on the length of the growing phase of the follicle, and of course, how often he visits a hair stylist. Baldness occurs if hair follicles die and no longer produce new hair. Thick hair grows out of large follicles; narrow follicles produce finer hair.

❧ Weird Words

Apocrine gland: A sweat gland found mostly in the armpits and pubic region.

Collagen: Strong skin fiber housed in the dermis.

Dermis: the layer of skin under the outer layer (epidermis).

Eccrine gland: a kind of sweat gland most prevalent in the forehead, palms, and soles of the feet.

Elastin: Elastic skin fiber housed in the dermis.

Epidermis: The protective top layer of skin.

Follicle: Sac-like pit in the skin from which a hair grows.

Keratin: Tough protein substance in hair and nails.

Keratinocyte: Skin cell that produces the protein keratin.

Skin, Hair, And Nails

Nails grow out of a deep fold in the skin of the fingers and toes. As epidermal cells below the nail root move up to the surface of the skin, they increase in number. The cells closest to the nail root become flattened, are tightly pressed together, and are then transformed into a thin plate. These plates are piled in layers to form the nail. As these cells accumulate, the nail is pushed forward, and grows in length.

Fingernails grow about three times as quickly as toenails. Like hair, nails grow more rapidly in summer than in winter. If a nail is torn off, its regrowth is possible if the matrix at the base of the nail is not severely injured. A fingernail can grow from its matrix to the tip of the finger in about six months; a toenail takes one to one-and-a-half years to grow from the matrix to the tip of a toe.

Diseases, Conditions, And Disorders

It's important to keep the skin, hair, and nails skin clean because many disease-causing organisms can infect them. Some of the more common diseases and conditions include:

Lunula: Whitish, crescent-shaped area of the nail.

Melanin: Black or dark brown coloring found in the skin and hair.

Melanocyte: Skin cell that produces melanin, which gives skin its color.

Nail plate: Large part of the nail.

Root: Soft, thickened bulb at the base of the hair embedded in the skin.

Sebaceous gland: Small gland in the skin that produces an oil called sebum.

Sebum: Oil that lubricates the skin and hair.

Shaft: The part of the hair that projects from the surface of the skin.

Subcutaneous tissue: The innermost layer of skin, which is made up of connective tissue, blood vessels, and cells that store fat.

Disorders Of The Skin

- Dermatitis is any inflammation of the skin. There are many different types of dermatitis, including:
    - *Atopic dermatitis,* also called eczema, is a common hereditary dermatitis that causes an itchy rash primarily on the cheeks, face, trunk, and the arms and legs. It usually develops in infancy, but can also occur in early childhood. It is often associated with other allergic diseases such as asthma and allergic rhinitis.
    - *Contact dermatitis* is an inflammation that occurs when the skin comes in contact with an irritating substance. One well-known cause of contact dermatitis is poison ivy, but there are many others, including chemicals found in laundry detergent, cosmetics, and perfumes. Metals like nickel found in inexpensive jewelry can also cause contact dermatitis.
    - *Seborrheic dermatitis,* common in newborns and adolescents, is caused by an overproduction of sebum from the sebaceous glands and results in a greasy rash on the scalp, face, chest, and sometimes groin area.

- Bacterial infections of the skin:
    - *Impetigo.* A condition that affects mostly kids and teens, impetigo is a bacterial infection that results in honey-colored crusted sores, which often appear on the face near the mouth and nose.
    - *Cellulitis.* Cellulitis is an infection of the skin and underlying tissue that often occurs when bacteria enter through a puncture, bite, or other break in the skin. The infected area is usually warm and tender, has some redness, and is painful.
    - *Streptococcal and staphylococcal infections.* In addition to being the main causes of cellulitis and impetigo, these bacteria are responsible for distinctive rashes on the skin, including the rashes associated with scarlet fever and toxic shock syndrome.

- Fungal infections of the skin:

Skin, Hair, And Nails

- ◊ *Candidal dermatitis.* A warm, moist environment, such as that found in the folds of the skin in the diaper area of infants, is perfect for growing the yeast *Candida*. Candidal dermatitis (yeast infection) is also a common vaginal infection in teen girls.
- ◊ *Tinea corporis* (ringworm). The same type of fungus that causes ringworm in the scalp (tinea capitis) can cause scaly, ring-like lesions anywhere on the body.
- ◊ *Tinea pedis* (athlete's foot) is an infection of the feet that's also caused by the same type of fungus that causes ringworm on the scalp and body. Athlete's foot is commonly found in teens and usually appears during warm weather.

- Other skin infections:
  - ◊ *Viral infections.* Many viruses cause characteristic rashes on the skin, including *Varicella* (chickenpox and shingles), *Herpes simplex* (which causes cold sores), *Papillomavirus* (which causes warts), measles, mumps, parvovirus, and many others.
  - ◊ *Infestations.* When the skin is infested by parasites (usually tiny insects or worms) that burrow into the skin, the result is often an itchy rash. Scabies (dust mites) and lice are examples of infestations. Both are highly contagious, especially among classmates.

- *Acne* (acne vulgaris). Acne is the single most common skin condition in kids and teens. Some degree of acne is seen in 85 percent of adolescents. Acne is the result of clogged sebaceous follicles—a condition that worsens with the hormonal changes of puberty. It is also seen in newborns, although the causes are unknown.

- *Skin cancer.* Though skin cancer is rare in kids and teens, it's crucial to take care of your skin when you're in the sun. The use of sunscreen and other sun protection measures can help prevent melanoma (a serious form of skin cancer that can spread to other parts of the body) later in life, especially among fair-skinned people who sunburn easily and live in very sunny areas.

Disorders Of The Scalp And Hair

- *Tinea capitis*, also known as ringworm, is not a worm at all but a type of fungal infection that forms a scaly, ringlike lesion in the scalp. It's fairly contagious and common among kids and teens in school.
- *Alopecia* is an area of hair loss. Ringworm is a common cause of alopecia in kids. Alopecia areata (rapid hair loss in round or oval patches on the scalp) is a rarer condition with unknown causes, although stress has been suggested as a contributing factor.

Disorders Of The Nail

- *Nail pitting* occurs occasionally in healthy nails, but deep, patterned pitting can be seen with certain chronic diseases. For example, psoriasis (pronounced: suh-rye-uh-sis) is a chronic skin disorder that commonly involves deep pits forming in the nail.
- *Nail biting* is a common habit that may last into adulthood. Nail biting is generally harmless, but can sometimes cause irritation or infections in the skin surrounding the cuticle or nail. Nail biting can be helped by applying foul-tasting substances (that can be purchased at your local pharmacy) made especially for this purpose to the nails.
- In *ingrown toenails*, which commonly affect the big toe, the nail pierces the skin surrounding it, causing pain and swelling. Shoes that don't fit properly, foot or toe injuries, and improper trimming of the nail can all lead to ingrown toenails. Treatment includes removal of part or all of the affected nail and antibiotics if there is an infection.
- *Subungual hematoma* is caused by injury (usually a hard direct blow, like a door shutting on a fingertip) to the nail, which results in pain, bleeding, and blood collection under the nail's surface. This can cause the nail to separate and sometimes fall off. Usually the blood needs to be drained from under the nail (this should be done by a health care professional as soon as possible) to prevent further damage to the tissues of the fingertip and to help prevent the nail from falling off.

Skin, Hair, And Nails

- Bacterial infections of the nail:
    - ◊ *Paronychia* (pronounced: par-oh-nick-ee-uh) is an infection behind the cuticle of the nail that can form an abscess (collection of pus). Paronychia can occur from nail biting, from going to nail salons that don't use sterile equipment, or from cuts on the cuticle. Treatment includes draining the abscess and taking antibiotics.
- Fungal infections of the nail:
    - ◊ *Tinea unguium* (pronounced: ung-gwee-um), or ringworm of the nail, is a fungal infection that can cause nails to become thick and discolored. It can be treated with antifungal medication and may take several months to disappear.

Chapter 2

Oily Skin, Dry Skin

Oily Skin

Heredity and hormones play the key role in whether or not you have oily skin. The most important thing you can do for oily skin is to work hard and consistently at keeping your skin clean using hot water and soap. Cleaning your face with astringent pads is also recommended if washing your face frequently is leaving your skin irritated. Use only water-based cosmetics if you have oily skin. If is extremely unlikely that your diet has anything to do with whether or not you have oily skin.

Dry Skin

Alternative Names

Dry skin; asteatosis; winter itch.

Definition

This symptom is a skin irritation caused by lack of moisture in the skin.

About This Chapter: The text in this chapter includes "Oily Skin" and "Skin — Dry," © 2002 A.D.A.M., Inc. Reprinted with permission. Available online at http://www.nlm.nih.gov/medlineplus/ency/article/002043.htm and http://www.nlm.nih.gov/medlineplus/ency/article/003250.htm.

Considerations

To help prevent dry skin, maintain moisture in the body and skin, especially during the winter.

Symptoms often associated with dry skin include:

- Skin feels dry, may have scales
- Itching (pruritus)
- Cracks in the skin
- Round patches of irritated skin
- Most common on the lower legs, arms, flanks, and thighs

> **Weird Words**
>
> Asteatosis: Medical term for dry skin.
>
> Pruritus: Medical term for itching.

Common Causes

Dry skin is extremely common, especially in the elderly. It is seen more often in the winter when cold air outside and heated air inside may cause a decrease in humidity. Use of a forced-air furnace increases the risk.

The skin loses moisture and may crack and peel, or become irritated and inflamed. Too frequent bathing, especially with harsh soaps, may contribute further to dry skin.

When To Call Your Health Care Provider

If dry skin is present and persists despite treatment, or if new symptoms develop, call your health care provider.

The medical history will be obtained, and a physical examination performed. Medical history questions documenting your dry skin in detail may include:

- Time pattern
    - ◊ When did it develop?
    - ◊ Has your skin always been dry?

- Location
    - ◊ Is all of the skin dry?
    - ◊ Is the dryness only in a specific location?
- Aggravating factors
    - ◊ What makes it seem worse?
    - ◊ What are your bathing habits?
- Relieving factors
    - ◊ What have you done to try to make it better?
    - ◊ How well has that worked?
- Other
    - ◊ What other symptoms are also present?

The physical examination will include special attention to examination of the skin. A diagnosis is made on the basis of your medical history and the appearance of the skin.

✔ **Quick Tip**

Home Care For Dry Skin

Decrease moisture loss by changing bathing habits. Short baths should be taken, with tepid (not hot) water. Minimize the use of soap; limit its use to face, armpits, and genitals if possible. Dry the skin gently. There may be a need to reduce the frequency of bathing.

Increase or maintain skin and body moisture. Bath oils or moisturizers may help, especially if used at least daily. Thick, greasy moisturizers work best. Use of a humidifier may help if the air is very dry.

Inflammation may be reduced by over-the-counter or prescribed cortisone creams or other antiinflammatory creams or lotions.

Chapter 3

Flushing And Blushing

Alternative Names

Blushing; flushing; red face.

Definition

A sudden reddening of the face, neck, and, occasionally, upper chest.

Considerations

Blushing is a normal response when one is embarrassed, angry, feeling guilty, or experiencing some other strong emotion. Flushing of the face may also be associated with certain medical conditions.

Common Causes

- Extremes of emotion
- Rapid changes in temperature
- Hot or spicy foods
- Rosacea
- High fever

About This Chapter: Text in this chapter is from "Skin Blushing/Flushing," © 2002 A.D.A.M., Inc. Reprinted with permission. Available online at http://www.nlm.nih.gov/medlineplus/ency/article/003241.htm.

- Alcohol abuse or alcohol intolerance
- Medications such as Diabinese® (for diabetics) and niacin (for lowering cholesterol; sometimes contained in high-potency vitamins)
- Menopause ("hot flush"; due to a drop in estrogen levels)
- Carcinoid syndrome

Home Care

Eliminate any triggers that you can identify. Try to avoid hot drinks, spicy food, extremes of temperature, and bright sunlight.

When To Call Your Health Care Provider

- There is continual and persistent flushing.
- Other symptoms, such as diarrhea, are present.

What To Expect

The medical history will be obtained and a physical examination performed. Medical history questions documenting your skin blushing/flushing in detail may include:

- Location
    ◊ Do you have facial flushing (blushing)?
    ◊ Does it affect the whole body?
- Quality
    ◊ Are you having hot flushes?
- Time pattern
    ◊ Do you have flushing attacks?
    ◊ How often do you have flushing or blushing?

> **✎ Weird Words**
>
> <u>Carcinoid syndrome</u>: Irregular blotching or flushing that results from cancer in the stomach or intestine spreading to the liver; other symptoms involve the heart, lungs, and brain.
>
> <u>Rosacea</u>: A persistent condition involving enlargement of blood vessels and pores in the skin of the nose and cheeks; varies from mild to severe.
>
> Source: Adapted from *Stedman's Medical Dictionary, 27th Edition*, © 2000. Lippincott Williams, and Wilkins. All rights reserved. Reprinted with permission.

       ◊ Are episodes getting worse?
       ◊ Are they getting more frequent?
- Aggravating factors
    ◊ Is it worse after alcohol intake?
- Other
    ◊ What other symptoms are also present?
    ◊ Is there diarrhea?
    ◊ Is there wheezing?
    ◊ Are there hives?
    ◊ Is there difficulty breathing?

Part 2

Managing The Appearance Of Skin, Nails, And Hair

Chapter 4

Clearing Away Confusion About Cosmetics

Cosmetics run the gamut from eye shadow to deodorant sprays. And consumers' concerns and questions are just as varied as the products themselves.

"Consumers are so confused by the products out there because they all do so many different things," says Lynn Reniers, a licensed cosmetologist with Elizabeth Arden. "So it's important to send them away with a very clear understanding of product usage."

When the U.S. Food and Drug Administration (FDA) surveyed 1,687 consumers ages 14 and older in 1994 about their use of cosmetics, many of the responses pertained to consumer perceptions about cosmetic labeling claims. For example, many said they expect a product to prevent or slow the formation of wrinkles if it makes such a claim on its packaging. And nearly half of those surveyed felt that a product claiming to be "natural" should contain all natural ingredients. But do these products live up to their labeling claims?

Not necessarily. John Bailey, Ph.D., director of FDA's Office of Cosmetics and Colors, says, "Image is what the cosmetics industry sells through its products, and it's up to the consumer to believe the claims or not."

About This Chapter: Taken from "Clearing Up Cosmetic Confusion," published originally in *FDA Consumer* in May–June 1998 and revised in May 1998 and August 2000; available in revised form at http://www.fda.gov/fdac/features/1998/398_cosm.html.

Behind the image, however, are real products, and consumers want to know what works and what doesn't.

An understanding of FDA's cosmetic responsibilities can help consumers make wise, rational decisions about the cosmetics they buy.

Regulatory Authority

The regulatory requirements governing the sale of cosmetics are not as stringent as those that apply to other FDA-regulated products. Under the Federal Food, Drug, and Cosmetic (FD&C) Act, cosmetics and their ingredients are not required to undergo approval before they are sold to the public. Generally, FDA regulates these products after they have been released to the marketplace. This means that manufacturers may use any ingredient or raw material, except for color additives and a few prohibited substances, to market a product without a government review or approval.

But some regulations do apply to cosmetics. In addition to the FD&C Act, the Fair Packaging and Labeling Act requires an ingredient declaration on every cosmetic product offered for sale to consumers. In addition, these regulations require that ingredients be listed in descending order of quantity. Water, for example, accounts for the bulk of most skin-care products, which is why it usually appears first on these products.

Although companies are not required to substantiate performance claims or conduct safety testing, if safety has not been substantiated, the product's label must read "WARNING: The safety of this product has not been determined."

"Consumers believe that 'if it's on the market, it can't hurt me,'" says Bailey. "And this belief is sometimes wrong."

♣ **It's A Fact!!**

Some products are both cosmetics and drugs. A few examples:

- Dandruff shampoos
- Fluoride toothpastes
- Antiperspirant deodorants
- Foundations and tanning preparations that contain sunscreen

Clearing Away Confusion About Cosmetics

FDA's challenge comes in proving that a product is harmful under conditions of use or that it is improperly labeled. Only then can the agency take action to remove adulterated or misbranded products from the marketplace.

The Fine Line Between Cosmetics And Drugs

The FD&C Act defines cosmetics as articles intended to be applied to the human body for cleansing, beautifying, promoting attractiveness, or altering appearance without affecting the body's structure or functions. This definition includes skin-care creams, lotions, powders and sprays, perfumes, lipsticks, fingernail polishes, eye and facial makeup, permanent waves, hair colors, deodorants, baby products, bath oils, bubble baths, and mouthwashes, as well as any material intended for use as a component of a cosmetic product.

Products that intend to treat or prevent disease or otherwise affect structure or function of the human body are considered drugs. Cosmetics that make therapeutic claims are regulated as drugs and cosmetics, and must meet the labeling requirements for both. A good way to tell if you're buying a cosmetic that is also regulated as a drug is to see if the first ingredient listed is an "active ingredient." The active ingredient is the chemical that makes the product effective, and the manufacturer must have proof that it's safe for its intended use. For products that are both drugs and cosmetics, the regulations require that active ingredients be listed first on these products, followed by the list of cosmetic ingredients in order of decreasing predominance.

Before products with both a cosmetic and drug classification can be marketed, they must be scientifically proven safe and effective for their therapeutic claims. If they are not, FDA considers them to be misbranded and can take regulatory action.

Reading Is Believing

The ingredient list on a cosmetic container is the only place where a consumer can readily find out the truth about what he or she is buying. Consumers can check the listing to identify substances they wish to avoid.

✔ **Quick Tip**

Beauty On The Safe Side

Serious injury from makeup is a rare occurrence, according to John Bailey, director of FDA's Office of Cosmetics and Colors. But it does happen. Good common sense and a few precautions can help consumers protect themselves against hazards associated with the misuse of cosmetics.

- *Never drive and apply makeup.* Not only does it make for dangerous driving, but hitting a bump in the road and scratching your eyeball can cause bacteria to contaminate the cut and could result in serious injury, including blindness.

- *Never share makeup.* Always use a new disposable applicator when sampling products at a cosmetics counter. Insist that salespersons clean container openings with alcohol before applying their contents to your skin.

- *Never add liquid to a product to bring back its original consistency.* Adding other liquids could introduce bacteria that can easily grow out of control.

- *Stop using any product that causes an allergic reaction.*

- *Throw away makeup if the color changes or an odor develops.* Preservatives degrade over time and may no longer be able to fight bacteria.

- *Do not use eye makeup if you have an eye infection.* Throw away all products you were using when you discovered the infection.

- *Keep makeup out of sunlight.* Light and heat can degrade preservatives.

- *Keep makeup containers tightly closed when not in use.*

- *Never use aerosol beauty products near heat or while smoking because they can ignite.* Hairsprays and powders may cause lung damage if inhaled regularly.

Clearing Away Confusion About Cosmetics

And becoming familiar with what cosmetics contain can help counter some of the alluring appeal showcased elsewhere on the product.

"Our best friend is the ingredient label," says beauty consultant and 14-year veteran consumer reporter Paula Begoun. "And spending the time to read it may be all that is needed to protect ourselves from hurting our skin."

But the ingredient list, although a mandatory requirement on cosmetics, is also the most difficult part of the label to understand. Bailey admits that most of us don't recognize the names of the ingredients listed because there are thousands available to chemists creating a wide variety of products. But there's no way to change that, he says, and still accurately identify the substances that are used.

Consumers can, however, obtain specific information about a cosmetic ingredient in various references, such as the *International Cosmetic Ingredient Dictionary and Handbook*, published by the Cosmetic, Toiletry, and Fragrance Association, available at many public libraries. FDA recognizes the association as a reliable source of facts on substances that have been identified as cosmetic ingredients, as well as their definitions and trade names.

Cosmetic ingredient declaration regulations apply only to retail products intended for home use. Cosmetic samples and products used exclusively by beauticians in salons are not required to include the ingredient declaration. However, these products must state the distributor, list the content's quantity, and include all necessary warning statements.

They Can Be Irritating

Almost all cosmetics can cause allergic reactions in certain individuals. Often the first sign of a reaction is a mild redness and irritation. There is no list of ingredients that can be guaranteed not to cause allergic reactions, so consumers who are prone to allergies should pay careful attention to what they use on their skin.

Nearly one-quarter of the people questioned in FDA's 1994 cosmetics survey responded "yes" to having suffered an allergic reaction to personal care products, including moisturizers, foundations, and eye shadows.

"Because of the almost limitless combinations in all sorts of mixtures and formulations, it is virtually impossible to know if, when, or how anyone's skin will react to any cosmetic," Begoun says. She advises consumers to "buy with a healthy dose of skepticism," and to stop using an offending product and return it to the place of purchase. "Returning the product gives the cosmetics company essential information about how these formulas are working."

What Lies Behind The Meaning

FDA has tried to establish official definitions for the use of certain terms such as "natural" and "hypoallergenic," but its regulations were overturned in court. So companies can use them on cosmetic labels to mean anything or nothing at all. Most of the terms have considerable market value in promoting cosmetic products to consumers, but dermatologists say they have very little medical meaning.

Some of the more common terms that consumers should be aware of include:

- *Natural*: implies that ingredients are extracted directly from

> ✔ **Quick Tip**
>
> ## Helping The Buyer Beware: Hydroxy Acids
>
> Despite many questions about their safety, alpha hydroxy acids (AHAs) and beta hydroxy acids (BHAs) have become widely used in recent years. AHAs are derived from fruit and milk sugars, and are among the popular ingredients that attract customers with their claims to reduce wrinkles and age spots, and help repair sun-damaged skin.
>
> FDA recommends that consumers take precautions with AHA and BHA products:
>
> - Test any AHA/BHA-containing product on a small area of skin before applying to a larger area.
> - Avoid the sun when possible.
> - Use an effective sunscreen when using an AHA-containing product, even if you haven't used the product that day.
> - Follow use instructions on the label.
> - Do not exceed recommended applications.
> - Do not use on infants and children.

plants or animal products as opposed to being produced synthetically. There is no basis in fact or scientific legitimacy to the notion that products containing natural ingredients are good for the skin.

- *Hypoallergenic*: implies that products making this claim are less likely to cause allergic reactions. There are no prescribed scientific studies required to substantiate this claim. Likewise, the terms "dermatologist-tested," "sensitivity tested," "allergy tested," or "nonirritating" carry no guarantee that they won't cause skin reactions.

- *Alcohol-free*: traditionally meant that certain cosmetic products do not contain ethyl alcohol (or grain alcohol). Cosmetic products, however, may contain other alcohols, such as cetyl, stearyl, cetearyl, or lanolin, which are known as fatty alcohols.

> ✔ **Quick Tip**
> "Natural" doesn't necessarily mean "safe." Poison ivy is "natural."

- *Fragrance-free*: implies that a cosmetic product so labeled has no perceptible odor. Fragrance ingredients may be added to a fragrance-free cosmetic to mask any offensive odor originating from the raw materials used, but in a smaller amount than is needed to impart a noticeable scent.

- *Noncomedogenic*: suggests that products do not contain common pore-clogging ingredients that could lead to acne.

- *Shelf life (expiration date)*: the amount of time for which a cosmetic product is good under normal conditions of storage and use, depending on the product's composition, packaging, preservation, etc. Expiration dates are, for practical purposes, a rule of thumb, and a product may expire long before that date if it has not been stored and handled properly.

- *Cruelty-free*: implies that products have not been tested on animals. Most ingredients used in cosmetics have at some point been tested on animals so consumers may want to look for "no new animal testing," to get a more accurate indication.

The list of ingredients, once again, can help consumers determine if there is any significant difference between products labeled with terms in the list and competing brands that don't make these claims.

Since the cosmetics industry often produces new, reworked versions of old ingredients, a wise consumer will take the time to read the labels to know what's in a product and how to use it safely. After all, consumers are likely to try other products with the same recognizable names. Once you have all the information, you can begin to make your own decisions about what products work best for you.

"There is really very little that's new under the sun," Bailey concludes, "and that certainly applies to cosmetics."

—by Carol Lewis

> ♣ **It's A Fact!!**
>
> **Prohibited Ingredients**
>
> The following ingredients, because of the dangers they impose, are either restricted or prohibited by regulation for use in cosmetics:
>
> - Bithionol
> - Mercury compounds
> - Vinyl chloride
> - Halogenated salicylanilides
> - Zirconium complexes in aerosol cosmetics
> - Chloroform
> - Methylene chloride
> - Chlorofluorocarbon propellants
> - Hexachlorophene
> - Methyl methacrylate monomer in nail products

Chapter 5

Skin Problems From Cosmetics

Cosmetics and skin care products are part of most people's daily grooming habits. The average adult uses at least seven different skin care products each day. These include fragrances, astringents, moisturizers, sunscreens, skin cleansers, hair care items, deodorants/antiperspirants, colored cosmetics, hair cosmetics, and nail cosmetics.

Most people experience few problems from these products. Dermatologists estimate that problems arise in only .021 percent of all people (about one in 5,000).

However, problems can arise either with the first few applications or after years of use. Most people know which product is causing the problem. Severe, chronic reactions may require the skills of a dermatologist. This article will help identify possible product-related problems and suggest solutions.

What Are The Possible Problems Associated With The Use Of Cosmetics And Skin Care Products?

Reactions to skin care products depend on the condition of the skin and the immune system. Uninjured skin is an excellent barrier to most substances

---

About This Chapter: From the brochure, "Solving Problems Related to the Use of Cosmetics and Skin Care Products," © 1999 American Academy of Dermatology. Available at http://www.aad.org/pamphlets/cosmetic.html. Reprinted with permission from the American Academy of Dermatology. All rights reserved.

found in cosmetics and skin care products. If skin is overly dry or injured, openings make that barrier less protective. This is the most common setting for problems related to the use of skin care or cosmetic products, which can be simple irritation or a true allergy.

What Is Irritant Contact Dermatitis?

Burning, stinging, itching, and redness may be signs that a product is irritating the skin. Bath soaps, detergents, antiperspirants, eye cosmetics, moisturizers, permanent hair-waving solutions, and shampoos are the most common skin irritants. Even water can irritate very dry skin. Irritant contact dermatitis is the most common problem seen with cosmetics and skin care products.

What Is Allergic Contact Dermatitis?

Some people are allergic to a specific ingredient or ingredients in a product. Symptoms include redness, swelling, itching, and fluid-filled blisters. People will usually react whenever they are exposed to the ingredient, although it could take up to several days for the symptoms to appear.

What Are Some Of The Ingredients That Cause Allergic Reactions?

Fragrances and preservatives, ingredients commonly found in skin care products and cosmetics, cause most skin problems.

Fragrances

Fragrances cause more allergic contact dermatitis than any other ingredient. More than 5,000 different fragrances are used in cosmetics and skin care products. Hypoallergenic fragrances have been developed to minimize the problem.

Remember that a product labeled "unscented" may in fact contain a fragrance to mask other chemical odors. A product must be marked "fragrance-free" or "without perfume" to indicate nothing has been added to make it smell good. Some fragrance reactions occur only when the skin is exposed to sunlight.

Skin Problems From Cosmetics

Preservatives

Preservatives in cosmetics and skin care products are the second most common cause of skin reactions. They prevent bacterial and fungal growths that can cause skin infections, and they protect products from oxygen and light damage. Cosmetics that contain water must include some type of preservative. Consumers who react to one preservative will not necessarily react to others. Examples of preservatives include paraben, imidazolidinyl urea, quaternium-15, DMDM hydantoin, phenoxyethanol, methylchloroisothiazolinone, and formaldehyde.

What Are Skin Care Products?

Skin care products are designed to maintain healthy skin. They include astringents, moisturizers, and sunscreens.

Astringents

Astringents remove oils and soap residue from the skin. They are generally drying and may contain water, alcohol, propylene glycol, witch hazel, or salicylic acid. Individuals with dry, sensitive, or irritated skin may experience itching, burning, or tingling following the use of astringents.

Moisturizers

Dry skin develops cracks and fine wrinkles, losing effectiveness as a barrier and causing pain and itching. Moisturizers prevent water loss by layering an oily substance over the skin to keep water in or by attracting water to the outer skin layer from the inner skin layer.

Substances that stop water loss include petrolatum, mineral oil, lanolin, and silicone. Substances that attract water to the skin include glycerin, propylene glycol, proteins, and some vitamins. People may be allergic to any of these.

Sunscreens

Sunscreens contain chemicals that absorb, reflect, or scatter light. Light-absorbing chemicals include the PABA esters, avobenzone, and the cinnamates. People can sometimes be allergic to these ingredients. Physical sunscreens contain fine powders of zinc oxide or titanium dioxide. There are no known allergies to physical sunscreens.

What Are Personal Care Products?

Personal care products that help keep skin and hair clean and fresh smelling include skin cleansers, shampoos, conditioners, and deodorants/antiperspirants.

Skin Cleansers

Soaps, detergents, and bubble baths remove dirt, body oils, and bacteria, while preventing odor and infection. Heavy use of these products can overdry the skin, causing flaking, itching, and irritation. People with dry skin should choose a mild cleanser, shower with cool water, minimize water contact, and apply a moisturizer immediately after bathing.

Soaps come in several different varieties. Deodorant soaps use an antibacterial agent to eliminate odors, but may be irritating. Beauty bar soaps are generally less drying and irritating.

> **Weird Words**
>
> <u>Dermatitis</u>: Inflammation of the skin.
>
> <u>Hypoallergenic</u>: A product formulated to reduce the likelihood of allergic reaction.
>
> <u>Nonacnegenic</u>: A product that does not cause or promote acne.
>
> <u>Noncomedogenic</u>: A product that does not cause or promote comedos, the medical term for blackheads and other acne lesions.

Shampoos

Shampoos remove dirt and oils from the scalp and leave the hair soft and shiny. Allergic reactions to shampoos are uncommon since their contact with the skin is brief, but they can irritate and dry the skin when rinsed over the body.

There are several types of shampoos. Mild baby shampoos don't irritate the eyes; conditioning shampoos cleanse lightly and leave hair soft; shampoos for oily hair remove oil; and shampoos for damaged hair are pH-adjusted to prevent more damage.

Skin Problems From Cosmetics

Conditioners

Conditioners are sometimes applied after shampooing to make hair shiny, easier to comb and style, and more manageable. They are not a common source of skin reactions.

Deodorants And Antiperspirants

Deodorants kill bacteria and leave a pleasant smell. Antiperspirants prevent sweating. The fragrance in deodorants and the aluminum salts in antiperspirants rarely cause problems. Skin irritation can occur if these products are used on already-irritated skin or right after shaving or if they are spread too widely around the armpit.

What Are Colored Cosmetics?

Colored cosmetics are applied to the face, eyes, and lips to beautify and adorn the body.

Facial Cosmetics

Facial cosmetics, or "makeup," are used to color the face. It is important to select makeup carefully since it remains in contact with the skin for a long time. Ideally, makeup should be hypoallergenic, noncomedogenic, and nonacnegenic—meaning it produces fewer allergies and won't plug pores or cause acne. Look for cosmetics with sunscreen, which will help prevent skin cancer and wrinkles.

Eye Cosmetics

Eyelids, the most sensitive skin on the body, need to be treated with care. Eye cosmetics include eye shadow, eyeliner, and mascara. Lighter colored, matte-finish, powered eye shadows are less irritating. Scrubbing or vigorous rubbing to remove eye cosmetics may irritate eyelids. Water-soluble (or washable) eye cosmetics are easier to remove. Remember that other irritating and allergenic substances can be introduced to the eye area by the fingers.

Eye cosmetics should never be shared with others, and they should be replaced every three to four months because of possible bacterial contamination.

Lip Cosmetics

Lip cosmetics, lipsticks, and lip balms moisturize dry, cracked lips and provide sun protection. Some long-wearing lip stains have been linked to allergic contact dermatitis.

What Are Hair Cosmetics?

The hair's appearance can be altered by changing its color through dyeing or its shape by permanent waving.

Dyes

Temporary hair dyes wash out after one shampoo. Gradual hair dyes produce a color change over a two- to three-week period. These dyes generally don't cause problems. Semipermanent hair dyes that wash out after four to six shampoos and permanent hair dyes that don't wash out can cause allergic reactions. These products should be tested on a small area of skin behind the ear or inside the elbow for 24 hours before use.

☞ **Remember!!**

Cosmetics and skin care products are part of grooming and daily hygiene. Problems rarely develop from the use of these products. If a problem is suspected, your dermatologist may suggest patch testing to help determine whether an allergy to ingredients in these products exists. Your dermatologist can also answer your questions and provide additional information on how to use cosmetics and skin care products safely.

Skin Problems From Cosmetics

Permanent hair dyes make hair lighter or darker. Ammonium persulfate, sometimes used to lighten hair, can cause contact dermatitis in some individuals. It can also cause an immediate allergic reaction of hives and wheezing.

Permanent Waving

"Permanents" make straight hair curly. A perm solution breaks the chemical bonds in straight hair to reform them in a curled position. The process can damage the hair. Hair should not be permed more often than every three months. If the perming solution is left on too long, is too strong, or is applied to hair already damaged by dyes, bleaches, or recent permanents, the hair can break. Scalp irritation may also occur.

What Are Nail Cosmetics?

Nail cosmetics are used to color nails, increase nail strength, or artificially add nail length.

Polishes

Nail polishes can cause allergic contact dermatitis. A person allergic to nail polish may develop a rash on the fingers or eyelids, face, and neck—places the nail polish may have touched while it was drying. People with nail polish allergies can try hypoallergenic varieties that are formaldehyde-free.

Cuticles prevent infection and protect nail-forming cells and should not be cut or removed.

Artificial Nails

The illusion of long nails can be created with plastic nails that cover the entire nail or nail tips. These artificial nails attach with glue that may contain methacrylate, a known allergen. Methacrylate-free glues may cause the underlying nail to peel and crack. Nail repair kits also use these glues.

Sculptured Nails

Long-term use of sculptured nails, custom-made to fit permanently over natural nails, can cause severe and painful reactions, including infection of the skin around the nail, loosening or loss of nails, and dermatitis.

Women who have worn artificial or sculptured nails for a long time may notice their real nails are thin, dull, and brittle. Dermatologists recommend that regular artificial nail users take them off every three months to allow natural nails to rest.

What Are Cosmeceuticals?

Cosmeceuticals are skin care products designed to go beyond strictly coloring and adorning the skin. These products actually improve the functioning of the skin and may be helpful in preventing premature aging. Examples of these substances are alpha hydroxy acids, such as glycolic acid, beta hydroxy acid, and salicylic acid. These hydroxy acids increase skin exfoliation (the removal of dead skin cells), making aging skin appear smoother and feel softer. Some vitamins, such as vitamin A (retinal), improve the appearance of aging skin by making the skin function better. Dermatologists know how to use these new cosmeceutical ingredients and can customize skin care routines for their patients to achieve healthy-looking skin.

Chapter 6

Brown Spots, Freckles, And Moles

Brown Spots And Freckles

Freckles, known in medical parlance as ephelides, are small flat brown marks arising on the face and other sun-exposed areas. They are seen in children and in fair-skinned people, especially those with red hair, who have an inherited predisposition for them on the face and other areas exposed to the sun. The characteristic color of freckles comes from the pigment melanin accumulating in the skin cells.

Ephelides are prominent in summer but fade considerably or disappear in winter as old skin cells are replaced by new cells. As the person ages, this type of freckle generally become less noticeable. Apart from sun protection, no particular treatment is necessary.

Larger flat brown spots on the face and hands arising in middle age also result from sun damage. Unlike freckles, they tend to persist for long periods and don't disappear in the winter (though they may fade). Commonly known as age spots or liver spots, the correct term for a single lesion is benign solar lentigo (plural, lentigines). Lentigines are common in those with fair skin

---

About This Chapter: These pages are reprinted from "Brown Spots and Freckles" and "Moles" with the permission of DermNet, the website of the New Zealand Dermatological Society. Visit www.dermnetnz.org for patient information on numerous skin conditions and their treatment. © 2002 New Zealand Dermatological Society.

but are frequently seen in those who tan easily or have naturally dark skin. Lentigines are due to accumulated pigment cells (melanocytic hyperplasia).

If the brown marks are scaly, they may be solar keratoses (sun damage) or seborrheic keratoses (senile warts). These are usually treated by cryotherapy.

It is important to distinguish the benign solar lentigo from an early malignant melanoma (a potentially fatal form of skin cancer), called a lentigo maligna. If the freckle has arisen recently, is made up of more than one color, or has irregular borders, or if you have any doubts, see your dermatologist for advice.

> ✔ **Quick Tip**
> **What To Do About Brown Spots?**
>
> Benign lentigines can be faded with careful sun protection and regular applications of anti-aging creams containing antioxidants, such as alpha hydroxy acids, vitamin C, retinoids, and azelaic acid.
>
> However, they can be removed even more effectively by chemical peels, cryotherapy, or certain pigment lasers, which produce either green or red light absorbed by melanin. Intense pulsed light (PhotoDerm) has a similar effect. Carbon dioxide and Erbium:YAG lasers vaporize the surface skin, thus removing the pigmented lesions. Results are variable but sometimes very impressive with minimal risk of scarring.
>
> With superficial resurfacing techniques, there is minimal discomfort and no downtime, but several treatments are often necessary. Unfortunately the treatment occasionally makes the pigmentation worse. Continued careful sun protection is essential, because the pigmentation is likely to recur next summer.
>
> Unsightly benign skin moles may be removed with traditional surgical techniques (excision biopsy or resurfacing laser).

Moles

Moles are common and usually harmless skin lesions. Correctly called melanocytic or pigmented nevi (singular, nevus), moles may be flat or protruding. They vary in color from pink flesh tones to dark brown or black. The number of moles a person has depends on genetic factors and on sun exposure; most individuals have 20 to 50 of them.

Melanocytic nevi may be present at birth (congenital) but more usually begin to grow during childhood, although new ones can appear at any age, sometimes in crops. Since early nevus cells form nests on the junction between the epidermis (outer layer of the skin) and the dermis (inner layer), they are known as junctional nevi. These are flat colorful moles. With maturity, nests of nevus cells can also form in the dermis (compound nevi) or may only be found in the dermis (intradermal nevi). These nevi are thickened and often protrude from the skin surface. Heavily pigmented dermal nevi appear blue (blue nevi).

Moles may darken following sun exposure or during pregnancy. During adulthood they often lose their pigmentation, and they may even disappear in old age.

> ### ✎ Weird Words
>
> Congenital: Present at birth.
>
> Cryotherapy: The use of extreme cold, usually in the form of liquid nitrogen, to remove tissue.
>
> Melanoma: A potentially fatal form of skin cancer that often begins as an abnormal mole. See Chapter 33 for more detail.
>
> Source: Adapted from *Stedman's Medical Dictionary, 27th Edition*, © 2000. Lippincott Williams, and Wilkins. All rights reserved. Reprinted with permission.

Types Of Moles

Congenital Pigmented Nevus

A mole present at birth is called a congenital pigmented nevus. One in 100 babies has a congenital pigmented nevus varying in size from a few millimeters in diameter to covering half the baby's skin. There may an increased risk of melanoma developing within congenital nevi, especially very large ones, so if any change has been noted, it should be checked by a doctor.

Halo Nevus

Sometimes the skin around a mole loses its color so the mole appears to be surrounded by a white ring. This halo nevus occurs most often in children and teenagers. It is harmless, and with time the central mole and the white ring disappear. Loss of color may also be seen in melanoma, so if in doubt, the mole should be checked by a dermatologist.

Atypical Nevi

Atypical nevi are moles that have unusual features, often resembling a cancerous mole (melanoma), but are actually benign. Because of their worrying appearance, they are often removed, although this is not always necessary. People with atypical nevi may have an increased risk of developing melanoma, especially if there has been a close family member who has had a melanoma.

> ✔ **Quick Tip**
>
> **Hairy Moles**
>
> The coarse hair that sometimes grows in a mole can be removed by shaving. Plucking may cause inflammation, resulting in a painful lump under the mole. The hair can only be removed permanently by electrolysis (destroying the hair follicle with an electric needle) or surgical removal of the whole mole.

Change In A Mole

Malignant melanoma is a cancerous growth occurring in melanocytes (pigment cells). A melanoma may look much like a harmless mole.

If a mole changes size, shape, or color, or if a new one develops in adult life, it should be evaluated by a doctor, preferably a dermatologist. It is not always possible to tell with the naked eye whether the lesion is a melanoma, so sometimes it is necessary to cut the mole out for pathological examination.

Removal Of Moles

Although most moles are harmless and can be safely left alone, moles may be treated under the following conditions:

Brown Spots, Freckles, And Moles

- Possible malignancy: a mole that has bled, has an unusual shape, is growing rapidly or changing color
- Nuisance moles: a mole that is irritated by clothing, comb, or razor
- Cosmetic reasons: a mole that is unsightly

Shave Biopsy

Treating a protruding mole is simple with a procedure called a shave biopsy. After numbing the skin with local anesthetic, the doctor removes the projecting part of the mole with a scalpel. The wound heals to leave a flat white mark, but sometimes the color remains the same as the original mole.

Excision Biopsy

Excision biopsy is necessary if the mole is flat or melanoma is suspected. The full thickness of the skin is removed and the wound is sutured (stitched). The specimen should always be sent to the laboratory for pathological examination. The resulting scar may be just a thin line, but it is sometimes more noticeable than the mole was.

Chapter 7

Birthmarks

Many babies have what are called birthmarks when they're born. In some cases they may appear within the first few weeks of life. They can be brown, tan, blue, pink, or red. More than 10 in every 100 babies have vascular birthmarks. These are made up of blood vessels bunched together in the skin. They can be flat or raised, pink, red, or bluish discolorations.

What Causes Birthmarks?

Why do vascular birthmarks occur? The exact causes are unknown. Most vascular birthmarks are not inherited, nor are they caused by anything that happens to the mother during pregnancy.

What Are The Different Types Of Vascular Birthmarks?

There are different kinds of vascular birthmarks. Sometimes, the birthmark must be watched for several weeks or months before the specific type can be identified. The most common types of vascular birthmarks are macular stains, hemangiomas, and port-wine stains. There are also many rare types of vascular birthmarks.

About This Chapter: From "Vascular Birthmarks," © 2001 American Academy of Dermatology. Reprinted with permission from the American Academy of Dermatology. All rights reserved.

Macular Stains

Your physician will call faint, mildly red marks macular stains. They are the most common type of vascular birthmarks. They are also called "angel's kisses" when they are located on the forehead or eyelids. When they're found on the back of the neck, they're called "stork bites." They may also occur on the tip of the nose, upper lip, or any other body location. They are pink and flat. Angel's kisses almost always go away by age two, but stork bites usually last into adulthood. These birthmarks are harmless and require no treatment.

Hemangiomas

The term *hemangioma* is used to describe many different kinds of blood vessel growths. Most dermatologists prefer to use hemangioma to refer to a common type of vascular birthmark. These marks do not usually appear immediately after birth, but become visible within the first few weeks of life. Hemangiomas are usually divided into two types: strawberry hemangiomas and cavernous hemangiomas.

A strawberry hemangioma is slightly raised, and bright red because the abnormal blood vessels are very close to the surface of the skin.

Cavernous hemangiomas have a blue color because the abnormal vessels are deeper under the skin. Hemangiomas are more common in females and in premature babies. They can occur anywhere on the face or body.

Usually, a child will have only one hemangioma, but sometimes there will be two or three. In rare cases, an infant may have many, or even some internally. Unlike other vascular birthmarks,

> ♣ **It's A Fact!!**
> Most of what are commonly called birthmarks are simply oddities in skin coloration. Physicians are more concerned with vascular birthmarks, which comprise blood vessels tangled or bunched together in the skin. Vascular birthmarks are relatively common, found on a little over 10 percent of newborns.

Birthmarks

hemangiomas can grow very rapidly. Growth generally begins during the first six weeks of life and continues for about one year. Most never get bigger than two or three inches in diameter, but some may be larger. After the first year, most hemangiomas will stop growing. They then begin to turn white and slowly shrink. Half of all hemangiomas are flat by age 5; 9 out of 10 are flat by age 9. Many will completely go away, but often a faint mark is left. It's impossible to know how big any hemangioma will grow or if it will completely disappear.

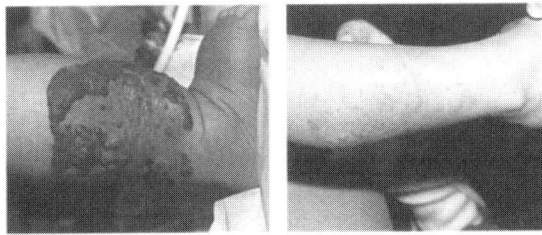

Figure 7.1. An untreated strawberry hemangioma at eight months of age (left) and two-and-a-half years (right). As is typical of this kind of vascular birthmark, the condition improves on its own.

Complications Of Hemangiomas

Occasionally, a hemangioma that's growing or shrinking rapidly can form an open sore or ulcer. These sores can be painful, and they can become infected. It's very important to see your dermatologist and keep this sore clean and covered with antibiotic ointment and/or a dressing.

A hemangioma located over the female genitals or rectum or near an eye, the nose, or mouth can cause special problems. These hemangiomas should be watched closely by your dermatologist, who will decide if further treatment is necessary.

Parents are often concerned that a hemangioma will bleed. These birthmarks do look as if they could bleed easily. However, this usually isn't a problem.

Bleeding usually occurs only after injury. If the hemangioma starts to bleed, it should be treated like any other injury—clean the area with soap and water or hydrogen peroxide and apply a gauze bandage. Apply firm, but not tight, pressure on the area for 5 to 10 minutes. If the bleeding has not stopped, call your doctor.

A hemangioma will rarely grow suddenly over one or two days. If this occurs, it's important to call your dermatologist. Also, if a bruise begins to develop, your dermatologist should be notified.

Treatment Of Hemangiomas

It's very important that a baby with a vascular birthmark be examined by a dermatologist as early as possible so that a correct diagnosis can be made and the need for treatment discussed.

It's not always easy for parents to watch a hemangioma grow, or wait for it to disappear, without doing anything. However, most hemangiomas do not require treatment. They eventually shrink by themselves, leaving very few signs.

There are several different types of treatments for hemangiomas that need care. No treatment is absolutely safe and effective. The potential benefits must be weighed against the possible risks.

The most widely used treatment for rapidly growing hemangiomas is corticosteroid medication, which is either injected or given by mouth. Long-term or repeated treatment may be necessary. Some of the risks of therapy include poor growth, elevated blood sugar and blood pressure, cataracts, and an increased chance of infection.

> ### ✎ Weird Words
>
> <u>Hemangioma</u>: A type of vascular birthmark characterized by abnormal blood vessel growth in the skin. Strawberry hemangiomas are slightly raised and bright red; cavernous hemangiomas are blue. Hemangiomas usually improve with age and require no treatment.
>
> <u>Macular stain</u>: Faint, mildly red, vascular birthmark. Macular stains are harmless and require no treatment.
>
> <u>Port-wine stain</u>: Flat vascular birthmarks of a red, pink, or purplish color; present at birth. Port-wine stains are permanent and are usually treated; sometimes they cause medical complications.

Birthmarks

Lasers can be used to both prevent growth of hemangiomas and remove hemangiomas. Hemangiomas with sores that will not heal can also be treated with lasers. New lasers are being developed and studied by dermatologists to treat this condition.

Port-Wine Stains

The port-wine stain is another type of vascular birthmark that occurs in 3 in every 1,000 infants. It is sometimes called a nevus flammeus or capillary hemangioma, but it should not be confused with a hemangioma.

Port-wine stains appear at birth. They are flat, pink, red, or purplish discolorations, found most often on the face, neck, arms, or legs. They can be any size. Unlike hemangiomas, port-wine stains grow only as the child grows. Over time, port-wine stains may become thick and develop small bumps or ridges. Port-wine stains do not go away by themselves. They last a lifetime.

Complications Of Port-Wine Stains

Port-wine stains, especially those on the face, can have emotional, social, and economic complications. Port-wine stains on the forehead, eyelids, or both sides of the face can be associated with glaucoma, increased pressure within the eye that, left untreated, can cause blindness. These complications occur in less than one-fourth of those with port-wine stains of the forehead and eyelids. All infants with a port-wine stain in those areas should have a thorough eye and brain examination.

Occasionally, there may be very gradual enlargement of tissues surrounding a port-wine stain. All children with large port-wine stains involving an arm or leg should be followed for any growth problems.

With time, port-wine stains can develop small blood vessel growths called pyogenic granulomas. These can bleed easily and should be removed.

Treatment Of Port-Wine Stains

The use of cover-up makeup has been a common treatment for port-wine stains. Your doctor can provide you with more information about products that are made to cover up birthmarks.

Various methods have been tried in the past to remove port-wine stains, but none have worked well. New types of lasers have shown the best results with the least amount of risk and side effects. Laser treatment of port-wine stains is FDA-approved and available at many centers around the country. For best results, treatment should begin as early as possible, even in infancy. Laser surgery is performed on an outpatient basis. Several treatments are usually required, given at two-month intervals. Younger patients often require fewer treatments than adults. In about one-fourth of the patients, lasers can totally clear up the port-wine stain. Seventy percent will look much better. For reasons that are not understood, a small number of patients will not respond well to laser therapy.

There are several risks of laser therapy. An increase or decrease in skin color can occur, leaving patchy tanning or whitening of the skin. In most cases this is not permanent. Swelling, crusting, or minor bleeding can occur. This is unusual and can be treated easily. Permanent scarring has happened, but is extremely rare. Laser therapy is uncomfortable, but not extremely painful. Anesthesia is not required for most adults. However, anesthesia is often important for toddlers and young children. If putting the child to sleep is required, there are some risks and higher costs.

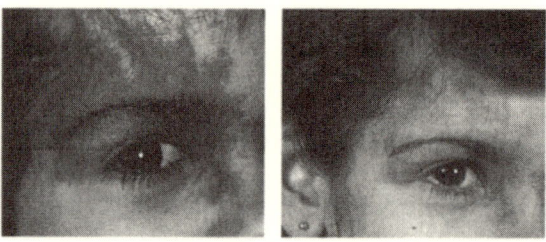

Figure 7.2. Treatment can reduce the severity of port-wine stains. The untreated birthmark appears on the left; the right-hand photo shows the effect of treatment.

Chapter 8

Stretch Marks

Your skin is usually fairly elastic, but when you grow or gain weight really quickly (like during puberty or pregnancy), you may get fine lines on your body called stretch marks. Stretch marks occur when the tissue under your skin tears from rapid growth or stretching. When the skin is overstretched, it produces too much collagen, which can form the "scars" called stretch marks.

Stretch marks often show up on places like your breasts, thighs, hips, and butt. Most girls and women have stretch marks, so if you have them, you're not alone.

Although they're more common in girls, guys can get stretch marks, too. Guys and girls who are bodybuilders are more prone to getting them because of the rapid body changes that bodybuilding can produce. Obesity can also lead to stretch marks. Stretch marks are also more likely to occur if a person uses steroid-containing (such as hydrocortisone) creams or ointments on his or her skin for a long time (more than a few weeks).

About This Chapter: This information was provided by KidsHealth, one of the largest resources online for medically reviewed information written for parents, kids, and teens. For more articles like this one, visit www.KidsHealth.org or www.TeensHealth.org. © 2001 The Nemours Center for Children's Health Media, a division of the Nemours Foundation. The original article, "What Are Stretch Marks?" is available online at http://www.kidshealth.org/teen/question/skin/stretch_marks.html.

> **♣ It's A Fact!!**
>
> The medical term for stretch marks is striae or, more completely, striae cutis distensae, which in Latin means "streaks of stretched skin."
>
> Source: Adapted from *Stedman's Medical Dictionary, 27th Edition*, copyright © 2000 Lippincott Williams & Wilkins. All rights reserved. Reprinted with permission

At first, stretch marks may show up as reddish or purplish lines, but they often will turn lighter (whitish or flesh-colored) and almost disappear over time. So if you're taking a trip to the beach this summer, you shouldn't stress out too much about them. Your stretch marks will usually fade and become less noticeable over time.

Although there are tons of products on the market that claim to eliminate stretch marks, the truth is you can't make them go away without the use of a form of plastic surgery called microdermabrasion. If you are concerned about your stretch marks, talk to a dermatologist.

Stretch marks are a totally normal part of puberty—try not to sweat them, and they'll start to fade before you know it.

Chapter 9

Cellulite: Is There Any Such Thing?

Cellulite is a term coined in European salons and spas to describe deposits of dimpled fat found on the thighs and buttocks of many women. Widespread promotion of the concept in the United States followed the 1973 publication of *Cellulite: Those Lumps, Bumps, and Bulges You Couldn't Lose Before*, by Nicole Ronsard, owner of a New York City beauty salon that specialized in skin and body care. Cellulite is alleged to be a special type of "fat gone wrong," a combination of fat, water, and "toxic wastes" that the body has failed to eliminate. Alleged "anticellulite" products sold through retail outlets, by mail, through multilevel companies, and over the Internet have included "loofah" sponges; cactus fibers; special washcloths; horsehair mitts; creams and gels to "dissolve" cellulite; supplements containing vitamins, minerals, and/or herbs; bath liquids; massagers; rubberized pants; exercise books; brushes; rollers; body wraps; and toning lotions. Many salons offer treatment with electrical muscle stimulation, vibrating machines, inflatable hip-high pressurized boots, "hormone" or "enzyme" injections, heating pads, and massage. Some operators claim that 5 to 15 inches can be lost in one hour. A series of treatments can cost hundreds of dollars.

Many years ago, Neil Solomon, M.D., conducted a double-blind study of 100 people to see whether cellulite differed from ordinary fat. Specimens of

About This Chapter: Reprinted with permission from "'Cellulite' Removers" © 2000 Quackwatch, Inc. Available online at http://www.quackwatch.org/01Quackery RelatedTopics/cellulite.html.

regular fat and lumpy fat were obtained by a needle biopsy procedure and given to pathologists for analysis and comparison. No difference between the two was found.

More recently, researchers at Rockefeller Institute used ultrasonography, microscopic examinations, and fat-metabolism studies to see if "affected" and unaffected skin areas differed in seven healthy adult subjects (five women, two men; four affected, three unaffected). The researchers concluded: certain characteristics of skin make women more prone than men to develop cellulite; the process is diffuse rather than localized; and there were no significant differences in the appearance or function of the fatty tissue or the regional blood flow between affected and unaffected sites within individuals.

♣ **It's A Fact!!**
"Cellulite" is not a medical term. Medical authorities agree that cellulite is simply ordinary fatty tissue. Strands of fibrous tissue connect the skin to deeper tissue layers and also separate compartments that contain fat cells. When fat cells increase in size, these compartments bulge and produce a waffled appearance of the skin.

Electrical Muscle Stimulators (EMS) And Iontophoresis Devices

Muscle stimulators are a legitimate medical device approved for certain conditions—to relax muscle spasms, increase blood circulation, prevent blood clots, and rehabilitate muscle function after a stroke. But many health spas and figure salons claim that muscle stimulators can remove wrinkles, perform face-lifts, reduce breast size, reduce a "beer belly," and remove cellulite. Iontophoresis devices are prescription devices that use direct electric current to introduce ions of soluble salts (i.e., medications) into body tissues for therapeutic or diagnostic purposes. The only approved use is for diagnosing cystic fibrosis.

The U.S. Food and Drug Administration (FDA) considers promotion of muscle stimulators or iontophoresis devices for any type of body shaping or contouring to be fraudulent. The most infamous of these devices, the Relax-A-Cizor®, claimed to reduce girth by delivering electric shocks to the muscles. More than 400,000 units were sold for $200 to $400 each before the FDA obtained an injunction in 1970 to stop its sale. At the trial, 40 witnesses testified that they had been injured while using the machine. The judge concluded that the device could cause miscarriages and aggravate many preexisting medical conditions, including hernias, ulcers, varicose veins, and epilepsy.

Body Wrapping

Many salons and spas exist where clients supposedly can trim inches off the waist, hips, thighs, and other areas of the body. These facilities use wraps or garments, with or without special lotions or creams applied to the skin. The garments may be applied to parts of the body or to the entire body. Clients are typically assured that fat will "melt away" and they can lose "up to 2 inches from those problem areas in just one hour." Suddenly Slender, which licenses body-wrap shops in the United States and Canada, claims that "wrapping works because cellulite is waterlogged fatty tissue." As part of its sales pitch to prospective owners, the company notes that free publicity may be obtainable. Its website states: "Because clients get dressed up as 'mummies' and then, almost miraculously, achieve major inch loss and startling improvements to their figures, local and national media have been overwhelmingly receptive to featuring presentations about the service."

Home-use systems are also being marketed through the Internet and through multilevel marketing. Many of the systems are claimed to "remove toxins." Some marketers suggest measuring a large number of body areas before and afterward and adding up the differences to get "total inches lost." Life Force International, for example, recommends adding the results of 17 measurements. This enables minor changes due to temporary effects or to measurement variations to appear to be large numbers.

No product taken by mouth can cause selective reduction of an area of the body. Although wrapping may cause temporary water loss as a result of perspiration or compression, any fluid will soon be replaced by drinking or eating. The idea that herbal wraps detoxify the body is absurd.

Cellasene®

An herbal product called Cellasene is being vigorously promoted as a cellulite remedy. The product was developed by an Italian chemist named Gianfranco Merizzi. Its ingredients are evening primrose oil, dried *Fucus vesiculosus* extract, gelatin, fish oil, glycerol, soya oil, grape seed, bioflavonoids, soya lecithin, fatty acids, dried sweet clover extract, dried *Ginkgo biloba* extract, and iron oxide. The product, to be taken twice daily (or three times per day for an "intensive" program) for two months and then once daily for maintenance, costs $1.50 to $2.00 per capsule. Here's what one Internet marketer says, followed by my comments in brackets:

- Dried *Ginkgo biloba* extract assists in blood circulation and stimulates the metabolism of fats. [Although *Ginkgo* can increase circulation, it does not stimulate fat metabolism. Even if it did, there is no reason why it would exert a localized effect.]

- Dried sweet clover extract can increase blood circulation and assist in removing fluid buildup. [This ingredient may have mild diuretic action, but "fluid buildup" is not a factor in the appearance or composition of fatty tissue.]

- Grape seed bioflavonoids are powerful antioxidants that protect cells and blood vessels from damage. [Whether antioxidant supplements help protect tissues is not scientifically settled. Regardless, any such mechanism has nothing to do with the quantity or appearance of fatty tissues.]

- Dried *Fucus vesiculosus* extract stimulates metabolism and can help reduce localized fats. [This herb contains significant amounts of iodine and could adversely effect the thyroid gland. The U. S. Recommended Daily Allowance (USRDA) for iodine is 150 micrograms. The average American woman ingests 170 micrograms per day from food (not including iodized salt). Each capsule of Cellasene contains 240 micrograms of iodine. If enough were taken to increase thyroid function, the result would be unhealthy.]

Cellulite: Is There Any Such Thing?

- Evening primrose oil and fish oil are rich in polyunsaturated fatty acids, a source of energy that increases metabolic levels and helps in diminishing saturated fatty acids. [The "energy" is simply the caloric value. Neither oil increases metabolism nor reduces the amount of other fats one eats.]
- Soya lecithin helps to break down fats. [The body makes all the lecithin it needs. Lecithin supplements do not cause the body to shed fat.]

Rexall Sundown, Inc. has been Cellasene's primary marketer in the United States. The company's website claimed:

> Cellasene works from within, nutritionally, to help fight cellulite at its source....
>
> Cellasene is a safe, clinically studied formula that works over time at the source of the problem—below the surface of the skin. This unique formula of plant extracts and other beneficial dietary supplements nourishes connective tissue from within and helps reduce cellulite. The herbal ingredients in Cellasene work to increase blood circulation, reduce fluid buildup, stimulate metabolism and reduce localized fats. CONVENIENT AND EASY TO USE....
>
> You do not need to change your diet and exercise routine for Cellasene to work. It is simple and effortless to incorporate the easy-to-swallow Cellasene softgels into your daily regimen.

On March 15, 1999, during an interview on CNBC-TV, Rexall's chief executive officer claimed that three clinical trials sponsored by the company had demonstrated a 90 percent success rate, but the results would not be submitted to scientific journals because Rexall did not want to reveal the amounts of each ingredient in its formula. This statement was preposterous because results could be published without revealing the exact amounts of each ingredient. Two weeks later, I searched Medline for "cellulite" and "Cellasene" and found no report that any product taken by mouth was proven useful against cellulite.

Near the end of May, apparently in response to criticism in the media, Rexall released various details on two of the studies and posted them to its

Science on Cellasene website. The first study was performed on 25 healthy female volunteers whose hip and thigh and ankle circumference were measured before and after eight weeks of daily consumption of the product. Although differences between the initial and final measurements were reported, no control group was used, so that it would not be possible to tell whether any changes were related to taking the products or to measurement variations. In addition, neither individual measurements nor weights were reported, so that it is not possible to judge from the data whether the reductions were related to weight loss, coincidental or otherwise.

The second study compared 25 people who took the product with 15 people who took a placebo for eight weeks. According to the report, the average weight of both groups varied little, but average hip and thigh circumference and skin thickness (measured with an ultrasound test) decreased. However, the experimental design was so seriously flawed that the findings should not be regarded as valid. The participants were not told whether they were receiving Cellasene or the placebo, but the investigators knew who was in each group because only the Cellasene group had blood drawn for testing. This could have influenced the way the measurements were performed, as well as the participants' motivation. No data were given to demonstrate whether the measurement process was accurate or whether the appearance or feel of the women's skin had changed. In addition, although measurements were made at the experiment's beginning, midpoint, and end, the midpoint measurements were not reported on Rexall's website.

It seems to me that a valid test should involve more participants, a longer initial investigative period plus monthly follow-up measurements for at least a year, standardization of the measurement technique, measurements taken by at least three investigators, blinding of the investigators about who received the Cellasene and who did not, measuring several times a week to see whether measurements tend to change or remain constant, weekly ratings of the appearance of the skin by both the participants and the experimenters, and release of the individual data in addition to the group averages. I have suggested these points to Rexall's chief executive officer.

A spokesperson for Cellasene's Italian manufacturer stated that a study involving 200 women would be done at the University of Miami with results expected in the fall of 1999. In June 2000, however, the lead researcher stated that the $400,000 study could not be completed because some of the participants had not come to the testing site to be measured. In the interim a British researcher reported finding no difference in hip and thigh measurements between 11 women taking Cellasene and 8 women using a placebo.

> ♣ It's A Fact!!
>
> The gold standard for medication and treatment research is the double-blind study. In a double-blind study, half the patients receive the medication or treatment, and half receive something else, which is called a placebo. The patients can't tell which is which, and the researchers themselves do not know who is receiving the medication or treatment and who is getting the placebo. Double-blind studies ensure objective measurement of the results of the medication or treatment.
>
> Source: Adapted from *Stedman's Medical Dictionary, 27th Edition*, © 2000. Lippincott Williams, and Wilkins. All rights reserved. Reprinted with permission.

Piggyback Attempt?

InHealth America, of Carlsbad, California, is competing with Rexall by marketing a similar product called CelluLean®. The company's website, which was registered during the week Rexall introduced Cellasene, states:

> CelluLean melts away cellulite by increasing your metabolism and blood circulation, breaking down the fats found in cellulite, and removing toxins from your body. The herbal extracts in CelluLean have been proven to be effective in reducing fatty deposits. Simply put, CelluLean helps your body to reach and break down cellulite, enabling your skin to regain its youthful smooth appearance.

One way to attract browsers to a website is to place "meta tags" into the site's source code. The words in the meta tags are not visible when you are looking at the page, but search engines use them as hints about the relevance of a site. For example, if a user searches for "cancer," and a website uses "cancer" as a meta tag, the search engine may consider the site to be relevant to the search, regardless of the site's actual content. InHealth America's "keywords" meta tag reads:

> Cellasene, Cellulean, selesene, neurosharp, cellesene, selasene, selleseen, cellasene, celesene, celasene, SlimRX, Rexall, cellulite, Cellulene, Cellutrim, Inhealth America, InHealthAmerica, In Health America, Pharmaceuticals, interactive, InHealth, In Health, America, Metabolife, Metabo, 356, Herbalife, Nu-way, MegaTrim, Mega Trim, Megatrim, Adaptogenol, Adaptagenol, Adaptogen, Adaptagen, Adaptotrim, Adaptatrim, Lipuramine, Liporimine, Arthranol, Artharanol, stress, Stress, health, liver, arthritis, San Diego, Carlsbad, California, NASA, diet, weight loss, heal, herbal, MLM, network marketing, marketing, unilevel, binary, multilevel marketing, interactive, business, home business, downline, sponsors, products, compensation, joints, business opportunity, remedy, pain, relief, natural, performance, endurance, mental, concentration, sleep, research, immune system, fatigue, weight gain, California, inflammation supplement, science, doctor, energy, recovery, future, Fat, Cortisol, eat, food, high fat, low fat

Thus people searching for any of the above topics may find a link to InHealth America's site.

Endermologie®

In 1998, the FDA approved a high-powered, handheld massage tool that consists of a treatment head and two motorized rollers with a suction device that compresses the affected tissue between the two rollers. The manufacturer is permitted to promote it for "temporarily improving the appearance of cellulite." The procedure—called Endermologie—usually takes 10 to 20 treatments to get the best results, and one or two maintenance treatments per month are required to maintain them. Without the maintenance, the benefits will soon be lost. The typical cost is $45 to $65 per session. A recently published study of 85 women between the ages of 21 to 61 found that 46 patients who completed seven sessions showed a mean index reduction in body circumference of 1.34 centimeter, while 39 patients who completed 14 sessions of treatments showed a mean index reduction in body circumference of 1.83 centimeter. However, another study, involving 52 women, found

Cellulite: Is There Any Such Thing?

no objective difference in thigh girth (at two points) or thigh fat depth (measured by ultrasound).

Enforcement Actions

The FTC has taken successful action against many marketers of alleged cellulite-reducing products:

- In 1991, Slender You, Inc., signed a consent agreement prohibiting unsubstantiated claims that its continuous passive motion (CPM) tables enable the user to lose weight, lose inches, remove cellulite, flush out toxins, tone and firm muscles, or achieve physical fitness benefits comparable or superior to those provided by rigorous exercise.

- In 1993, a similar action was taken against Fleetwood Manufacturing, Inc., of Mesa, Arizona, and its owner, Thomas A. Fleetwood.

- In 1993, Nature's Cleanser, based in Beverly Hills, California, and Donald Douglas-Torry agreed not to make unsubstantiated claims that its herbal tablets would promote weight loss by "cleansing" the bowel. The company had claimed that weight could be immediately controlled by without dieting or watching calories by eliminating waste such as fatty tissues, cellulite, toxins, mucus, hardened fecal matter, and harmful drug residues.

- In 1993, Revlon, Inc., and its subsidiary, Charles Revson, Inc., signed a consent agreement not to make unsubstantiated claims that their Ultima II ProCollagen® anticellulite body complex would: significantly reduce cellulite, help disperse toxins and excess water from areas where cellulite appears; reduce skin's bumpy texture, ripples or slackness caused by cellulite; help disperse toxins and excess water from areas where cellulite appears; and increase subskin tissue strength and tone.

- In 1993, Synchronal Corp agreed to stop unsubstantiated claims for its Anuska Bio-Response Body Contouring Program® cellulite cream and to pay $3.5 million in consumer redress.

- In 1993, National Media Corp./Media Arts International, Ltd., agreed to a consent agreement and $275,000 in consumer redress in connection with infomercials claiming that its Cosmetique Français® would substantially reduce or eliminate cellulite, was more effective than diet or exercise, and would prevent recurrence if used once or twice a week.

- In 1995, a federal judge in California permanently banned Silueta Distributors, Inc., a Chatsworth, California-based company, and its president, Stanley Klavir, from deceptively claiming that their Sistema Silueta® cream and tablets would reduce cellulite. The judge concluded that Sistema Silueta was nothing more than moisturizer and diuretic tablets, neither of which would cause cellulite loss. The defendants were also ordered to pay $169,339 in consumer redress.

- In 1995, European Body Concepts and its president James Marino signed a consent agreement prohibiting it from making unsubstantiated claims that its body-wrapping system would cause the user to lose inches, pounds, and cellulite quickly and easily, without dieting or exercising, and that the system could reduce the size of specific areas of the body.

☞ Remember!!

The amount of fat in the body is determined by the individual's eating and exercise habits, but the distribution of fat in the body is determined by heredity. In most cases, reduction of a particular body part can be accomplished only as part of an overall weight-reduction program. Endermologie may temporarily improve the appearance of dimpled areas, but the procedure is time-consuming and expensive.

Cellulite: Is There Any Such Thing?

- In 1995, National Dietary Research, Inc., (NDR) and its owner William H. Morris agreed to pay $100,000 to settle FTC charges of deceptively advertising Food Source One (FS-1)® as a weight-loss and cholesterol-reducing product. The product was a compressed tablet made largely from plant fiber. The consent agreement included a clause that prohibited unsubstantiated claims of cellulite reduction.

- In 1998, an Australian federal judge ordered the Swiss Slimming and Health Institute and its director to pay $1.47 million in penalties and interest, some of which would be refunded to defrauded clients.

- In 1999, the Iowa attorney general obtained an order prohibiting Lipo Slim, Inc., of New York City from continuing to marketing its Lipo Slim Briefs® in Iowa. Ads said wearing the briefs would "get rid of your cellulite" and "dissolve fat and hydric deposits that accumulate in your hips, stomach, buttocks and thighs." An ad in the *National Enquirer* said that "thousands of thermo-active micropore cells" in the briefs "produce a gentle massage that destroys deep fat particles and liquid molecules which are the cause of excess fat." The order required the company to offer full refunds to its Iowa buyers and pay $12,000 to the state consumer education fund.

- In 1999, the FDA ordered Cellulite Reduction of New York to stop suggesting that Endermologie could have more than a temporary effect on cellulite.

- In July 2000, the FTC charged Rexall Sundown, Inc., with making false and unsubstantiated claims for Cellasene.

— by Stephen Barrett, M.D.

Chapter 10

Body Piercing: A Guide For Teens

Many different cultures have pierced their bodies for centuries. If you look in a history book, you will find that Egyptians, Greeks, and Romans did body art, such as piercing and tattooing. People pierced their bodies for decoration to show the person's importance in a group, or because they thought it protected them from evil. Today, we know much more about the risks of body piercing. Body piercing is a serious decision. Before you decide what you want to do, ask your friends, parents, and trusted adults what they think.

What Are Teens Saying About Body Piercing Today?

Ask other teens who have been pierced what they thought of the whole experience. How much did it cost? Was it painful? How long did it take to heal? If they had the chance to do it over again, would they?

What Are The Risks With Body Piercing?

The most serious risks are infections, allergic reactions, bleeding, and damage to nerves or teeth. Infections may be caused by hepatitis, HIV, tetanus,

---

About This Chapter: This information is reprinted with permission from the Center for Young Women's Health, Children's Hospital of Boston, 333 Longwood Avenue, 5th floor, Boston, MA 02115; (617) 355-2994 (voice), (617) 232-3136 (fax), cywh@tch.hardvard.edu (e-mail). For additional information, visit the Center's website at www.youngwomenshealth.org. © 2000 Center for Young Women's Health.

bacteria, and yeast. If the piercer washes his or her hands and uses gloves and sterile equipment and you take good care of your piercing, the risk of infection is lowered (but still exists).

Another cause of problems from piercings is the wrong kind of jewelry for the area pierced. If the jewelry is too small, it can actually cut off the blood supply to the tissue, causing swelling and pain. If the jewelry is either too thin or too heavy, or if you are allergic to the metal, your body can sometimes reject the jewelry (your body reacts against the jewelry because it is a "foreign object").

Know the risks before you have your body pierced:

- Bacterial infection (where you had the piercing)
- Excessive (a lot of) bleeding
- Allergic reactions (especially to certain kinds of jewelry)
- Damage to nerves (for example, you may lose feeling at the area that gets pierced)
- Keloids (thick scarring at the piercing site)
- Dental damage (swelling and infection of tongue, chipped and broken teeth, choking on loose jewelry)

Does It Matter Where On My Body I Get Pierced?

Healing time is different depending on where on your body you get pierced. Some places are more likely to get infected or have problems. Piercings on your ear lobes usually take about six to eight weeks to heal. But piercings on the side of your ear, which is cartilage, can take anywhere from four months to one year to heal. The reason for this is that the type of tissue in each area is different and the amount of pressure on the pierced area while you are sleeping is different.

Tongue piercings swell a lot at first but heal fairly quickly if the right type of jewelry is used. However, metal jewelry in the tongue piercing may damage gums and chip the enamel surface on your teeth. In fact, the ADA, which stands for the American Dental Association (a group of dentists that set professional standards for dentists in the United States), is against any type of oral piercings because of all the risks.

In some cases, nipple piercings can damage some of the milk-producing glands in a young woman's breasts. This can cause infections or problems later if the woman decides to breast-feed her baby. Some pierced areas, like navel (belly button) piercings, are more likely to become infected because of irritation from tight clothing. A pierced site needs air to help the healing process.

Table 10.1   Healing Time For Body Piercings

Pierced Body Part	Time It Takes To Heal
Ear lobe	six to eight weeks
Ear cartilage	four months to one year
Eyebrow	six to eight weeks
Nostril	two to four months
Nasal septum	six to eight months
Nasal bridge	eight to ten weeks
Tongue	four weeks
Lip	two to three months
Nipple	three to six months
Navel	four months to one year
Female genitalia	four to ten weeks
Male genitalia	four weeks to six months

If I Decide That A Piercing Is Important To Me, Where Should I Go?

You should ask friends and relatives with piercings where they went and if they liked the place. Look for a place that does a lot of piercings and that only employs piercers with piercing licenses. Some states make piercers get a license, while other states do not. So there are actually people who are doing body piercings with very little training! As you can imagine, this can be very dangerous for you. However, the APP, which stands for the Association of Professional Piercers (a professional organization of piercers), makes safety rules for people who do piercings. Make sure that there is a certificate on the wall that says the piercer is registered with the APP. You may need to bring a copy of your birth certificate. If you are under 18 years old, you will need your parents' or guardians' permission. Your parent or guardian will need to go with you to the piercing salon and sign a consent form.

Since the law is different from state to state, you will need to find out what the law in your area says about whether or not you need parental permission to have a piercing.

What Should I Look For In A Piercing Salon?

When you go into a salon, look around. Is the place clean? The shop should be kept clean and sanitary. The lighting should be good so the piercers can see well while working. Do they wash their hands and use sterile gloves and instruments? All the instruments should either be brand new and disposable (meant to be thrown away after one use) or be sterilized in pouches. If the piercer uses disposable needles, you should see him or her open sealed packages of the needles! The piercers should throw away the needles in a biohazard container after using them.

♣ **It's A Fact!!**

You should know that:

- You *can* get or spread a serious infection, including HIV, if the piercing equipment hasn't been sterilized properly. Infections caused by bacteria getting into the puncture of the piercing may also happen later, even after the piercing has healed.

- If the studio uses a piercing "gun" to do body piercings, *leave*! Piercing guns cannot be sterilized and should *not* be used for body piercing.

What Kind Of Jewelry Should I Buy?

It is best to use surgical stainless steel when you first have your piercing done. It is least likely to produce a foreign body reaction or infection in the skin. Other choices for when you first have your piercing done are metals like gold (at least 18K), titanium, or niobium. All of these cost more than surgical steel. For people who are extremely sensitive to metal, Teflon or nylon piercings may be used.

Look for a salon that has a large choice of jewelry. The salon should not tell you to use a certain type of jewelry just because it's the only kind they have.

What's Up With All The Different Kinds Of Jewelry?

- Bars, which are the type of jewelry used in some piercings like the tongue, are measured in length (how long the bar is). When the piercing is first done, a longer bar will be used. When the piercing heals, a shorter bar is used.
- Ring jewelry is measured by diameter, or how wide the ring is.
- Gauge means the thickness of the jewelry. The smaller the gauge number, the thicker the jewelry. The APP says that jewelry no greater than 14 gauge should be used below the neck. This is because of the risk of a foreign body reaction and the possibility of the ring cutting the skin.

How Are Piercings Done?

An experienced piercer uses a hollow needle to create a hole by passing the needle through the body part you want pierced. The body jewelry is then inserted through the hole. Sometimes there can be a small amount of bleeding. You should not take aspirin or any pain medication that contains aspirin the week before any piercing is done, since these medicines may cause you to bleed a little bit more than usual. Remember, piercing guns should *never* be used since they can damage tissue and cause infection.

How Much Will A Piercing Cost?

There are actually two costs with piercings: the site cost and the jewelry cost. The site cost depends on where on your body you get pierced. For example, ear and nose piercings usually cost less than tongue, nipple, or genital piercings. Gold jewelry costs more than stainless steel or another metal. You should shop around and check prices at different piercing salons before you decide on where to have your piercing done.

How Should I Clean My New Piercing?

Follow these steps to prevent infection:

1. Wash your hands first with soap and water before touching or cleaning the pierced area. (Don't let anyone else touch the pierced area until it is healed.)
2. Remove any crusty skin from the site and from the jewelry with warm water.
3. Gently wash the area around the piercing with antibacterial soap (liquid soap works the best).
4. Gently rinse off all of the soap and crusty discharge.
5. Gently dry the area with a paper towel or plain white napkin. (Bacteria can stay in cloth towels.)
6. Do steps 1–5 twice a day until the skin heals. (Overwashing or overscrubbing can irritate the area.)
7. Do *not* use antibacterial ointments because they don't allow air to get to the area and they trap bacteria.

> ✔ **Quick Tip**
>
> Some tips teens have passed along to us:
>
> - *You* do *not* have to pierce your body to "belong."
> - *You* can *always* change your mind or *wait* if you are not sure.
> - If *you* do decide to have your body pierced, *never* pierce your own body or let a friend do it because you can get very serious health problems.

How Can I Prevent Infections After I Get Pierced?

Preventing infections is really not hard. It shouldn't take a lot of your time to keep your piercing clean. The good news is that you won't have to worry about complications if you keep the piercing clean.

Body Piercing: A Guide For Teens

- Do *not* use alcohol or peroxide to clean the area. (Both products will dry out your skin.) Other strong solutions, such as Betadine®, will discolor gold jewelry.
- Rinse the pierced skin after exercising since sweat may irritate the piercing.
- Keep the pierced area from coming in contact with other people's body fluids, such as saliva and sweat. (Do not have oral sexual contact for four to six weeks if you have a tongue, lip, or genital piercing).
- Keep things clean that come in contact with the pierced body part. For example, keep your phone clean if you have an ear piercing, keep your glasses clean for ear and eyebrow piercings, cover your ear lobe with a tissue if you use hair spray, and try not to apply makeup close to piercing sites.
- Wear clean clothing with soft fabric for navel piercings. Avoid wearing jeans because the material can be irritating.
- Don't wear pantyhose, leotards, belts, or tight clothing while a navel piercing is healing.
- Wear loose-fitting clothing with a navel piercing to let the air help with healing.
- Check your jewelry many times during the day to see if any parts have become loose, especially if you have a tongue piercing. If a bar becomes loose, you can accidentally swallow it or damage a permanent tooth.
- Do *not* use a hot tub or swim in public pools until your piercing has healed.
- Use an antibacterial mouthwash (for example, Listerine® or Glyburide®) or a salt-water rinse if you have a tongue or lip piercing, especially after all meals and snacks.
- See your dentist for regular checkups and if you think you have a problem. Studies have shown that people who have piercings in their mouth are much more likely to have injuries to their teeth and gums.

- Eat healthy foods. Foods rich in vitamins and minerals help your body heal.

- Be on the lookout for signs of infection that may include one or more of the following: redness, swelling, discharge, bad smell, or rash at or around the piercing site, or a fever.

- If you think you have an infection, don't try to take care of it by yourself. Make an appointment to see your health care provider.

—by Phaedra Thomas, R.N., B.S.N.;
Traci Brooks, M.D.; Estherann Grace, M.D.;
and Lara Hauslaib, B.A.

☞ Remember!!

Body piercing is a big decision. After understanding the risks, we hope that this information will help you make a decision that's best for you. If you do decide to get a body piercing, we hope that you will follow the guidelines in this information sheet. Go to a reliable salon/piercer, buy good jewelry, keep the site clean and away from irritating materials, and see your health care provider if you have symptoms of an infection!

Chapter 11

Tattoos And Permanent Makeup

The inks used in tattoos and permanent makeup (also known as micropigmentation) and the pigments in these inks are subject to U. S. Food and Drug Administration (FDA) regulation as cosmetics and color additives. However, FDA has not attempted to regulate the use of tattoo inks and the pigments used in them and does not control the actual practice of tattooing. Rather, such matters have been handled through local laws and by local jurisdictions.

But with the growth in popularity of tattooing and permanent makeup, FDA has begun taking a closer look at related safety questions. Among the issues under consideration are tattoo removal, adverse reactions to tattoo colors, and infections that result from tattooing.

Another concern is the increasing variety of pigments and diluents being used in tattooing—more than 50 different pigments and shades, and the list continues to grow. Although a number of color additives are approved for use in cosmetics, none is approved for injection into the skin. Using an unapproved color additive in a tattoo ink makes the ink adulterated. Many pigments used in tattoo inks are not approved for skin contact at all. Some

---

About This Chapter: Excerpted from "Tattoos and Permanent Makeup," Office of Cosmetics and Colors Fact Sheet, Center for Food Safety and Applied Nutrition, U. S. Food and Drug Administration, November 29, 2000; available at http://vm.cfsan.fda.gov/~dms/cos-204.html.

are industrial-grade colors that are suitable for printers' ink or automobile paint.

Nevertheless, many individuals choose to undergo tattooing in its various forms. For some, it is an aesthetic choice or an initiation rite. Some choose permanent makeup as a time saver or because they have physical difficulty applying regular, temporary makeup. For others, tattooing is an adjunct to reconstructive surgery, particularly of the face or breast, to simulate natural pigmentation. People who have lost their eyebrows due to alopecia (a form of hair loss) may choose to have "eyebrows" tattooed on, while people with vitiligo (a lack of pigmentation in areas of the skin) may try tattooing to help camouflage the condition.

Whatever their reason, consumers should be aware of the risks involved in order to make an informed decision.

What Risks Are Involved In Tattooing?

The following are the primary complications that can result from tattooing:

- *Infection.* Unsterile tattooing equipment and needles can transmit infectious diseases, such as hepatitis. The risk of infection is the reason the American Association of Blood Banks requires a one-year wait between getting a tattoo and donating blood. It is extremely important to make sure that all tattooing equipment is clean and sterilized before use. Even if the needles are sterilized or never have been used, it is important to understand that in some cases the equipment that holds the needles cannot be sterilized reliably due to its design. In addition, the person who receives a tattoo must be sure to care for the tattooed area properly during the first week or so after the pigments are injected.

- *Removal problems.* Despite advances in laser technology, removing a tattoo is a painstaking process, usually involving several treatments and considerable expense. Complete removal without scarring may be impossible.

- *Allergic reactions.* Although allergic reactions to tattoo pigments are rare, when they happen they may be particularly troublesome because the pigments can be hard to remove. Occasionally, people may develop an allergic reaction to tattoos they have had for years.

- *Granulomas.* These are nodules that may form around material that the body perceives as foreign, such as particles of tattoo pigment.

- *Keloid formation.* If you are prone to developing keloids—scars that grow beyond normal boundaries—you are at risk of keloid formation from a tattoo. Keloids may form any time you injure or traumatize your skin, and according to Office of Cosmetics and Colors (OCAC) dermatologist Ella Toombs, M.D., tattooing or micropigmentation is a form of trauma. *Micropigmentation: State of the Art*, a book written by Charles Zwerling, M.D., Annette Walker, R.N., and Norman Goldstein, M.D., states that keloids occur more frequently as a consequence of tattoo removal.

- *MRI complications.* There have been reports of people with tattoos or permanent makeup who experienced swelling or burning in the affected areas when they underwent magnetic resonance imaging (MRI). This seems to occur only rarely and apparently without lasting effects. There also have been reports of tattoo pigments interfering with the quality of the image. This seems to occur mainly when a person with permanent eyeliner undergoes MRI of the eyes. Mascara may produce a similar effect. The difference is that mascara is easily removable. The cause of these complications is uncertain. Some have theorized that they result from an interaction with the metallic components of some pigments. However, the risks of avoiding an MRI when your doctor has recommended one are likely to be much greater than the risks of complications from an interaction between the MRI and tattoo or permanent makeup. Instead of avoiding an MRI, individuals who have tattoos or permanent makeup should inform the radiologist or technician of this fact in order to take appropriate precautions, avoid complications, and assure the best results.

The Most Common Problem: Dissatisfaction

According to Dr. Toombs, the most common problem that develops with tattoos is the desire to remove them. Removing tattoos and permanent makeup can be very difficult.

Skill levels vary widely among people who perform tattooing. According to an article by J. K. Chiang, S. Barsky, and D. M. Bronson in the June 1999 issue of the *Journal of the American Academy of Dermatology*, the main complication with eyelid tattooing is improperly placed pigment. You may want to ask the person performing the procedure for references and ask yourself how willing you are to risk permanently wearing someone else's mistake.

Although tattoos may be satisfactory at first, they sometimes fade. Also, if the tattooist injects the pigments too deeply into the skin, the pigments may migrate beyond the original sites, resulting in a blurred appearance.

Another cause of dissatisfaction is that the human body changes over time, and styles change with the season. The permanent makeup that may have looked flattering when first injected may later clash with changing skin tones and facial or body contours. People who plan to have facial cosmetic surgery are advised that the appearance of their permanent makeup may become distorted. The tattoo that seemed stylish at first may become dated and embarrassing. And changing tattoos or permanent makeup is not as easy as changing your mind.

> ✔ **Quick Tip**
> ### Reporting Adverse Reactions
>
> FDA urges consumers and healthcare providers to report adverse reactions to tattoos and permanent makeup, problems with removal, or adverse reactions to temporary tattoos. The agency operates the Cosmetics Adverse Reaction Monitoring (CARM) system to monitor problems consumers experience with cosmetic products and ingredients, including color additives. Consumers and healthcare providers can register complaints by contacting their FDA district office. A list of FDA district office consumer complaint coordinators is available online at www.fda.gov/opacom/backgrounders/complain.html or see the blue pages of your local phone directory. Written reports of adverse reactions can be sent to:
>
> Office of Cosmetics and Colors
> HFS-106
> Center for Food Safety and Applied Nutrition
> Food and Drug Administration
> 5100 Paint Branch Parkway
> College Park, MD 20740-3835

Tattoos And Permanent Makeup

Removal Techniques

Methods for removing tattoos include laser treatments, abrasion, scarification, and surgery. Some people attempt to camouflage an objectionable tattoo with a new one. Each approach has drawbacks:

- *Laser treatments* can lighten many tattoos, some more easily and effectively than others. Generally, several visits are necessary over a span or weeks or months, and the treatments can be expensive. Some individuals experience hypopigmentation—a lightening of the natural skin coloring—in the affected area. Laser treatments also can cause some tattoo pigments to change to a less desirable shade. Unfortunately, knowing what pigments are in your tattoo or permanent makeup has always been difficult and has become more so as the variety of tattoo inks has multiplied. Inks are often sold by brand name only, not by chemical composition. Because the pigments are sold to tattoo parlors and salons, not on a retail basis to consumers, manufacturers are not required by law to list the ingredients on the labels. Furthermore, because manufacturers may consider the identity and grade of their pigments "proprietary," neither the tattooist nor the customer may be able to obtain this information. There also have been reports of individuals suffering allergic reactions after laser treatments to remove tattoos, apparently because the laser caused allergenic substances in the tattoo ink to be released into the body.

- *Dermabrasion* involves abrading layers of skin with a wire brush or diamond fraise (a type of sanding disk). This process itself may leave a scar.

- *Salabrasion*, in which a salt solution is used to remove the pigment, is sometimes used in conjunction with dermabrasion, but has become less common.

- *Scarification* involves removing the tattoo with an acid solution and creating a scar in its place.

- *Surgical removal* sometimes involves the use of tissue expanders (balloons inserted under the skin, so that when the tattoo is cut away, there is less scarring). Larger tattoos may require repeated surgery for complete removal.

- *Camouflaging* a tattoo entails the injection of new pigments to either form a new pattern or cover a tattoo with skin-toned pigments. Dr. Toombs notes, however, that injected pigments tend not to look natural because they lack the skin's natural translucence.

What About Temporary Tattoos?

Temporary tattoos, such as those applied to the skin with a moistened wad of cotton, fade several days after application. Most contain color additives approved for cosmetic use on the skin. However, the agency has issued an import alert for several foreign-made temporary tattoos.

According to OCAC Consumer Safety Officer Allen Halper, the temporary tattoos subject to the import alert are not allowed into the United States because they don't carry the FDA-mandated ingredient labels or they contain colors not permitted by FDA for use in cosmetics applied to the skin. FDA has received reports of allergic reactions to temporary tattoos.

In a similar action, FDA has issued an import alert for henna intended for use on the skin. Henna is approved only for use as a hair dye, not for direct application to the skin. Also, henna typically produces a reddish brown tint, raising questions about what ingredients are added to produce the varieties of colors labeled as "henna," such as "black henna" and "blue henna."

Chapter 12

Making Decisions About Tattooing And Body Piercing

History Of Tattooing And Body Piercing

Throughout history, tattooing and body piercing have been practiced by many cultures. The body of a 4,000-year-old tattooed man was discovered in a glacier on the Austrian border in 1992. Egyptians in the period from 4000–2000 B.C. identified tattooing with fertility and nobility. During the 17th and 18th centuries, European sailors traveling through the Polynesian islands saw extensive tattooing on both men and women. Since the fifth century B.C. the Japanese have used tattooing for ornamental, cosmetic, and religious purposes as well as for identification and punishment of criminals. In the late nineteenth century, tattooed royalty in England and European countries were fashionable. Lady Randolph Churchill (Winston's mother) had a snake tattooed around her wrist.

Like tattooing, body piercing has been practiced in many cultures for many centuries. Body piercing was often identified with royalty and portrayed courage and virility. Egyptian pharaohs pierced their navels as a rite

---

About This Chapter: Adapted from "Tattooing and Body Piercing: Decision Making for Teens," Virtual Hospital, University of Iowa Health Care, http://www.vh.org/Patients/IHB/Derm/Tattoo/#1, November 1998. Revised by David A. Cooke, M.D., November 6, 2002. Copyright-protected material used with permission of the author and the University of Iowa's Virtual Hospital.

♣ It's A Fact!!
Tattooing And Body Piercing As A Risk-Taking Behavior

Myrna L. Armstrong, Ed.D, R.N., F.A.A.N., professor of nursing at the Texas Tech University Health Sciences Center, has researched and written on tattooing as a risk-taking behavior in adolescents. She has identified body piercing as another risk-taking behavior that is gaining wide acceptance in the adolescent population.

Her research and articles studied the prevalence of tattooing in the last four years with two surveys conducted in urban high schools in 1993 and 1995. These surveys revealed an increasing number of adolescents engaging in tattooing at a younger age. A 1993 study of 642 adolescents from six suburban high schools in Texas revealed 8.6 percent had a tattoo, with the youngest being 11 years old when the tattoo was obtained. Very few markings were identified as gang markings, and 65 percent of the students with tattoos reported academic grades of A's and B's. Gender distribution of the 105 adolescents with tattoos were 65 percent male and 35 percent female.

Two years later the study was repeated in eight high schools across the United States to document a nationwide perspective with 1,762 students responding. The proportion of adolescents with a tattoo was higher, at 9 percent, with the youngest being only eight years old at the time the tattoo was obtained. Gang affiliation was reported, and 60 percent of the students with tattoos reported grades of A's and B's. The average age of first tattoo dropped from 16 years in the 1993 study to 14.5 years. In 1995, 55 percent of the adolescents expressed an interest in tattooing, compared to 33 percent in the 1993 study. Gender distribution of tattooed adolescents in the second study was not available.

No studies were found on the incidence of body piercing in adolescents. School nurses are beginning to see more students with health problems associated to piercing of various body parts. Armstrong has suggested that school nurses can become important resources to assist adolescents in becoming informed about the risks of body piercing.

Making Decisions About Tattooing And Body Piercing

of passage. Roman soldiers pierced their nipples to show their manhood. Mayans pierced their tongues as a spiritual ritual, and both sexes of Victorian royalty chose nipple and genital piercing.

In recent times tattoos have been most common among motorcyclists, criminals, gang members, individuals with psychiatric problems, and military personnel. Members of these groups often obtained tattoos to show loyalty to their group. Today the number of musicians and sports stars who are tattooed or body pierced has skyrocketed. Cher and Dennis Rodman are two of the most outspoken stars wearing tattoos. Many of these figures serve as role models for teenagers.

Thinking About Getting A Tattoo Or Body Piercing?
You Might Want To Know

- Unsterile tattooing and piercing equipment and needles can spread serious infection: hepatitis, tetanus, or possibly even HIV.
- Asking a friend to apply a tattoo may ruin a friendship if the tattoo doesn't look the way you thought it would.
- Tattoo removal is very expensive. A tattoo that costs $50 to apply may cost over $1,000 and more to remove.
- The law in many states prohibits the tattooing of minors.
- Tattoos are not easy to remove and in some cases may cause permanent discoloration. Think carefully before getting a tattoo. You can't take it back if you don't like it.
- Some people are allergic to the tattoo dye. Their bodies will work to reject the tattoo.
- Blood donations cannot be made for a year after getting a tattoo, body piercing, or permanent makeup.

Questions To Ask Friends

- First:
    - ◊ Talk to your friends or others who have been tattooed or pierced.

- ◊ Ask them about their experience, the cost, pain, healing time, and so forth.
- ◊ Ask them what they would do if they had a chance to do it over again.
- Second:
    - ◊ Understand that you do not have to tattoo or pierce your body to belong.
    - ◊ Remember that you are directly involved in decisions that affect your health and body.
    - ◊ You can always change your mind or wait if you are not sure.
- Third:
    - ◊ If you decide to have a tattoo or body piercing, never tattoo or pierce your own body or let a friend do it because of potential complications.

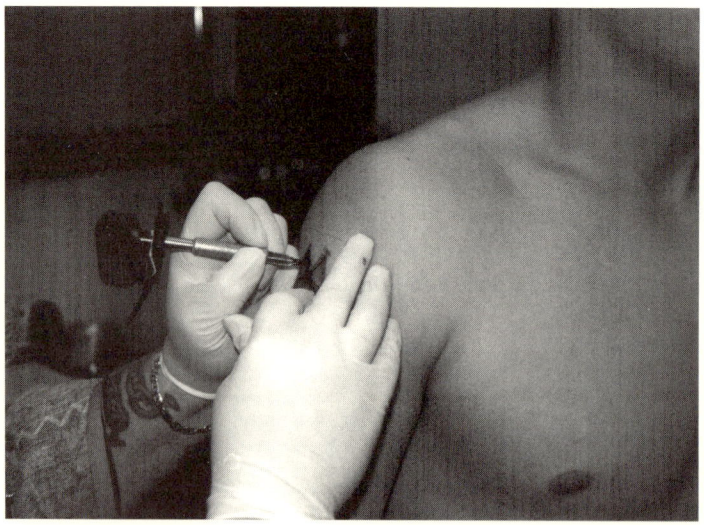

Figure 12.1. Good sterile procedure must be followed to reduce the risk of acquiring a blood-borne infection such as hepatitis or HIV from a tattoo. Tattoo equipment must be sterilized properly, and the tattooist should wear latex gloves.

Making Decisions About Tattooing And Body Piercing

How To Choose A Tattooist Or Piercing Artist

Visit several piercers or tattooists. The work area should be kept in a clean and sanitary condition and have good lighting. If they refuse to discuss cleanliness and infection control, go somewhere else.

Consent forms (which the customer must fill out) should be handled before tattooing. Reputable piercing and tattoo studios will not serve a minor without signed consent from parents. Check the laws in your state about tattooing of minors if you are under 18.

The tattooist/piercer should have an autoclave—a heat sterilization machine used to sterilize equipment between customers. Most tattooists/piercers are proud of their sterilization equipment.

Packaged, sterilized tattoo needles should be used only once and then thrown away in a special biohazard container.

Leftover tattoo ink should be thrown away after each procedure. Ink should never be poured back into the bottle. Needles should never be inserted into the bottle.

Immediately before tattooing/piercing, the tattooist/piercer should wash and dry his or her hands and put on latex gloves. The gloves should be worn at all times during the tattoo or piercing procedure. If the tattooist/piercer leaves the procedure and touches other objects such as the phone, new gloves should be used.

A piercing gun should not be used because it cannot be sterilized properly. Only jewelry made of a noncorrosive metal, such as surgical stainless steel, niobium, titanium, or solid 14K gold is safe for a new piercing. Gold-plated jewelry should not be used.

Does It Hurt?

Tattoo Procedure

Adolescents can acquire either a "professional" or amateur tattoo depending upon the law in their state. Typically, the "professional" tattoo is applied by an unlicensed artist using non–FDA-approved pigments at a studio. The tattoo may have been applied with or without consent from their parent or guardian. Tattoo artists use an electrically powered, vertical vibrating instrument to inject the tattoo pigment 50 to 3,000 times per minutes into the second layer of the skin (dermis), at a depth of 1/64 to 1/16 of an inch. A single needle outlines the tattoo, and the design is then filled in with five to seven needles in a needle bar. State regulations of tattooing range from prohibition of tattooing to no regulation at all. In some states with no regulation, local cities set up their own standards. The law for each specific state may be obtained from state, county, or local health departments.

The second method of obtaining a tattoo is from an amateur. More frequently teens obtain their tattoos from friends or self-inflict their own tattoos. These tattoos are done in unclean conditions with objects such as pencils, pens, straight pins, or needles. Pigments injected include India ink, carbon, soot, mascara, charcoal, and dirt. These tattoos are often placed on easy-to-reach parts of the body such as thighs, ankles, forearms, backs of hands, and the tops of fingers.

Both types of tattooing carry the risk of catching a blood-borne disease or infection. Needles must be sterilized before use and should not be reused. Leftover dye should not be returned to the bottle after use and the needles should not be placed directly into the bottle. The tattooist should wear latex gloves and should change gloves if the tattooing procedure is interrupted for other activities such as answering the phone or leaving the room.

Body Piercing Procedure

Teens obtain body piercings from either a studio piercer or an amateur. Earlobe and ear cartilage are the most frequently pierced sites. Other body parts pierced include eyebrow, lip, nose, tongue, nipple, navel, and various genital sites. A hollow needle is passed through the body part followed by the insertion of the body jewelry in the hole. A small amount of bleeding may occur as a result of the piercing. A piercing gun should not be used because it crushes the tissues that are pierced and it cannot be properly resterilized.

The type of jewelry inserted will depend on the body part. For example, a short barbell in the tongue will lead to problems when the tongue starts to

Making Decisions About Tattooing And Body Piercing

swell. The type of jewelry used must accommodate the swelling that follows the piercing procedure. Piercers recommend nontoxic metals such as surgical steel, 14K gold, niobium, or titanium to avoid infections and allergic reactions.

As Table 12.1 shows, healing times for body piercing vary with the site.

Table 12.1. Healing Times By Piercing Site

Site	Healing Time
Ear lobe	6 to 8 weeks
Ear cartilage	4 months to 1 year
Eyebrow	6 to 8 weeks
Nostril	2 to 4 months
Nasal septum	6 to 8 months
Nasal bridge	8 to 10 weeks
Tongue	4 weeks
Lip	2 to 3 months
Nipple	3 to 6 months
Navel	4 months to 1 year
Female genitalia	4 to 10 weeks
Male genitalia	4 weeks to 6 months

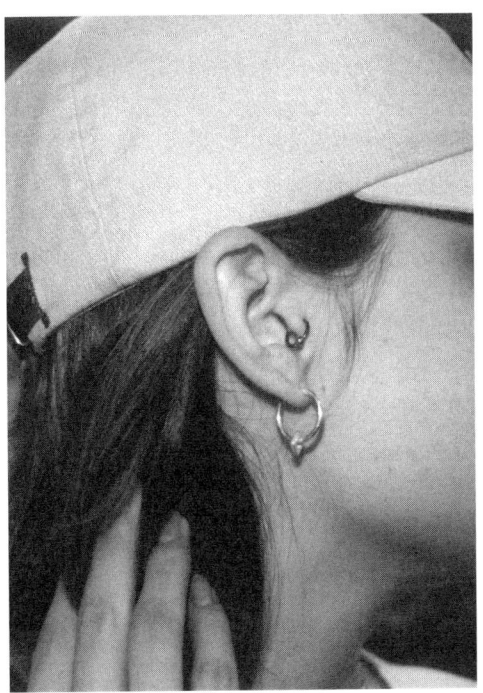

Figure 12.2. How long a body piercing takes to heal depends upon the site of the piercing. The piercing through the ear cartilage may take up to a year to heal, while the nearby lobe piercing will be completely healed within eight weeks.

How Do I Take Care Of A New Tattoo Or Body Piercing?

Tattoos

Tattoo site care is similar to skin care used for a minor burn. The area must be kept clean and moisturized until the tattoo has healed. Here are the basic guidelines:

- Keep the tattoo covered with the bandage for 2 to 12 hours or overnight. Touch the area as little as possible and do not allow others to touch the new tattoo.

- Remove the bandage by first wetting the gauze in the shower. Do not rebandage the tattoo.

- Wash the tattoo with antibacterial soap such as (Jergens®, Dial®, or Lever 2000®) and water to remove all Vaseline® and blood. Rinse thoroughly and pat dry with a soft towel. Do not use alcohol or peroxide. They dry out the tattoo.

- With clean hands, apply a light coat of an antibiotic ointment such as Neosporin®, Bacitracin®, or Mycitracin® at least three times a day. Rub it into the tattoo like lotion. The scab will stay soft and won't get hard and crack. Antibiotic ointment can be purchased at any drug store. Ask the pharmacist if you have questions and especially if you are allergic to antibiotics. Do not apply Vaseline or petroleum jelly. It has no healing abilities and will cause a heavy scab to form and the tattoo will become dull.

- If a rash occurs, stop using the antibiotic ointment and use A & D Ointment® or your regular hand lotion.

- After five days you may stop using an antibiotic ointment and switch to a gentle body lotion such as (Dermassage Lotion® or Curel®). The brand you use should be a cream-based moisturizer and not greasy. Do not use lotions with perfumes and color additives. Within 7 to 10 days your tattoo should stop feeling tender. Continue to apply the lotion for at least two weeks.

- Avoid exposure to direct sunlight for four weeks. Five minutes of direct sunlight on any part of a healing tattoo may trigger an allergic

Making Decisions About Tattooing And Body Piercing

reaction. A strong (30 SPF) waterproof sunscreen is recommended forever.

- Do not use a tanning bed during the healing process. Even after the tattoo has healed, always wear a bandage over the tattoo in a tanning bed.

- Soaking in a hot tub, swimming, or taking hot baths can ruin a tattoo. Avoid these activities until the peeling has stopped.

Body Piercings

The area around the new piercing must be kept clean to allow the body to heal around the jewelry. Piercing sites that are covered by clothes such as nipple, navel, or genitals may become infected because of perspiration and rubbing of clothing. Piercers stress the importance of not fingering the jewelry to prevent infection.

Here are the basic guidelines:

- Clean the piercing area with an antibacterial soap (such as Jergens, Dial, Lever 2000) twice a day. This is enough to keep the piercing clean and allow the body to heal. Gently wash the area surrounding and including the piercing with the soap. Remove all crusty formations from the piercing and jewelry. Rinse off the soap, making sure that all the soap and crust formations are gone.

- Salt water soaks are good to loosen up crusty formations. You can make salt water by adding one-quarter teaspoon of salt to one cup of clean water.

- You do not need strong cleaning agents if the area is infection-free. Do not use alcohol or peroxide to clean the area at any time. They will dry out your skin. Betadine® will discolor gold jewelry.

- Wash your hands with soap before touching or cleaning the pierced part during the healing process. Don't let anyone else touch the pierced part during the healing period.

- Avoid contact with other people's body fluids (saliva, sweat, and so forth). Even your own sweat may irritate the piercing. Be sure to rinse the area after all exercise to remove all sweat.

♣ It's A Fact!!
D-TAG—Tattoo Removal Program For Gang Members Who Want Out!

In Dallas, Texas a volunteer program called D-TAG helps teenage gang members to get out of gang life by sponsoring their tattoo removal. This program, which was started by a school nurse, uses family and community support to redirect the teen's life style away from gang activities in addition to sponsoring the removal of the tattoo.

Gang members often apply tags or marks to show that they belong to a gang. Most tags are acquired during the middle high school years as a part of gang initiation and involvement. Specific groupings of color and clothing and tattooing are examples of tagging. Tattoos are usually applied by fellow gang members.

As the gang members grow older, they may want to get out of the gang. This often comes at a time when the teen wants to get a job. Potential employers may not hire a person with a visible tattoo especially if it is related to a gang. Removal of the tattoo will also send the message that this person is no longer the property of a specific gang.

For admission into the D-TAG program, the teen must be enrolled in school or a gang intervention program. If the applicant is not enrolled in school, GED enrollment is required. The applicant must provide three letters of recommendation from supportive adults. One of these adults must agree to serve as a mentor for the teen to monitor school attendance and grades. The mentor will also monitor the 10 hours of community service that the teen is required to perform. A home visit with parents is made to discuss the procedure, obtain consent, and discuss the after-care needs of the teen. Parents are required to attend the first treatment

A private group of dermatologists provides the tattoo removal services, and a medical company that owns various types of laser equipment provides equipment. An advisory committee made up of community members and health providers oversees the program, and the school continues to identify teens who want to have their tattoos removed.

Other programs like D-TAG are starting in major cities in the U.S. If a teen gang member wants to leave gang life and have a tattoo removed, contact a school nurse or probation officer who may know about such a program.

Source: Excerpted from "Tattooing and Body Piercing: Decision Making for Teens," Virtual Hospital, University of Iowa Heath Care, http://www.vh.org/Patients/IHB/Derm/Tattoo#1, November 1998. Revised by David A. Cooke, M.D., November 6, 2000. Copyright-protected material used by permission of the author and the University of Iowa's Virtual Hospital.

Making Decisions About Tattooing And Body Piercing

- Always wear clean clothing and change bedsheets every week during healing. If the piercing is an ear piercing, clean your telephone and sun or eye glasses with Lysol® spray or alcohol. Wash the part of eyeglasses that touch your ear with soap and water.

- Check any threaded jewelry in your mouth (such as barbells) twice a day to make sure the ends are tight. You may swallow the barbell or damage a tooth if it comes loose.

- For ear and cartilage piercings, avoid makeup and powders around your face and neck during the healing process. Cover the pierced part with a tissue when using hair spray.

- No tight clothes. For navel piercing, don't wear large belts, stockings, or body suits, and do not sleep on your stomach. Good air circulation is important for healing.

- Be careful where you swim. Avoid public pools and hot tubs until the piercing has healed.

- For mouth care following tongue or lip piercing, choose an antibacterial mouthwash that does not contain alcohol and rinse your mouth after all meals and snacks. If you notice bad breath and an off-colored tongue, the mouthwash may have killed the mouth's own bacteria. If this happens, switch to salt water rinses instead of mouthwash.

What Can Go Wrong?

Tattoo Troubles

Tattooing carries the risk of acquiring HIV (although none has been reported), hepatitis B and C, and tetanus. Years ago, other infections such as TB and syphilis were reported due to use of fluids such as urine and saliva in the tattooing process. Blood cannot be donated for one year after a person has obtained a new tattoo. If the tattoo was obtained at a studio, the tattooist may provide instructions for the care of the new tattoo. Without proper cleaning and protection from sun, the new tattoo may become a source of infection and the body may work to reject the tattoo. Hypersensitivity to a pigment may result in an allergic response. Tattoo-mediated severe allergic contact dermatitis (severe skin irritation) has been reported with the use of certain pigments. Also reported are sarcoid-like granulomas called keloids (large thick scars) developing at the site of the tattoo. Iron oxide used in some eyeliner tattoos has caused tissue injury when the person had a special x-ray study called magnetic resonance imaging (MRI testing).

Piercing Problems

Complications from body piercings relate to the body part pierced. Ear cartilage piercings do not heal as quickly as lobe piercings because of the different type of tissue and pressure on the piercing area during sleep. Tongue piercings initially swell a large amount but heal quickly because of the tongue's great blood supply. However, tooth damage can occur from large tongue barbells, and retained food inside the piercing hole can be a problem. Nipple piercings may burrow through some of the milk-producing ducts and cause infection or problems if a woman wishes to breastfeed an infant later in her life. Navel piercings become infected easily because tight-fitting clothes do not allow enough air to circulate and allow moisture to collect around the piercing site. The teen may have healing problems if the selected jewelry is not the correct jewelry for the pierced area. If the jewelry is too thin or too heavy, the body may reject the jewelry and work to expel it like a splinter. If the jewelry is too small in diameter, the jewelry may cut off the blood supply and cause a lot of swelling and pain.

I've Changed My Mind. Now What Do I Do?

Tattoo Removal

Until the recent development of the Q-switched lasers, tattoos were removed by destroying the epidermis and dermis (first and second layers of skin), depending on the depth of the tattoo. Salabrasion—the removal of the tattoo by rubbing salt into the tattoo—and dermabrasion—the scrapping of the skin down to the dermis (second layer of skin) to remove the tattoo—both left extensive scarring at the site. The carbon dioxide laser removed the top layers of skin to expose the tattoo. The tattoo particles were then removed with chemicals such as urea. This method also resulted in scarring.

Making Decisions About Tattooing And Body Piercing

Three Q-switched lasers are designed for tattoo removal. The Q-switched ruby laser is used in removing blue-black and green pigments. The Q-switched Nd-YAG laser removes blue-black and red pigments. The Q-switched alexandrite laser removes blue-black pigments. The Q-switched laser radiation enters the skin layer where the tattoo granules reside. The energy of the laser breaks down the fibrous capsule around the pigment. Waste products from this reaction are either scattered into the air or removed by the body's elimination system. The procedure is slightly painful, with the sensation described as the snap of a thin rubber band or specks of hot bacon grease on the skin. Local anesthetics may be used to reduce the pain during the procedure. The removal of a "professional" tattoo may require five to six treatments and the removal of an amateur tattoo may require two to four treatments. The number of treatments depends on the amount and type of ink or pigment used and the depth of the ink in the skin. Dark (blue or black) inks and red inks fade the best. Oranges and purples usually respond well. Green and yellow inks are the most difficult to remove. In some cases, even though the tattoo ink is removed, a permanent, pale-white outline of the tattoo may remain. The cost of laser removal is quite expensive and not covered by insurance. A tattoo that costs $50 to $100 to obtain may cost $1,200 to $1,500 to remove by laser.

Chapter 13

Healing Body Piercings

Ear Piercing Of The Pinna (Above The Lobe)

- Always wash hands thoroughly before contact with piercing.

- Do not use rubbing alcohol or hydrogen peroxide. Both slow the healing of the piercing by drying and killing new healthy cells.

- Because of decreased vascularization in the upper pinna of the ear, it will take longer than the ear lobe to heal, generally between 12 and 16 weeks.

- Because it is important to not irritate the ear, it is recommended that you sleep on the opposite side from the pierced ear and use the unpierced ear for talking on the telephone.

- To clean the pierced ear use mild antiseptic products such as benzalkonium chloride, (Bactine® or Johnson's No More Ouchies®). Dilute 50/50 with water if soap is too harsh.

    ◊ Twice a day saturate a cotton swab with the cleaning solution.

    ◊ Remove any dried matter.

    ◊ Work the solution into the piercing; rotate the jewelry.

About This Chapter: Reprinted with permission from "Body Piercing: Cleaning and Healing," University Health Services, University of California, Berkeley, 2001. Available online at http://www.uhs.berkeley.edu/HealthInfo/EdHandouts/bodypiercing.htm.

Pierced Belly Buttons Or Nipples

- Always wash hands thoroughly before contact with piercing.
- Do not use rubbing alcohol or hydrogen peroxide. (Both slow the healing of the piercing by drying and killing new healthy cells.)
- Do not use bacitracin or other ointments. (Ointments try to heal piercing and stop the breathing of the tissue.)
- Use salt soaks for best care.
- Use a cup cleaned with antibacterial soap. Mix one teaspoon salt with one cup warm water. Make suction seal between cup and belly button by leaning over cup and then lie down to towel. Do this two or three times daily. Rinse with plain water. Dry with plain cotton swab.
- Wear loose-fitting clothing. (Some clear, pink, or slightly bloody discharge is normal for several days after piercing.)

Cheek And Lip Piercing

- Always wash hands thoroughly before contact with piercing.
- Do not use rubbing alcohol or hydrogen peroxide. (Both slow the healing of the piercing by drying and killing new health cells.)
- No oral contact of any kind for six weeks. (No wet kissing or oral sex without a barrier.)
- Suck on ice or popsicles the first 24 to 48 hours to minimize swelling and pain.
- Reduce intake of warm beverages, hot or spicy foods, tobacco, alcohol, and anything irritating to your mouth.
- Rinse with mouthwash for 30 to 60 seconds after consumption of anything other than water. If Listerine® is too harsh, it may be diluted, or use one-quarter teaspoon sea salt to an 8-ounce glass of water.

> ♣ **It's A Fact!!**
> Rubbing alcohol and hydrogen peroxide should never be used to clean piercings. They dry the skin and kill new cells as they appear.

Healing Body Piercings

- Use Gly-Oxide® or Peroxyl® twice daily following the instructions on the bottle. Afterwards you may rinse with water or salt water.
- The outer opening of the piercing is best treated with ear care antiseptic or Bactine.® If Bactine is too harsh, it may be slightly diluted with water. Apply liberally with a cotton swab while rotating jewelry. Do this two or three times daily.
- Continue this care regimen for six to eight weeks.

Tongue Piercing

- Always wash hands thoroughly before contact with piercing.
- Do not use rubbing alcohol or hydrogen peroxide. (Both slow the healing of the piercing by drying and killing new healthy cells.)
- Healing time six to eight weeks.
- No oral contact of any kind for six weeks. (No wet kissing or oral sex without a barrier.)
- Suck on ice or popsicles the first 24 to 48 hours to minimize swelling and pain.
- Reduce intake of warm beverages, hot or spicy foods, tobacco, alcohol, and anything irritating to your mouth.
- Rinse with mouthwash for 30 to 60 seconds after consumption of anything other than water. If Listerine is too harsh it may be diluted, or use one-quarter teaspoon sea salt to an 8-ounce glass of water.
- Use Gly-Oxide or Peroxyl twice daily following the instructions on the bottle. Five drops on top, five underneath; let foam and spit. (This is very important.) Afterwards you may rinse with water or salt water.
- The size of the stud is important in the healing process. It is best to use a post one-quarter inch longer than the thickness of your tongue. When the swelling has gone down, the post can be downsized to a slightly shorter but still roomy length. After six to eight weeks you can wear a stud the length of the piercing.

Genital Piercing

- Always wash hands thoroughly before contact with piercing.
- Do not use rubbing alcohol or hydrogen peroxide. (Both slow the healing of the piercing by drying and killing new healthy cells.)
- To clean, use warm water with a cleansing agent of antibacterial soap (for example, Phisoderm®, Johnson's No More Germies®, or liquid antibacterial soaps such as Dial®, Lever 2000®, or Softsoap®).
- Remove any dried matter from the surface of the ring and around the opening of the piercing.
- Apply a small amount of cleansing agent on the piercing; lather up and work the ring back and forth through the piercing half a dozen times.
- Leave the cleanser on the skin for three minutes.
- Rinse under running water while working the ring back and forth at least six times.
- Urinate to totally cleanse the area of soap. (Urine is sterile.)
- Keep the new piercing clean.
- Never touch it with dirty hands.
- During sexual contact, use barriers to keep saliva and other body fluids out of your piercing.
- Use condoms for intercourse.

Chapter 14

Fingernails: Looking Good, Playing Safe

With the ease that comes from years of practice, Julie Le, of Nails R Us in Alexandria, Virginia, sets out to remake customer Natalie Harris's nails. She buffs, files, snips, clips, smoothes, and then, with a nod from Harris, paints on ruby-red polish.

It's a process repeated every day throughout the country as thousands of women like Harris—and men, too—strive for beautiful nails. They seek the services of nail and beauty salons or manicure their nails themselves with a host of nail products available on the market.

The reason, said Kim Siridavong, owner of Nails R Us, is simple: "Everybody wants to look good."

But achieving that look is not without potential hazard. Infections and allergic reactions can occur with some nail services and products. Some chemicals in nail products, if ingested, are poisonous. Many are flammable.

Relying on nail and beauty salons is not risk-free, either. They use the same products, and they may present a greater risk for disease transmission.

Federal and state regulations help reduce the risks, but consumers also need to take care that their pursuit of beautiful nails ensures healthy nails.

> About This Chapter: This article, originally entitled "Fingernails: Looking Good While Playing Safe," was published in *FDA Consumer* in December 1995; available at http://www.fda.gov/fdac/features/095_nail.html. Reviewed and revised by David A. Cooke, M.D., on October 11, 2002.

Selecting A Safe Nail Salon

✔ **Quick Tip**

To help you decide if a salon provides sanitary nail services, nail and public health experts suggest considering the following:

- *Is the salon licensed?* Licenses often are posted. If you don't see one, ask.

- *Are the nail technicians licensed?* These licenses also are usually posted. Ask if you don't see one for your technician.

- *How are nail implements sanitized?* Autoclaving (heat sterilization) is best, says Ralph Daniel, M.D., a dermatologist in Jackson, Mississippi. But most states allow chemical sterilizing as long as the implements are immersed in the solution for at least 10 minutes between customers. Ask the technician what the salon's practices are. If they're using a chemical solution, check the product's label for words like "germicidal" to indicate that it is strong enough to kill bacteria. If in doubt, bring your own implements, Daniel suggests.

- *Is there a pre-service scrub?* Both the nail technician and the client should wash their hands with an antimicrobial soap before nail work begins.

- *Is each customer given a fresh bowl of soapy water to soak his or her nails in, and is a new nail file used for each customer?* Both practices should be followed.

- *Is the facility neat and clean?* Paul Kechijian, M.D., a clinical associate professor of dermatology and chief of the nail section at New York University, compares selecting a salon to selecting a restaurant. "Ask yourself when you walk in: Would you want to eat there?" he says.

- *Is there a strong smell of fumes?* If there is, it's a sign that the facility is poorly ventilated, says John Bailey, Ph.D., acting director of FDA's Office of Cosmetics and Colors. Inhaling the fumes from nail products can make you sick.

If you have a complaint about a salon providing nail services, contact your state board of cosmetology.

Fingernails: Looking Good, Playing Safe

Growth Of An Industry

With the increased use of nail services and products in recent years has come growing concern about safety. According to *Nails 1995 Fact Book*, U.S. consumers will spend an estimated $5.2 billion on nail services in 1995, half a billion more than in 1994. They can choose from 34,852 freestanding nail salons across the country—nearly 2,000 more than a year ago—or hundreds of thousands of beauty salons that offer nail services.

The most requested service, according to the *Fact Book*, is artificial nails. Manicures are number 2. Other popular services include nail jewelry and nail art.

Because of the variety of nail services, the preferred term for a person who provides nail services is "nail technician" rather than manicurist, said Suzette Hill, managing editor for *Nails*, a magazine for professionals and students.

"Twenty years ago, they mainly did manicures," she said. "Now, they're doing so much more."

They use a range of products, including polishes, paints, artificial nails, glues, and laminates, many of which are available for home use, too.

Nail Products As Cosmetics

Nail products for both home and salon use are regulated by the Food and Drug Administration (FDA). Under the Federal Food, Drug, and Cosmetic Act, these products are considered cosmetics because they are "articles other than soap which are applied to the human body for cleansing, beautifying, promoting attractiveness, or altering the appearance."

By law, nail products sold as cosmetics in the United States must be free of poisonous or deleterious substances that might injure users under the usual or customary conditions of use intended by the manufacturer. These uses are printed on the package or on a package insert. Many nail products contain poisonous substances, such as acetonitrile in glue removers, but are allowed on the market because they are not harmful when used as directed. They're poisonous only when ingested, which is not their intended use.

Products sold for home use also must be labeled properly, with the names of the ingredients listed in descending order of predominance.

FDA does not review or approve nail products and other cosmetics before they go on the market. However, the agency inspects cosmetic manufacturers and samples and analyzes cosmetics as needed. If a safety problem arises, the agency can take legal action against the product.

FDA also tracks safety problems through its Cosmetic Voluntary Registration Program, in which cosmetic manufacturers voluntarily report to FDA the types of adverse reactions their customers have reported to them. FDA uses this information to determine a baseline reaction rate for specific product categories, such as cuticle softeners, nail extenders (artificial nail ends), and nail polishes. The agency gives this information to participating companies so they can compare their adverse reaction rates to FDA's determined baseline.

FDA also learns about potentially harmful products from manufacturers' competitors, consumers, doctors, and nail technicians, who report adverse reactions directly to the agency.

Salon Safety

The salons and their technicians are regulated by the states, usually their cosmetology boards. Lois Wiskur, past president of the National Interstate Council of State Cosmetology Boards, said that as far as she knows, every state has some type of licensing requirements for nail salons, nail technicians, or both.

> ♣ **It's A Fact!!**
> From current consumer habits, one might surmise that the main function of nails is to look good. But nails serve several physiological purposes: They enhance fine touch and fine motor skills and protect the fingers and toes. Doctors also may examine them for indications of serious underlying diseases; for example, clubbed nails (a condition in which fingers or toes thicken and the nails wrap around them) is a classic sign of chronic lung and heart disorders.

Under these requirements, salons providing nail services usually must meet certain requirements, such as:

- Employing nail technicians who have had a minimum number of hours of classroom and practical training.

- Properly sterilizing manicure implements. The preferred methods are autoclaving (heat sterilization) or chemical sterilization.
- Undergoing a state inspection periodically.
- Maintaining sufficient equipment, such as at least one manicure table and one sink that runs hot and cold water.
- Making sure that employees wash their hands before beginning work on a customer.

To prevent blood-borne infections, such as HIV and hepatitis, the national Centers for Disease Control and Prevention (CDC) recommended similar sanitary practices for salon employees in guidelines issued in 1985. The guidelines targeted, among others, personal-service workers, such as manicurists and pedicurists. To date, there have been no reports of transmission of blood-borne diseases to or from a personal service worker, according to CDC.

Nail Infections

More common nail problems, dermatologists report, are infections from bacteria, such as *Staphylococcus*; fungi, such as *Candida* (also known as yeast); and skin viruses, such as warts.

Bacterial and fungal infections frequently result from artificial nails, whether applied at home or in a salon. A bump or knock to a long artificial nail may cause it to lift from the natural nail at the base, leaving an opening for dirt to get in. If the nail is reglued without proper cleaning (with rubbing alcohol, for example), bacteria or fungi may grow between the nails and spread into the natural nail.

Also, as the natural nail grows, an opening develops between the natural nail and artificial nail. If this space is not filled in regularly, it can increase the chances for infection.

A fungal infection can take hold when an acrylic nail is left in place too long—such as three months or more—and moisture accumulates under the nail.

Bacterial, fungal, and viral infections also can occur from using unsanitary nail implements, especially in a salon, where the same implements are used on many people.

Unclean implements are especially dangerous if the skin around the nail is broken. This can occur with overzealous manicuring—if, for example, too much of the cuticle is cut or pushed back too far. If the cuticle is cut or separated from the fingernail, infectious agents can get into the exposed area. This is why dermatologists recommend leaving cuticles intact.

Symptoms of an infection include pain, redness, itching, and pus in or around the nail area. Yellow-green, green, and green-black nail discolorations are signs of a *Pseudomonas* bacterial infection. A blue-green discoloration signals a fungal infection.

If an infection appears while you are wearing artificial nails, they should be removed and the area cleaned thoroughly with soap and water. If symptoms persist, you should consult a doctor, who may prescribe a topical or oral anti-infective medicine.

There are no approved nonprescription products to treat fungal nail infections, and over-the-counter (OTC) products to treat other types of fungal infections should not be used for nail infections. In a review of OTC antifungal products, FDA found that fungal infections of the nails respond poorly to topical therapy, partly because of the nail's thickness. So, in 1993, the agency ruled that any OTC product labeled, represented, or promoted as a topical antifungal to treat fungal infections of the nail is a new drug and must be approved by FDA before marketing. This rule, which went into effect in 1994, does not include prescription antifungal products.

Despite the rule, some companies continue to sell unapproved OTC nail products, such as nail glues, with antifungal claims. FDA has warned these companies it might take legal action if they don't stop selling the products.

It is also worth being aware that artificial nails can transmit infections to others. A variety of harmful bacteria are known to grow underneath artificial nails. Because of this problem, many hospitals and health care businesses now ban the wearing of artificial nails to work. If you work in a health care setting, it may be best to leave these cosmetics at home, as they can potentially infect patients.

Allergies And Other Hazards

Other common problems associated with nail products are allergic reactions, such as contact dermatitis, a skin rash characterized by redness and itching and sometimes tiny blisters that ooze.

Certain nail ingredients are known for their tendency to cause allergic reactions. Residual traces of the basic building blocks of acrylic resins ("acrylics") used in artificial nails, for example, can cause redness, swelling, and pain in the nail bed. In some cases, the reaction is so severe that the natural nail separates from the nail bed, and although a new nail usually grows in, it may be imperfect if the nail root has been damaged.

Nail strengtheners that contain "free formaldehyde" may cause an irritation or reaction, as can certain other chemicals in nail glues and polishes.

In the late 1970s, use of methyl methacrylate, then a common ingredient in artificial nail products, resulted in FDA receiving a number of reports of injuries and allergic reactions, including damage and deformity of

---

✔ Quick Tip
Precautions For Artificial Nails

- If there is any question about sensitivity to the materials in artificial nails, have one nail done as a test and wait a few days to see if a reaction develops.

- Never apply an artificial nail if the natural nail or skin around it is infected or irritated. Let the infection heal first.

- Read the directions for do-it-yourself nails before applying them, and follow the directions carefully. Save the ingredient list for your doctor in case you have an allergic reaction or other injury.

- Treat your artificial nails with care. They may be stronger than your own, but they still can break and separate. Try not to bump or knock them. Find new ways to do ordinary tasks, like using a pencil to dial or depress the numbers on the phone.

- If an artificial nail separates, dip the fingertip into rubbing alcohol to clean the space between the natural and artificial nails before reattaching the artificial nail. This will help prevent infection.

- Never use household glues for nail repairs. Use only products intended for nail use, and follow directions.

- Don't wear artificial nails for longer than three months at a time. Remove them for one month to give nails a rest.

- Keep nail glues and other poisonous substances out of the reach of children.

fingernails and contact dermatitis. The ingredient now is rarely used because of legal action against a former manufacturer of methyl methacrylate–containing products and numerous seizures and recalls of such products. Methyl methacrylate has since been replaced with other chemicals, such as ethyl methacrylate. However, according to John Bailey, Ph.D., acting director of FDA's Office of Cosmetics and Colors, the replacement chemicals have never been fully studied for safety, and they may be as harmful as methyl methacrylate.

"Our current guidance is that products containing ethyl methacrylate should be used only by trained nail technicians under conditions that minimize exposure and skin contact because of their potential to cause allergies," he said.

Whatever the cause, allergic reactions usually take place where the product has been applied or where it has inadvertently come in contact with other skin surfaces, such as the face, eyelids, and neck.

When the offending agent is no longer used, reactions clear up. Sometimes, the user can identify the chemical causing the allergic reaction and avoid it.

Though rare, some nail products can cause illness and even death, particularly if ingested by children. In 1987, a 16-month-old toddler died of cyanide poisoning after swallowing a mouthful of solvent used to remove sculptured artificial fingernails. At least one other youngster was rushed to the emergency room for intensive care after swallowing a similar product. These products contained acetonitrile, a chemical that breaks down into cyanide when swallowed. Since 1990, the Consumer Product Safety Commission has required household glue removers containing more than 500 milligrams of acetonitrile in a single container to carry child-resistant packaging. This includes glue removers for artificial nails.

Nail products also can be dangerous if they get in the eyes. And they can easily catch on fire if exposed to the free flame of the pilot light of a stove, a lit cigarette, or even the heating element of a curling iron.

Consumers should read labels of nail products carefully and heed any warnings.

With proper care and precautions, nails can be both healthy and attractive.

—by Paula Kurtzweil

Chapter 15

Head Off Hair-Care Disasters

It's never a good sign when the hairdresser panics. That's what happened to Barbara Cabrera-Avila, 38, when she returned to the salon about six weeks after having her hair straightened a couple of years ago. The cause for alarm: several bald spots in the back of her head.

The Adelphi, Maryland, resident began having her curls straightened at the age of six so her hair would be easier to comb and style. She says overprocessed hair likely played a role in her hair loss, and stress could have been a factor. What's certain is that three dermatologists advised her to take a break from hair straighteners, also known as relaxers.

Barbara says giving up the straight hair she had grown comfortable with wasn't easy. After all, people's personal preferences about how they want to look tie into self-esteem—a fact that makes for good sales in the hair business. In addition to paying for trims and cuts to achieve a certain look, consumers spend millions of dollars each year to get hair that's different from what nature intended—whether it's to tame tight curls, give flat hair a boost, or get rid of the gray.

About This Chapter: Originally published as "Heading Off Hair-Care Disasters: Use Caution With Relaxers and Dyes," *FDA Consumer*, January–February 2001. Available online at http://vm.cfsan.fda.gov/~dms/fdahdye.html and http://www.fda.gov/fdac/features/2001/101_hair.html.

Hair Color And Cancer

♣ It's A Fact!!

Over the years, some studies have indicated a possible link between hair dye use and cancer, while others have not. In February 1994, FDA and the American Cancer Society released an epidemiologic study involving 573,000 women. Researchers found that women who had ever used permanent hair dyes showed decreased risk of all fatal cancers combined and also of urinary system cancers. The study also revealed that women who had ever used permanent hair dyes showed no increased risk of any type of hematopoietic cancer (cancer of the body's blood-forming systems).

This research, published in the Journal of the National Cancer Institute (NCI), did suggest that prolonged use (20 years or more of constant use) of black hair dye may slightly increase the occurrence of non-Hodgkin's lymphoma and multiple myeloma, but these cases represented a small fraction of hair dye users. This study followed previous NCI studies that raised concern about the use of hair dyes and higher rates of non-Hodgkin's lymphoma.

In another study, published in the October 5, 1994, issue of the *Journal of the National Cancer Institute*, researchers from Brigham and Women's Hospital in Boston followed 99,000 women and found no greater risk of cancers of the blood or lymph systems among women who had ever used permanent hair dyes.

Then in 1998, scientists at the University of California at San Francisco questioned 2,544 people about their use of hair-color products. After integrating the results of this study with those of animal and other epidemiologic studies, they concluded that there was little convincing evidence linking non-Hodgkin's lymphoma with normal use of hair-color products in humans. The study was published in the December 1998 issue of the *American Journal of Public Health*.

FDA continues to follow research in this field.

Head Off Hair-Care Disasters

According to the Food and Drug Administration's (FDA) Office of Cosmetics and Colors, hair straighteners and hair dyes are among its top consumer complaint areas. Complaints range from hair breakage to symptoms warranting an emergency room visit. Reporting such complaints is voluntary, and the reported problem is often due to incorrect use of a product rather than the product itself. FDA encourages consumers to understand the risks that come with using hair chemicals, and to take a proactive approach in ensuring their proper use. The agency doesn't have authority under the Federal Food, Drug, and Cosmetic Act to require premarket approval for cosmetics, but it can take action when safety issues surface.

When The Product Is The Problem

When consumers notify FDA of problems with cosmetics, the agency evaluates evidence on a case-by-case basis and determines if follow-up is needed, says Allen Halper, an FDA consumer safety officer. FDA looks for patterns of complaints or unusual or severe reactions. The agency may conduct an investigation, and if the evidence supports regulatory action, FDA may request removal of a cosmetic from the market.

Take the example of two popular hair relaxer products by World Rio Corporation—the Rio Naturalizer System (Neutral Formula) and the Rio Naturalizer System with Color Enhancer (Black/Licorice). After receiving complaints about these products in November and December 1994, FDA warned the public against using them. Consumers complained of hair loss, scalp irritation, and discolored hair.

In December 1994, the World Rio Corporation, Inc., of Los Angeles, California, announced that it stopped sales and shipments of the product. But reports indicated that the company continued to take orders, and the California Department of Health also stepped in to stop sales. In January 1995, the U.S. Attorney's Office in Los Angeles filed a seizure action against these products on behalf of FDA. By then, the agency had received more than 3,000 complaints about the Rio products.

Although most relaxers are alkaline, this product was formulated to be acidic. In the resulting consent decree of condemnation and permanent injunction, FDA alleged that the products were potentially harmful or injurious when used as intended, that they were more acidic than declared in the labeling, and that the labeling described the products as "chemical free" when "allegedly they contained ingredients commonly understood to be 'chemicals.'"

Safer Straightening

FDA has received complaints about scalp irritation and hair breakage related to both lye and "no lye" relaxers. Some consumers falsely assume that compared to lye relaxers, "no lye" relaxers take all the worry out of straightening.

"People may think because it says 'no lye' that it's not caustic," says FDA biologist Lark Lambert. But both types of relaxers contain ingredients that work by breaking chemical bonds of the hair, and both can burn the scalp if used incorrectly. Lye relaxers contain sodium hydroxide as the active ingredient. With "no lye" relaxers, calcium hydroxide and guanidine carbonate are mixed to produce guanidine hydroxide.

Research has shown that this combination in "no lye" relaxers results in less scalp irritation than lye relaxers, but the same safety rules apply for both. They should be used properly, left on no longer than the prescribed time, carefully washed out with neutralizing shampoo, and followed up with regular conditioning. For those who opt to straighten their own hair, it's wise to enlist help simply because not being able to see and reach the top and back of the head makes proper application of the chemical and thorough rinsing more of a challenge.

Some stylists recommend applying a layer of petroleum jelly on the scalp before applying a relaxer because it creates a protective barrier between the chemical and the skin. Scratching, brushing, and combing can make the scalp more susceptible to chemical damage and should be avoided right before using a relaxer. Parents should be especially cautious when applying chemicals to children's hair and should keep relaxers out of children's reach. There have been reports of small children ingesting straightening chemicals and suffering injuries that include burns to the face, tongue, and esophagus.

How often to relax hair is a personal decision. According to Pearl Freier, an instructor at the International Academy of Hair Design in South Daytona, Florida, relaxing at intervals of six to eight weeks is common, and the frequency depends on the rate of a person's hair growth. Leslie F. Safer, M.D., a dermatologist in Albany, Georgia, who has treated women with scalp irritation from relaxers, says straightening every six weeks is too frequent, in his opinion. Relaxers can cause hair breakage in the long term, he says, and blow drying and curling can do more damage.

Consumers should be aware that applying more than one type of chemical treatment, such as coloring hair one week and then relaxing it the next, can increase the risk of hair damage. "The only color we recommend for relaxed hair is semi-permanent because it has no ammonia and less peroxide," compared with permanent color, Freier says.

Hair Dye Reactions

As with hair relaxers, some consumers have reported hair loss, burning, redness, and irritation from hair dyes. Allergic reactions to dyes include itching, swelling of the face, and even difficulty breathing.

Coal tar hair dye ingredients are known to cause allergic reactions in some people, FDA's Lambert says. Synthetic organic chemicals, including hair dyes and other color additives, were originally manufactured from coal tar, but today manufacturers primarily use materials derived from petroleum. The use of the term "coal tar" continues because historically that language has been incorporated into the law and regulations.

The law does not require that coal tar hair dyes be approved by FDA, as is required for other uses of color additives. In addition, the law does not allow FDA to take action against coal tar hair dyes that are shown to be harmful, if the product is labeled with the prescribed caution statement indicating that the product may cause irritation in certain individuals, that a patch test for skin sensitivity should be done, and that the product must not be used for dyeing the eyelashes or eyebrows. The patch test involves putting a dab of hair dye behind the ear or inside the elbow, leaving it there for two days, and looking for itching, burning, redness, or other reactions.

> ### ✔ Quick Tip
>
> **Look Out For Your Eyes**
>
> Whether applying hair chemicals at home or in a hair salon, consumers and beauticians should be careful to keep them away from the eyes. FDA has received reports of injuries from hair relaxers and hair dye accidentally getting into eyes. And while it may be tempting to match a new hair color to eyebrows and eyelashes, consumers should resist the urge. The use of permanent eyelash and eyebrow tinting and dyeing has been known to cause serious eye injuries and even blindness. There are no color additives approved by FDA for dyeing or tinting eyelashes and eyebrows.
>
> The law does not require that coal tar hair dyes be approved by FDA, as is required for other uses of color additives. In addition, the law does not allow FDA to take action against coal tar hair dyes that are shown to be harmful, if the product is labeled with the following caution statement: "Caution — This product contains ingredients which may cause skin irritation on certain individuals and a preliminary test according to accompanying directions should first be made. This product must not be used for dyeing the eyelashes or eyebrows; to do so may cause blindness."

"The problem is that people can become sensitized—that is, develop an allergy—to these ingredients," Lambert says. "They may do the patch test once, and then use the product for 10 years" before having an allergic reaction. "But you're supposed to do the patch test every time," he says, even in salons.

And what about ending up with something other than the exact shade of strawberry blonde on the shelf? "Don't think the color on the box is the color you'll get," says Freier, the cosmetology instructor. "There are so many variables, like what chemicals are already in your hair and what your natural color is, that go into how your hair will turn out."

When using all hair chemicals, it's critical to keep them away from children to prevent ingestion and other accidents, and to follow product directions carefully. It sounds basic, but some people don't do it, says FDA's Halper. "If it says leave on hair for five minutes, seven minutes doesn't make it better," he says. "In fact, it could do damage."

—by Michelle Meadows

Chapter 16

The Luster In Your Locks

Having a good hair day doesn't just happen by chance. It happens when taking care of your hair becomes just as important as taking care of your skin. But what do you do when your hair has been damaged by every-day styling, and chemical processing, dyeing, or perming? Is there any solution for fly-away hair, dullness, and faded color? Understanding how hair damage can occur is the best defense against both preventing it and repairing it.

Speaking today at the American Academy of Dermatology's 2002 Annual Meeting in New Orleans, dermatologist Zoe Diana Draelos, M.D., clinical associate professor, Department of Dermatology, Wake Forest University, Winston-Salem, North Carolina, spoke about how to get and maintain the strength, shine, and softness of healthy hair.

"Hair damage results from both mechanical and chemical trauma that alters the physical structures of the hair," said Dr. Draelos. "There is no easy fix for hair that has become dull, brittle, and porous, but there are certainly products and tips that can help individuals minimize the damage that occurs to the hair every day."

About This Chapter: Text in this chapter is from "Keeping the Luster in Your Locks: The Four Most Common Hair Concerns," a press release dated February 25, 2002 © American Academy of Dermatology. Reprinted with permission from the American Academy of Dermatology. All rights reserved.

The hair has three basic layers, the cuticle, the cortex and the medulla. The cuticle is the outer layer of protective scales. It is the main hair structure and is responsible for the strength, shine, smoothness, softness, and manageability of healthy hair. There is also a layer of sebum, an oily substance secreted by the hair follicles, which coats the cuticles and adds shine and manageability to the hair. The cortex provides strength to the hair shaft, and determines the color and texture of hair. The medulla is the innermost core of the hair where the body and strength of the hair is determined.

The cuticle can be damaged by chemical or mechanical means, such as dyeing or blow-drying. Environmental factors, such as exposure to sunlight, air pollution, wind, seawater, and chlorinated swimming pool water can also cause damage to occur. When the cuticle is damaged by such means, the protective scales are peeled away and the rest of the hair shaft is exposed. In some cases, even the innermost layer—the medulla—is exposed for further damage.

> ### 🕮 Weird Words
>
> <u>Cortex</u>: The second layer of the hair, and the one that determines color and texture.
>
> <u>Cuticle</u>: The outermost layer of the hair, made up of protective scales.
>
> <u>Medulla</u>: The core of the hair.
>
> <u>Sebum</u>: An oily substance that is produced by sebaceous glands in the skin and coats the hair, making it shiny.
>
> <u>Trichoptilosis</u>: The technical name for split ends.

"The best way to improve the cosmetic value of the damaged or weathered hair shaft is to use conditioners, which cannot repair the hair shaft, but can increase shine, decrease static electricity, improve hair strength, and provide ultraviolet (UV) radiation protection," stated Dr. Draelos. "These are four factors which are very important for a healthy head of hair."

Shine

Shiny hair has always been equated with healthy hair, even though the health of a hair follicle cannot be determined due to its location deep within the scalp. The shine comes from light reflected by the smooth surface of the individual hair shafts. Conditioners containing polymer film-forming agents can increase hair shine by helping the cuticle "scales" lie flat against the hair shaft for a smoother appearance.

Static Electricity

Combing or brushing the hair allows the individual hair shaft to become negatively charged, creating static electricity and preventing the hair from lying smoothly in a given style. Fine hair is more susceptible to static electricity than coarse hair due to the greater surface area of the cuticle. Conditioners with the ingredient quaternary ammonium can minimize static electricity by imparting cationic properties, or positively charged ions, to the hair to neutralize the static.

Strength

Increasing the hair's strength can be attempted by using conditioners with ingredients such as hydrolyzed proteins or hydrolyzed human hair keratin proteins, which have a low molecular weight. They can easily penetrate the hair shaft to replenish the hair's nutrients, providing a high degree of improvement.

These proteins can also be used to smooth down split ends, also known as trichoptilosis. "Split ends develop after the protective cuticle has been stripped away from the end of hair fibers as a result of chemical or physical trauma," stated Dr. Draelos, "but it can also be a result of vigorous brushing." While there is no way to reverse split ends, trims every four weeks and deep-conditioning treatments can keep strands supple and flexible.

Photoprotection

While the hair is made up of nonliving materials and cannot develop cancerous qualities, its cosmetic value can be diminished through excessive exposure to the sun. UV exposure can induce oxidation of the sulfur molecules within the hair shaft, which are important for hair strength. If this oxidation occurs, the hair can become weak, dry, rough, faded, and brittle.

Individuals who bleach or lighten their natural hair color may also notice slight color changes in their hair when it is exposed to UV rays. Blonde hair may develop "photoyellowing," a process where chemicals in the hair shaft react to UV exposure, causing yellowing, fading, and a dull appearance. Even natural brunette hair tends to develop reddish hues due to the photo-oxidation of melanin pigments in the hair shaft.

To protect your hair from the damaging rays of the sun, look for a leave-in conditioner that contains zinc oxide. Wearing a hat made of a solid material is another form of protection. When selecting a hat for sun protection, choose carefully. Some hats, especially straw hats that may be fashionable and look nice, have open spaces, which cannot give you much protection.

"It's important to take care of the hair to prevent obvious damage," recommends Dr. Draelos. "Hair truly is the crowning glory on every person, and it only takes a few extra moments to add proper hair care to a daily routine."

✔ **Quick Tip**

Use A Conditioner

Hair conditioners are the single most effective measure for keeping hair looking good. They make hair shinier and stronger, reduce static electricity, and protect against damage from sunlight.

Chapter 17

Losing Your Hair

It's kind of weird how we sometimes define how we look by our hair. "Having a bad hair day" says it all, doesn't it?

Balding or hair loss may seem like something only adults need to worry about. But when teens begin to lose more than the usual amount of hair, it can mean that something is going on. It could mean you're sick, or maybe you're just not eating right. Whatever the cause, unusual hair loss means you should see a doctor. And if you're undergoing cancer treatment and you've lost your hair, there are ways to cope.

Hair Basics

First, a lesson on hair. Each hair on your head—or on your body, for that matter—is made of a hard protein called keratin. A single hair consists of a hair shaft (the part that shows), a root below the skin, and a follicle, from which the hair root grows.

The hair root is alive and is nestled in the follicle, which produces the hair shaft. The shaft consists of two or three concentric—or circular—layers

---

About This Chapter: "Hair Loss." This information was provided by KidsHealth, one of the largest resources online for medically reviewed information written for parents, kids, and teens. For more articles like this one, visit www.KidsHealth.org or www.TeensHealth.org. © 2001 The Nemours Center for Children's Health Media, a division of the Nemours Foundation.

of keratin. At the lower end of the follicle is the hair bulb, where pigment, or melanin, is produced and it colors the hair shaft—giving you black, blonde, brunette, red, or some other color hair.

Here's something interesting about hair: There's a link between hair color and the number of hairs on your head. For example, people with naturally blonde hair tend to have more hair on their heads than redheads.

Another fun fact: there are only three places on your entire body where the skin lacks hair follicles and hair doesn't grow. Where? Your lips, the palms of your hands, and the soles of your feet.

✎ Weird Words

<u>Alopecia</u>: The medical term for baldness or hair loss.

<u>Alopecia areata</u>: A disease of the immune system that results in hair loss, particularly on the scalp, eyebrows, and, in men, the bearded portion of the face. See Chapter 51 for more information.

<u>Anorexia</u>: A psychological disorder characterized by purposeful starvation and characterized by an extreme fear of obesity. Also known as anorexia nervosa.

<u>Bulimia</u>: A psychological disorder characterized by binges of uncontrolled eating followed by fasting, the use of laxatives or diuretics, self-induced vomiting, or extreme exercise to prevent weight gain. Also known as bulimia nervosa.

<u>Lupus</u>: A severe inflammatory disease that can affect the skin and hair, joints, lungs, heart, kidneys, and bloodstream.

<u>Trichotillomania</u>: A psychological disorder in which the individual repeatedly pulls out his or her hair.

Source: Adapted from *Stedman's Medical Dictionary, 27th Edition*, © 2000. Lippincott Williams, and Wilkins. All rights reserved. Reprinted with permission.

Losing Your Hair

What Is Hair Loss?

The medical term for hair loss is alopecia (pronounced: al-oh-pee-shah).

Most people lose about 50 to 100 hairs a day, and the hairs are replaced—in the same spot on your head. This amount of hair loss is totally normal and no cause for worry. If you're losing more than that, though, something may be wrong.

"It is not normal for teens of any age to lose their hair. They should get help," says Lynn Drake, M.D., a dermatologist in Cambridge, Massachusetts.

Hair loss can be caused by many things, and although sometimes the hair grows back, sometimes it doesn't. So if a teen is experiencing hair loss, she should see a doctor who can determine why the hair is falling out and suggest treatment, if necessary.

What Causes Hair Loss?

Although there are many reasons for hair loss, almost 95 percent of people who lose their hair suffer from common baldness or androgenetic alopecia (pronounced: an-dro-jeh-net-ick al-oh-pee-shah). This condition is caused by several factors—getting older, hormones called androgens, and genetics.

Hair loss can also be caused by certain illnesses or medical conditions, including endocrine (hormonal) abnormalities such as diabetes or thyroid disease. Also, kidney and liver diseases and lupus can cause hair loss.

There is also a condition called alopecia areata (pronounced: al-oh-pee-shah air-ee-ah-tah), a skin disease that results in hair loss on the scalp and sometimes elsewhere on the body. It affects 1.7 percent of the population, including more than 4 million people in the United States. Alopecia areata is thought to be an autoimmune disease, in which the hair follicles are damaged by a person's own immune system. In autoimmune diseases, the immune system mistakenly attacks the cells, tissues, and organs of a person's own body.

Alopecia areata usually starts as one or more small, round bald patches on the scalp and can progress to total hair loss, but this only happens in a small number of cases. Both guys and girls can get it, and it often begins in childhood. The hair usually grows back in six months to two years, but not always.

Stacianna Sitts, an Olympic swimmer, developed alopecia areata when she was 12. Over the years, she has learned to cope with her baldness—including thoughtless comments from people who don't understand her situation. She swam in the 2000 Olympics in Sidney, Australia.

Another medical condition that causes baldness is called trichotillomania (pronounced: trik-oh-till-oh-may-nee-uh), a psychological disorder in which kids and teens repeatedly pull their hair out. It results in areas of baldness and damaged hairs of different lengths. Teens with trichotillomania need to get help to stop pulling their hair out.

Another reason why teens may lose their hair is because of medications they may be taking. Beta blockers, which are taken for heart problems, and diet medications that contain amphetamines can cause hair loss. Also, isotretinoin, an acne medicine, and lithium, which is used to treat bipolar disorder, can cause hair to fall out, Dr. Drake says. In fact, Dr. Drake says there are more than 300 medications that can cause hair loss. If this happens to you, talk to your doctor to see if there is a different medication you can take.

Chemotherapy drugs for cancer are probably the most well-known medications that cause hair loss, but some cancers including leukemia and lymphoma can cause hair loss even before treatment begins.

There are cosmetic causes for hair loss as well. Having your hair chemically curled, getting a perm, or getting your hair colored, bleached, or straightened can cause damage and make your hair fall out. If you get these procedures done too often or if they are done incorrectly, you may see bald spots.

Another kind of baldness, called traction alopecia, is caused by wearing your hair in braids that are too tight, which causes the hair to break. This often affects black girls, and occurs mostly at the edges of their hairlines.

Poor nutrition can also cause hair loss. Eating disorders such as anorexia and bulimia contribute to hair loss because the body is not getting enough protein, vitamins, and minerals to sustain hair growth. Also, some teens who are vegetarians lose their hair because they may not get enough protein if they don't structure their diet properly, Dr. Drake says.

Some athletes such as runners are at higher risk for hair loss because they may be more likely to develop iron-deficiency anemia, Dr. Drake says.

Hair loss can be brought on by an alteration in the hair cycle that is caused by a major event, like having a baby, having a high fever, undergoing anesthesia, or following an episode of heavy bleeding. This type of hair loss corrects itself.

Catastrophic Hair Loss

Teens who have cancer and lose their hair because of chemotherapy treatments go through a difficult time, especially girls.

"The guys generally don't have as much sadness about hair loss and will get a crew cut before it falls out," says Lee Lucas, a clinical social worker in Wilmington, Delaware, who provides counseling to kids going through cancer treatments.

It's important that teens be given as much control over their appearance as possible when they're losing their hair. There are options such as wearing wigs, hair wraps, hats, and baseball caps. Often, hair loss is the first outward sign that a person is sick, which can be really scary. But the hair will return. And being bald means the chemotherapy is working on the bad cells because you can see how it's working on the good cells.

What Can The Doctor Do?

If you're concerned about hair loss, you should see a doctor. The doctor will check your scalp and may take hair samples. He or she may also test you for certain medical conditions that can cause hair loss. It may be recommended that you see a nutrition expert.

If medication is causing hair loss, ask the doctor if a different drug can be substituted. If your hair loss is due to an endocrine condition, like diabetes or thyroid disease, proper treatment and control of the underlying disorder is important to reduce or prevent hair loss. Using a product like minoxidil that can discourage hair loss and speed up hair growth also may be helpful, Dr. Drake says. Alopecia areata can be helped by corticosteroids.

Taking Care Of Your Hair

Eating a balanced, healthy diet is important for a lot of reasons, and it really benefits your hair. Also, treat your hair well. For example, some doctors recommend using baby shampoo, shampooing no more than once a day, and lathering gently.

Also, consider putting away the blow dryer and air-drying your hair instead. Don't rub too vigorously with a towel, either. If you can't live without your blow dryer, try using it on a lower setting.

Style your hair when it's dry. Styling your hair while it's wet can cause it to stretch and break. And try to avoid teasing your hair, which can also cause damage. Perm and color carefully to avoid mistakes that can cause your hair to break or fall out.

Chapter 18

Removing Hair You Don't Want

Hair where hair oughtn't be, according to the current dictates of American fashion, raises many an eyebrow. And so, for cosmetic reasons, millions of women, and a growing number of men, spend millions of dollars each year on products and services that promise smooth, silky skin free of "unsightly," "excessive" body hair.

For do-it-yourselfers, a variety of home-use hair removal products are available over the counter. These include shaving creams, foams, and gels; waxes; chemical depilatories; and electrolysis devices. Professionals at beauty and skin care salons and in dermatologists' offices provide waxing, electrolysis, and, most recently, laser treatments to remove hair. On April 3, 1995, the U.S. Food and Drug Administration (FDA) cleared the first laser for this use.

The cost, safety, effectiveness, and ease of use of the various methods, as well as the area and amount of hair growth to be treated, are some factors to weigh in choosing a method and deciding whether to go to a professional. Often, different methods are better suited for different areas.

FDA's Office of Cosmetics and Colors in the Center for Food Safety and Applied Nutrition regulates chemical depilatories, waxes, and shaving creams

> About This Chapter: Taken from "Hair Today, Gone Tomorrow," published originally in the September 1996 *FDA Consumer*; available at http://www.fda.gov/fdac/features/796_hair.html and at http://vm.cfsan.fda.gov/~dms/cos-hrem.html. Reviewed and revised by David A. Cooke, M.D., on October 11, 2002.

and gels. (The Consumer Product Safety Commission regulates razors.) These products, says John E. Bailey Jr., Ph.D., acting director of the office, are classified as cosmetics, defined as substances applied to the body to alter the appearance, promote attractiveness, cleanse, or beautify.

The agency's Center for Devices and Radiological Health regulates electrolysis equipment and lasers.

Shaving

Shaving is by far the most common method of hair removal for both men and women. Men have been shaving their beards and mustaches for thousands of years, but cosmetic hair removal in women was relatively uncommon until after World War I. Now, many American women routinely shave their legs and underarms.

A clean razor with a sharp blade is essential for a safe and comfortable shave. Skin should never be shaved dry; wet hair is soft, pliable, and easier to cut. Contrary to what many believe, shaving does not change hair's texture, color, or rate of growth.

Depilatories

"Depilatories act like a chemical razor blade," Bailey says. Available in gel, cream, lotion, aerosol, and roll-on forms, they contain a highly alkaline chemical—usually calcium thioglycolate—that dissolves the protein structure of the hair, causing it to separate easily from the skin surface.

"It's very important to carefully follow the use directions for depilatories and to do a preliminary skin test both for allergic reaction and sensitivity," Bailey says. "Hair and skin are similar in composition," he explains, "so chemicals that destroy the hair can also cause serious skin irritations—possibly even chemical burns—if left on too long."

"The concentration of calcium thioglycolate is generally kept as weak as possible to avoid skin irritation, yet strong enough to work in a reasonable amount of time," says Stanley R. Milstein, Ph.D., special assistant to the cosmetics and colors director. "Contact with the skin is kept to somewhere between 4 and 15 minutes, depending on how fine or coarse the hair is."

Consumers should be sure to read the product label and select the formulation appropriate for the intended use, because skin sensitivity varies on different parts of the body. Some depilatories are for use only on the legs, for example, while others are safe for more sensitive areas, such as the bikini line, underarms, and face.

Depilatories should not be used for the eyebrows or other areas around the eyes, or on inflamed or broken skin. To minimize the chance of skin irritation, they should not be applied more often than recommended on the product label.

Although cosmetics are not subject to pre-market approval, FDA can take action against products that are found to cause harm.

"If we find an adverse reaction is occurring under recommended use conditions, and not because of misuse by the consumer, we can pursue any number of actions, depending on the severity and prevalence of the problem," says Bailey.

For example, he says, "A depilatory might cause second- or third-degree burns, and possibly scarring, if its formula is too strong or if an inactive ingredient in the product heightens its effect. In that case, FDA may, after evaluating the problem, initiate regulatory action such as seizure or injunction against the product or the firm to stop further manufacture."

Growth Retardants

Recently, a new kind of product for controlling excess hair growth was introduced. The medication, eflornithine cream, is marketed under the trade name Vaniqa, and it is approved by the FDA for control of excess facial hair. Unlike the other products described in this article, it does not actually remove hair. Rather, it slows the growth of new hair considerably, so that more time can pass between hair removal sessions. According to the manufacturer, eflornithine cream slows hair growth by about 50 percent. In other words, if waxing or tweezing were required every three weeks before eflornithine, six weeks may be often enough after.

Eflornithine is applied as a cream to the affected skin twice daily. It may take four to eight weeks of use before its effects are apparent. The most common side effects are burning sensations and irritation of the skin where it is applied. This medication is available only by prescription.

Tweezing And Waxing

While depilatories remove hair at the skin's surface, "epilatories," such as tweezers and waxes, pluck hairs from below the surface. Waxing and tweezing may be more painful than using a depilatory, but the results are longer lasting. Because the hair is plucked at the root, new growth is not visible for several weeks after treatment.

Tweezing is impractical for large areas, however, because it is such a slow process. Women mostly use tweezers for shaping eyebrows and removing facial hair.

Waxing, too, is mostly done to shape the eyebrows and remove hair on the chin and upper lip, says Brenda Ruffner, a cosmetologist in Rockville, Maryland, although, she says, many women also have their legs, underarms, and bikini line waxed.

"Men usually come in for treatment on their chest or back," Ruffner says. "I have male clients who are bodybuilders and want their skin to look smooth for competitions. And some men are uncomfortable with the hair on their back or are embarrassed by it," she says.

Epilatory waxes are also available over the counter for home use. They contain combinations of waxes, such as paraffin and beeswax, oils or fats, and a resin that makes the wax adhere to the skin. There are "hot" and "cold" waxes.

With hot waxing, a thin layer of heated wax is applied to the skin in the direction of the hair growth. The hair becomes embedded in the wax as it cools and hardens. The wax is then pulled off quickly in the opposite direction of the hair growth, taking the uprooted hair with it.

Cold waxes work similarly. Strips pre-coated with wax are pressed on the skin in the direction of the hair growth and pulled off in the opposite direction. The strips come in different sizes for use on the eyebrows, upper lip, chin, and bikini area.

Labeling of over-the-counter waxes cautions that these products should not be used by people with diabetes and circulatory problems, who are particularly susceptible to infection. Waxing—and tweezing as well—can leave the skin sore and open to infection. Waxes should not be used over varicose veins, moles, or warts. They should not be used on the eyelashes, inside the nose or ears, on the nipples or genital areas, or on irritated, chapped, sunburned, or cut skin. A small area should be tested for sensitivity or allergic reaction before treating the entire area. Some hair removal experts recommend professional waxing for the best results.

Electrical Epilators

Two types of devices use electric current to remove hair: the needle epilator and the tweezers epilator.

"Needle epilators introduce a very fine wire close to the hair shaft, under the skin, and into the hair follicle," explains Anthony Watson, a materials engineer in FDA's Center for Devices and Radiological Health. "An electric current travels down the wire and destroys the hair root at the bottom of the follicle. The loosened hair is then removed with tweezers. Every hair is treated individually."

Needle epilators are used in electrolysis. Because this technique destroys the hair follicle, it is considered a permanent hair removal method. The hair root may persist, however, if the needle misses the mark or if insufficient electricity is delivered to destroy it.

"Also," Watson adds, "the stimulus for hair growth in an area is never permanently removed. For instance, you can't control hormonal changes that cause new growth. Most people would probably define permanent as 'never comes back,' but from a medical standpoint that may not be practical."

Successful electrolysis usually requires considerable time and money. Mona Wexler, an electrologist in Bethesda, Maryland, says she is careful to explain the process to her clients at their first appointment.

"Electrolysis requires a series of treatments over a period of time. It's not just a one-, two- or three-time thing," she says. "For example, the process for

> **☞ Remember!!**
> Cosmetic hair removal can be quick and easy or time-consuming and somewhat uncomfortable. It can be costly or inexpensive. But, for just about anyone who so desires, there's a way to get rid of the hair you don't want.

a forearm takes a series of appointments once a week for about a year. You may have a first clearing of both forearms in about eight hours of treatment over two months. After that, you have to catch the hairs that are coming in on a different cycle of growth. For the best results, you want to treat each hair during its active growing stage."

Electrolysis may not always be the best approach, Wexler adds: "Some men who begin electrolysis to get rid of the hair on their back soon stop, because it can be a huge, costly, and very time-consuming job, depending on the amount of hair."

More often, she says, men are treated for the area between the eyebrows, around the outside of the ears, and the shoulders.

"Women mostly come in for facial hair—the lip, chin, eyebrows, and neck—but I also do a tremendous amount of body work—bikini line, abdomen, breast, forearms, underarms," says Wexler.

The major risks of electrolysis are electrical shock, which can occur if the needle is not properly insulated; infection from an unsterile needle or other infection control problem; and scarring resulting from improper technique.

There are no uniform standards governing the practice of electrology. Only 31 states require electrologists to be licensed, and, among those, the licensure requirements vary.

"Training requirements vary from as few as 120 hours to 1,100 hours," says Trudy Brown, president of the International Guild of Professional

Electrologists. "Some states may require continuing education classes, others not, and there are no national standards for testing," she adds.

Two organizations—the American Electrology Association and the Society of Clinical and Medical Electrologists—have certification programs, however, both based on a written exam, Brown says. A list of licensed and certified electrologists is available from the International Guild of Professional Electrologists, 202 Boulevard St., Suite B, High Point, North Carolina 27262; (800) 830-3247.

Home-use electrolysis devices work the same way as those for professional use and carry the same health risks. The risks are not very great, however, FDA's Watson says, because the voltages and currents for the home-use devices are not very high. Neither the home-use nor the professional devices use great amounts of current, he adds.

The American Medical Association's Committee on Cutaneous Health and Cosmetics says the success of electrolysis self-treatment depends largely on the condition of the hair and skin, the equipment, and the level of skill developed. The committee recommends limiting self-treatment to readily accessible areas, such as the lower parts of the arms and legs. Because working on facial hair requires use of a mirror, and, therefore, reversed movements, this area is best done by a professional.

Like needle epilators, tweezers epilators use electric current to remove hair. The tweezers grasp the hair close to the skin, and applied current travels down the hair shaft to the root. And, like needle epilators, electric shock is possible if the tweezers touch the skin instead of grabbing the hair. Tweezers epilator manufacturers can claim permanent hair removal if they can provide supporting data.

"Tweezers epilators are relatively new," Watson says, having been brought into the market only about 20 years ago. "Because they don't use a needle, they are supposed to be less painful than the older devices, which have been around for more than a hundred years," he says.

Needle epilators are exempt from pre-market notification; tweezers epilator manufacturers, however, must submit to FDA data showing their devices are substantially equivalent to similar devices already on the market. FDA is currently reviewing this policy.

"On Aug. 14, 1995, FDA published a Federal Register notice requesting manufacturers of tweezers epilators to submit safety and effectiveness data," Watson says. "After the information is analyzed, the agency will decide what kind of clearance will be required for these devices."

Laser

Hair removal entered the "laser age" last year when FDA cleared the ThermoLase Softlight laser, manufactured by Thermotrex Corporation, based in San Diego.

"The Softlight is essentially a standard dermatological laser similar to others already on the market for treating skin lesions and removing tattoos," says Richard Felten, a senior reviewer in FDA's Center for Devices and Radiological Health.

> **Weird Words**
>
> Laser: A device that concentrates high energies into an intense, narrow beam of single-wavelength electromagnetic radiation. Lasers are used for a variety of medical purposes besides removing hair, including surgery, cauterization (sealing cut blood vessels), and diagnosis.
>
> Source: Adapted from *Stedman's Medical Dictionary, 27th Edition*, © 2000. Lippincott Williams, and Wilkins. All rights reserved. Reprinted with permission.

With the ThermoLase method, a proprietary topical black-colored solution is applied to the treatment area before the laser is scanned across it.

"The solution penetrates the hair follicles, and the black material in it preferentially absorbs the laser wavelength, which heats and destroys the follicles," Felten explains.

Three-month clinical trials of the ThermoLase process showed at least a 30 percent reduction of hair on treated areas in 60 to 70 percent of people treated. Manufacturers must limit claims of laser treatment permanence to results substantiated by the clinical data. Thermotrex, therefore, can claim that its laser process causes hair reduction for up to three months after treatment.

Some side effects can be expected whenever a laser is used to treat the skin, Felten says. These include redness, caused by heating the tissue; possibly some darkening of light-complexioned skin and lightening of dark-complexioned skin; and a risk of some scarring in some patients.

"Usually the treated area is covered to prevent infection during the healing period, and then kept covered with a moist solution for a period of time," Felten says, adding that sunlight should be avoided during healing also, to avoid a change in pigment.

—by Marian Segal

Part 3

Acne:
Understanding Its Causes And Treatments

Chapter 19

The Skinny On Acne

What Is Acne?

Acne is a disorder resulting from the action of hormones on the skin's oil glands (sebaceous glands), which leads to plugged pores and outbreaks of lesions commonly called pimples or zits. Acne lesions usually occur on the face, neck, back, chest, and shoulders. Nearly 17 million people in the United States have acne, making it the most common skin disease. Although acne is not a serious health threat, severe acne can lead to disfiguring, permanent scarring, which can be upsetting to people who are affected by the disorder.

How Does Acne Develop?

Doctors describe acne as a disease of the pilosebaceous units (PSUs). Found over most of the body, PSUs consist of a sebaceous gland connected to a canal, called a follicle, that contains a fine hair. These units are most numerous on the face, upper back, and chest. The sebaceous glands make an oily substance called sebum that normally empties onto the skin surface through

---

About This Chapter: Adapted from "Questions and Answers About Acne," National Institute of Arthritis and Musculoskeletal and Skin Diseases, October 2001; available electronically at http://www.niams.nih.gov/hi/topics/acne/acne.htm and in hard copy as NIH Publication No. 01-4998 from the National Arthritis and Musculoskeletal and Skin Diseases Information Clearinghouse, NIAMS, National Institutes of Health, 1 AMS Circle, Bethesda, Maryland 20892-3675.

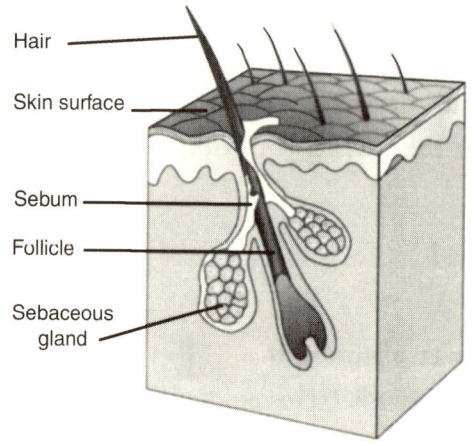

Figure 19.1. Normal pilosebaceous unit.

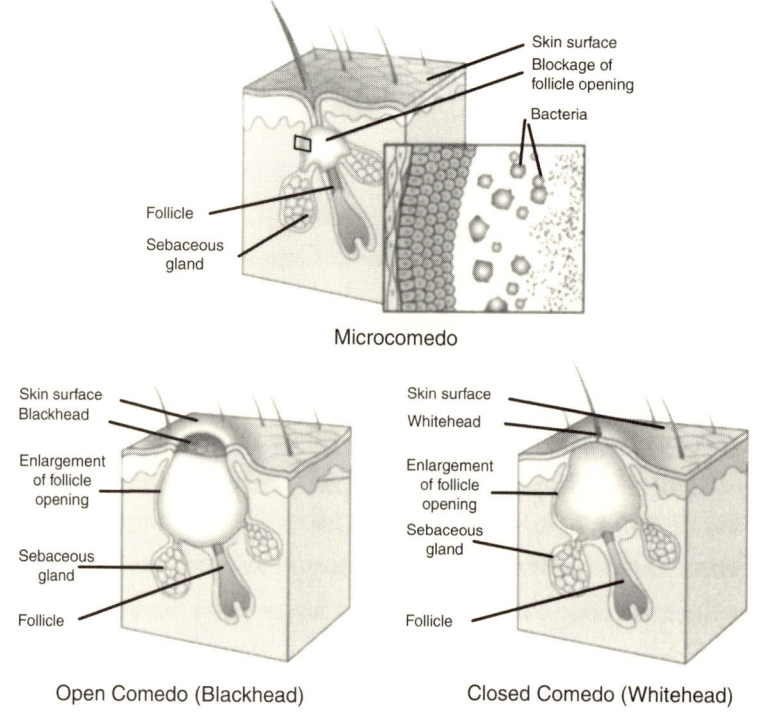

Figure 19.2. Three basic types of acne lesions.

the opening of the follicle, commonly called a pore. Cells called keratinocytes line the follicle.

The hair, sebum, and keratinocytes that fill the narrow follicle may produce a plug, which is an early sign of acne. The plug prevents sebum from reaching the surface of the skin through a pore. The mixture of oil and cells allows bacteria called *Propionibacterium acnes* (*P. acnes*) that normally live on the skin to grow in the plugged follicles. These bacteria produce chemicals and enzymes and attract white blood cells that cause inflammation. (Inflammation is a characteristic reaction of tissues to disease or injury and is marked by four signs: swelling, redness, heat, and pain.) When the wall of the plugged follicle breaks down, it spills everything into the nearby skin—sebum, shed skin cells, and bacteria—leading to lesions or pimples.

People with acne frequently have a variety of lesions, some of which are shown in the diagrams on page 136. The basic acne lesion, called the comedo (pronounced "KOM-e-do"), is simply an enlarged and plugged hair follicle. If the plugged follicle, or comedo, stays beneath the skin, it is called a closed comedo and produces a white bump called a whitehead. A comedo that reaches the surface of the skin and opens up is called a blackhead because it looks black on the skin's surface. This black discoloration is not due to dirt. Both whiteheads and blackheads may stay in the skin for a long time.

Other troublesome acne lesions can develop, including the following:

- Papules—inflamed lesions that usually appear as small, pink bumps on the skin and can be tender to the touch

> ### ✎ Weird Words
>
> Pilosebaceous unit: An anatomical structure in the skin consisting of a sebaceous (oil) gland, a hair follicle, and a hair.
>
> Comedo: An enlarged, plugged hair follicle; the basic acne lesion. The plural of comedo is comedos or comedones.
>
> Androgen: A male sex hormone. Androgens are produced by females as well as males.
>
> Noncomedogenic: A cosmetic formulated in a way that does not tend to promote the development of comedones.

- Pustules (pimples)—papules topped by pus-filled lesions that may be red at the base

- Nodules—large, painful, solid lesions that are lodged deep within the skin

- Cysts—deep, painful, pus-filled lesions that can cause scarring.

What Causes Acne?

The exact cause of acne is unknown, but doctors believe it results from several related factors. One important factor is an increase in hormones called androgens (male sex hormones). These increase in both boys and girls during puberty and cause the sebaceous glands to enlarge and make more sebum. Hormonal changes related to pregnancy or starting or stopping birth control pills can also cause acne.

Another factor is heredity or genetics. Researchers believe that the tendency to develop acne can be inherited from parents. For example, studies have shown that many school-age boys with acne have a family history of the disorder. Certain drugs, including androgens and lithium, are known to cause acne. Greasy cosmetics may alter the cells of the follicles and make them stick together, producing a plug.

Factors That Can Make Acne Worse

Factors that can cause an acne flare include:

- Changing hormone levels in adolescent girls and adult women two to seven days before their menstrual period starts

- Friction caused by leaning on or rubbing the skin

- Pressure from bike helmets, backpacks, or tight collars

- Environmental irritants, such as pollution and high humidity

- Squeezing or picking at blemishes

- Hard scrubbing of the skin

♣ **It's A Fact!!**
Acne is the most common skin disease. It affects both sexes and all races, and it is most prevalent between the ages of 12 and 24.

Myths About The Causes Of Acne

There are many myths about what causes acne. Chocolate and greasy foods are often blamed, but foods seem to have little effect on the development and course of acne in most people. Another common myth is that dirty skin causes acne; however, blackheads and other acne lesions are not caused by dirt. Finally, stress does not cause acne.

Who Gets Acne?

People of all races and ages get acne. It is most common in adolescents and young adults. Nearly 85 percent of people between the ages of 12 and 24 develop the disorder. For most people, acne tends to go away by the time they reach their thirties; however, some people in their forties and fifties continue to have this skin problem.

How Is Acne Treated?

Acne is often treated by dermatologists (doctors who specialize in skin problems). These doctors treat all kinds of acne, particularly severe cases. Doctors who are general or family practitioners, pediatricians, or internists may treat patients with milder cases of acne.

The goals of treatment are to heal existing lesions, stop new lesions from forming, prevent scarring, and minimize the psychological stress and embarrassment caused by this disease. Drug treatment is aimed at reducing several problems that play a part in causing acne: abnormal clumping of cells in the follicles, increased oil production, bacteria, and inflammation. Depending on the extent of the person's acne, the doctor will recommend one of several over-the-counter (OTC) medicines or prescription medicines that are topical (applied to the skin) or systemic (taken by mouth). The doctor may suggest using more than one topical medicine or combining oral and topical medicines.

Treatment For Blackheads, Whiteheads, And Mild Inflammatory Acne

Doctors usually recommend an OTC or prescription topical medication for people with mild signs of acne. Topical medicine is applied directly to the acne lesions or to the entire area of affected skin.

Benzoyl peroxide, resorcinol, salicylic acid, and sulfur are the most common topical OTC medicines used to treat acne. Each works a little differently. Benzoyl peroxide is best at killing *P. acnes* bacteria and may reduce oil production. Resorcinol, salicylic acid, and sulfur help break down blackheads and whiteheads. Salicylic acid also helps cut down the shedding of cells lining the follicles of the oil glands. Topical OTC medications are available in many forms, such as gel, lotion, cream, soap, or pad.

In some patients, OTC acne medicines may cause side effects such as skin irritation, burning, or redness. Some people find that the side effects lessen or go away with continued use of the medicine. Severe or prolonged side effects should be reported to the doctor.

OTC topical medicines are somewhat effective in treating acne when used regularly. Patients must keep in mind that it can take eight weeks or more before they notice that their skin looks and feels better.

Treatment For Moderate To Severe Inflammatory Acne

Patients with moderate to severe inflammatory acne may be treated with prescription topical or oral medicines, alone or in combination.

Prescription Topical Medicines

Several types of prescription topical medicines are used to treat acne, including antibiotics, benzoyl peroxide, tretinoin, adapalene, and azelaic acid. Antibiotics and azelaic acid help stop or slow the growth of bacteria and reduce inflammation. Tretinoin, a type of drug called a retinoid that contains an altered form of vitamin A, is an effective topical medicine for stopping the development of new comedones. It works by unplugging existing comedones, thereby allowing other topical medicines, such as antibiotics, to enter the follicles. The doctor may also prescribe newer retinoids or retinoid-like drugs, such as tazarotene or adapalene, that help decrease comedo formation.

Like OTC topical medicines, prescription topical medicines come as creams, lotions, solutions, or gels. The doctor will consider the patient's skin type when prescribing a product. Creams and lotions provide moisture and tend to be good for people with sensitive skin. Gels and solutions are generally alcohol-based and tend to dry the skin. Therefore, patients with very oily skin or those who live in hot, humid climates may prefer them. The doctor will tell the patient how to apply the medicine and how often to use it.

Some people develop side effects from using prescription topical medicines. Initially, the skin may look worse before improving. Common side effects include stinging, burning, redness, peeling, scaling, or discoloration of the skin. With some medicines, like retinoids, these side effects usually decrease or go away after the medicine is used for a period of time. Patients should report prolonged or severe side effects to their doctor. Between four and eight weeks will most likely pass before patients see their skin improve.

Prescription Oral Medicines

For patients with moderate to severe acne, the doctor often prescribes oral antibiotics (taken by mouth). Oral antibiotics are thought to help control acne by curbing the growth of bacteria and reducing inflammation. Prescription oral and topical medicines may be combined. For example, benzoyl peroxide may be combined with clindamycin, erythromycin, or sulfur. Other common antibiotics used to treat acne are tetracycline, minocycline, and doxycycline. Some people have side effects when taking these antibiotics, such as an increased tendency to sunburn, upset stomach, dizziness or lightheadedness, and changes in skin color. Tetracycline is not given to pregnant women, nor is it given to children under eight years of age because it might discolor developing teeth. Tetracycline and minocycline may also decrease the effectiveness of birth control pills. Therefore, a backup or another form of birth control may be needed. Prolonged treatment with oral antibiotics may be necessary to achieve the desired results.

Treatment For Severe Nodular Or Cystic Acne

People with nodules or cysts should be treated by a dermatologist. For patients with severe inflammatory acne that does not improve with medicines such as those described above, a doctor may prescribe isotretinoin (Accutane®), a retinoid. Isotretinoin is an oral drug that is usually taken once or twice a day with food for 15 to 20 weeks. It markedly reduces the size of the oil glands so that much less oil is produced. As a result, the growth of bacteria is decreased.

Advantages Of Isotretinoin (Accutane)

Isotretinoin is a very effective medicine that can help prevent scarring. After 15 to 20 weeks of treatment with isotretinoin, acne completely or almost completely goes away in up to 90 percent of patients. In those patients where acne recurs after a course of isotretinoin, the doctor may institute another course of the same treatment or prescribe other medicines.

Disadvantages Of Isotretinoin (Accutane)

Isotretinoin can cause birth defects in the developing fetus of a pregnant woman. It is important that women of childbearing age are not pregnant and do not get pregnant while taking this medicine. Women must use two separate effective forms of birth control at the same time for one month before treatment begins, during the entire course of treatment, and for one full month after stopping the drug. They should ask their doctor when it is safe to get pregnant after they have stopped taking Accutane.

Some people with acne become depressed by the changes in the appearance of their skin. Changes in mental health may be intensified during treatment or soon after completing a course of medicines like Accutane. A doctor should be consulted if a person feels unusually sad or has other symptoms of depression, such as loss of appetite or trouble concentrating.

Other possible side effects include dry eyes, mouth, lips, nose, or skin; itching; nosebleeds; muscle aches; sensitivity to the sun; and, sometimes, poor night vision. More serious side effects include changes in the blood, such as an increase in triglycerides and cholesterol, or a change in liver function. To make sure Accutane is stopped if side effects occur, the doctor monitors blood studies that are done before treatment is started and periodically during treatment. Side effects usually go away after the medicine is stopped.

Treatments For Hormonally Influenced Acne In Women

Clues that help the doctor determine whether acne in an adult woman is due to an excess of androgen hormones are hirsutism (excessive growth of hair in unusual places), premenstrual acne flares, irregular menstrual cycles, and elevated blood levels of certain androgens. The doctor may prescribe one of several drugs to treat women with this type of acne. Low-dose estrogen birth control pills help suppress the androgen produced by the ovaries. Low-dose corticosteroid drugs, such as prednisone or dexamethasone, may suppress the androgen produced by the adrenal glands. Finally, the doctor may prescribe an antiandrogen drug, such as spironolactone (Aldactone®). This medicine reduces excessive oil production. Side effects of antiandrogen drugs may include irregular menstruation, tender breasts, headache, and fatigue.

Other Treatments For Acne

Doctors may use other types of procedures in addition to drug therapy to treat patients with acne. For example, the doctor may remove the patient's comedones during office visits. Sometimes the doctor will inject cortisone directly into lesions to help reduce the size and pain of inflamed cysts and nodules.

Early treatment is the best way to prevent acne scars. Once scarring has occurred, the doctor may suggest a medical or surgical procedure to help reduce the scars. A superficial laser may be used to treat irregular scars. Another kind of laser allows energy to go deeper into the skin and tighten the underlying tissue and plump out depressed scars. Dermabrasion (or microdermabrasion), which is a form of "sanding down" scars, is sometimes combined with the subsurface laser treatment. Another treatment option for deep scars caused by cystic acne is the transfer of fat from one part of the body to the face.

How Should People With Acne Care For Their Skin?

Clean Skin Gently

Most doctors recommend that people with acne gently wash their skin with a mild cleanser, once in the morning and once in the evening and after heavy exercise. Some people with acne may try to stop outbreaks and oil production by scrubbing their skin and using strong detergent soaps and rough scrub pads. However, scrubbing will not improve acne; in fact, it can make the problem worse. Patients should ask their doctor or another health professional for advice on the best type of cleanser to use. Patients should wash the face from under the jaw to the hairline. It is important that patients thoroughly rinse their skin after washing it. Astringents are not recommended unless the skin is very oily, and then they should be used only on oily spots.

Doctors also recommend that patients regularly shampoo their hair. Those with oily hair may want to shampoo it every day.

Avoid Frequent Handling of the Skin

People who squeeze, pinch, or pick their blemishes risk developing scars or dark blotches. People should avoid rubbing and touching their skin lesions.

Shave Carefully

Men who shave and who have acne can test both electric and safety razors to see which is more comfortable. Men who use a safety razor should use a sharp blade and soften their beard thoroughly with soap and water before applying shaving cream. Nicking blemishes can be avoided by shaving lightly and only when necessary.

Avoid Sunburn Or Suntan

Many of the medicines used to treat acne can make a person more prone to sunburn. A sunburn that reddens the skin or suntan that darkens the skin may make blemishes less visible and make the skin feel drier. However, these benefits are only temporary, and there are known risks of excessive sun exposure, such as more rapid skin aging and a risk of developing skin cancer.

Choose Cosmetics Carefully

People being treated for acne often need to change some of the cosmetics they use. All cosmetics, such as foundation, blush, eye shadow, and moisturizers, should be oil free. Patients may find it difficult to apply foundation evenly during the first few weeks of treatment because the skin may be red or scaly, particularly with the use of topical tretinoin or benzoyl peroxide. Oily hair products may eventually spread over the forehead, causing closed comedones. Products that are labeled as noncomedogenic (do not promote the formation of closed pores) should be used; in some people, however, even these products may cause acne.

What Research Is Being Done On Acne?

Medical researchers are working on new drugs to treat acne, particularly topical antibiotics to replace some of those in current use. As with many other types of bacterial infections, doctors are finding that, over time, the bacteria that are associated with acne are becoming resistant to treatment with certain antibiotics. Research is also being conducted by industry on the potential side effects of isotretinoin and the long-term use of medicines used for treating acne.

Scientists are working on other means of treating acne. For example, researchers are studying the biology of sebaceous cells and testing a laser in laboratory animals to treat acne by disrupting sebaceous glands. Scientists are also studying the treatment of androgenic disorders, including acne, in men by inhibiting an enzyme that changes testosterone to a more potent androgen.

☞ **Remember!!**

Here are the basic ingredients to acne care.

1. Clean skin gently.

2. Avoid frequent handling of the skin.

3. Shave carefully.

4. Avoid sunburn or suntan.

5. Choose cosmetics carefully.

Chapter 20

The Psychological And Social Effects Of Acne

Acne can have profound social and psychological effects. These are not necessarily related to the disease's clinical severity. Even mild acne can be significantly disabling. Acne can affect people of all ages, but it predominantly occurs during the teenage years. Approximately 85 percent of people between the ages of 12 and 25 develop acne.

The psychological and social impacts of acne are a huge concern especially because the disease affects adolescents at the time when they are developing their personalities. During this time, peer acceptance is very important to the teenager, and unfortunately it has been found that physical appearance and attractiveness are highly linked with peer status.

The Problems Acne Causes

In recent years, open discussions between patients and medical professionals have revealed the impact acne has on the psyche. The following are some of the problems that patients with acne may face:

About This Chapter: This page is reprinted with the permission of DermNet, the website of the New Zealand Dermatological Society. Visit www.dermnetnz.org for patient information on numerous skin conditions and their treatment. © 2002 New Zealand Dermatological Society.

- Self-esteem and body image
    - ◊ Some embarrassed acne patients avoid eye contact.
    - ◊ Some acne sufferers grow their hair long to cover the face. Girls tend to wear heavy makeup to disguise the pimples, even though they know this sometimes aggravates the condition. Boys often comment, "Acne is not such a problem for girls because they can wear makeup."
    - ◊ Acne on the trunk of the body can reduce participation in sports such as swimming or rugby because of the need to disrobe in public changing rooms.
- Social withdrawal and relationship building
    - ◊ Acne, especially when it affects the face, provokes cruel taunts from other teenagers.
    - ◊ Some find it hard to form new relationships, especially with the opposite sex.
    - ◊ At a time when teenagers are learning to form relationships, those with acne may lack the self-confidence to go out and make these bonds. They become shy and even reclusive. The main concern is a fear of negative appraisal by others. In extreme cases a social phobia can develop.
- Education and work
    - ◊ Some refuse to go school, leading to poor academic performance and possibly future unemployment.
    - ◊ Some take "sick days" from work, risking their jobs or livelihoods.
    - ◊ Acne may reduce career choices, ruling out occupations such as modeling that depend upon personal appearance.
    - ◊ Acne patients are less successful in job applications; their lack of confidence is as important as potential employers' reaction to their spotty skin.
    - ◊ More people who have acne are unemployed than people who do not have acne.

The Psychological And Social Effects Of Acne

◊ Many young adults with acne seek medical help as they enter the workforce, where they perceive that acne is unacceptable and that they "should have grown out of it by now."

Acne And Depression

In some patients the distress of acne may result in depression. This must be recognized and managed. Signs of depression include:

- Loss of appetite
- Lethargy
- Mood disturbance
- Behavioral problems
- Wakefulness
- Spontaneous crying
- Feelings of unworthiness

> **Weird Words**
>
> Isotretinoin: A highly effective prescription medication used for severe acne. See Chapter 25 for more information.
>
> Social Phobia: A psychological disorder that results in extreme fear of social settings, like church, work, and school.
>
> Source: Adapted from *Stedman's Medical Dictionary, 27th Edition*, © 2000. Lippincott Williams, and Wilkins. All rights reserved. Reprinted with permission.

In teenagers depression may manifest as social withdrawal (retreat to the bedroom or avoidance of peers) or impaired school performance (lower grades or missed assignments). Worse still, severe depression from acne has resulted in attempted suicide and, unfortunately, successful suicide. Worrying statements include "I don't want to wake up in the morning"; "I'd be better off dead"; "I'm worthless"; "You'd be better off without me." Parents, friends, and school counselors need to take heed when they start to hear these types of comments.

Rarely, depression can be associated with acne treatment, particularly isotretinoin. There is considerable doubt that the drug has caused the problem, and it seems much more likely that depression results from the acne and its psychological disturbances.

Regardless of the cause, depression must be recognized and managed early. If you think you may be depressed, contact your dermatologist or family doctor urgently for advice.

Dysmorphophobic Acne

Some individuals with only minor acne suffer from disturbed body image. Even in the absence of lesions, they consider their acne severe and may suffer many of the psychological and social symptoms associated with the disease. Such patients are said to have dysmorphophobic acne because of the distortion in body image. If this distortion is the only abnormal behavioral symptom, patients respond well to oral isotretinoin therapy. A low dose of the medication may be required long term as even slight recurrence of oily skin may unduly concern the patient. Some severe cases of dysmorphophobia signal a more global mental disorder similar to anorexia nervosa; they require expert dermatological and psychiatric assistance.

> ☞ **Remember!!**
>
> Depression is an illness that can nearly always be treated effectively. Suitable treatments may include:
>
> - Antidepressant medication such as fluoxetine (Prozac®), paroxetine (Aropax®), citalopram (Cipramil®), dothiepin (Prothiaden®, Dopress®), moclobemide (Aurorix®)
>
> - Psychological treatments to overcome the negative thinking, anxiety, and avoidance that often accompany depression
>
> - Counseling to help build confidence and rebuild self-esteem
>
> - Group therapy

> 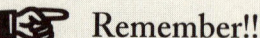 **Quick Tip**
>
> ## Seeking Help
>
> If your acne is interfering significantly with your life, seek help promptly from your family physician or dermatologist. Tell your doctor all your concerns so that he or she will take your acne seriously. Most cases of acne can be controlled and sometimes cured with one or more of the following preparations:
>
> - Over-the-counter topical acne creams, lotions, or gels for mild cases
>
> - Prescription medications, both topical and oral, that are available only through a physician

Chapter 21

Acne Scarring

Causes Of Acne Scars

In the simplest terms, scars form at the site of an injury to tissue. They are the visible reminders of injury and tissue repair. In the case of acne, the injury is caused by the body's inflammatory response to sebum, bacteria, and dead cells in the plugged sebaceous follicle.

When tissue suffers an injury, the body rushes its repair kit to the injury site. Among the elements of the repair kit are white blood cells and an array of inflammatory molecules that have the task of repairing tissue and fighting infection. However, when their job is done, they may leave a somewhat messy repair site in the form of fibrous scar tissue or eroded tissue.

White blood cells and inflammatory molecules may remain at the site of an active acne lesion for days or even weeks. In people who are susceptible to scarring, the result may be an acne scar. The occurrence and incidence of scarring is still not well understood, however. There is considerable variation in scarring between one person and another, indicating that some people are more prone to scarring than others. Scarring frequently results from severe inflammatory nodulocystic acne that occurs deep in the skin. But scarring also may arise from more superficial, inflamed lesions.

> About This Chapter: Adapted from "Acne Scarring," http://www.skincarephysicians.com/acnenet/scarring.html. Reprinted with permission from the American Academy of Dermatology, © 2002. All rights reserved.

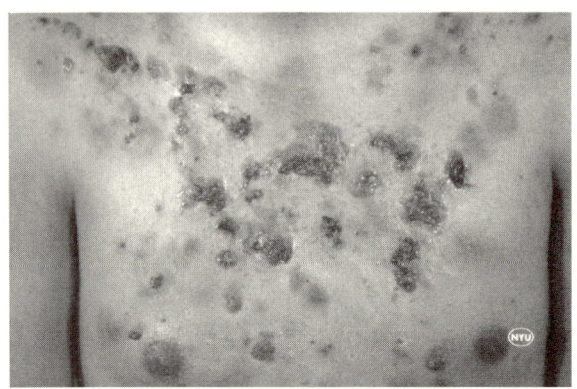

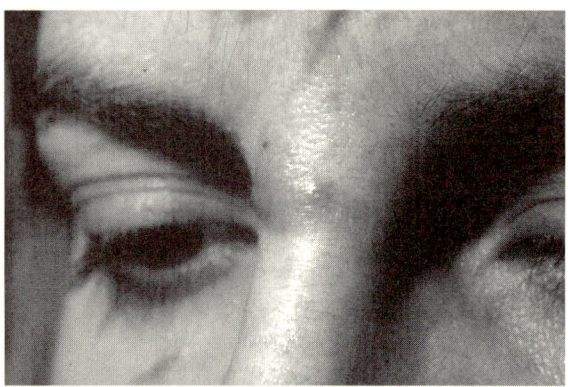

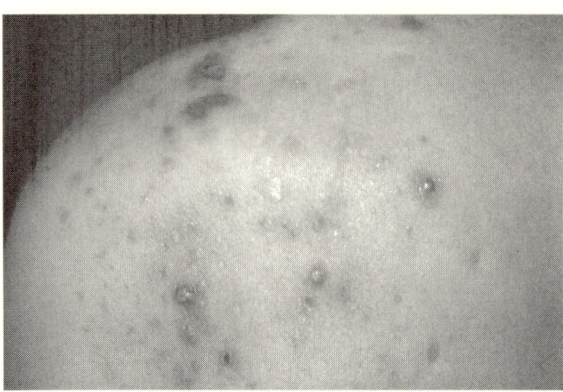

Figure 21.1. These three photos show the kind of severe, nodulocystic acne that is most likely to result in scars.

Acne Scarring

The life history of scars also is not well understood. Some people bear their acne scars for a lifetime with little change, but in other people the skin undergoes some degree of remodeling and acne scars diminish in size.

People also have differing feelings about acne scars. Scars of more or less the same size that may be psychologically distressing to one person may be accepted by another person as "not too bad." The person who is distressed by scars is more likely to seek treatment to moderate or remove the scars.

Prevention Of Acne Scars

As we have seen, the occurrence of scarring is different in different people. It is difficult to predict who will scar, how extensive or deep scars will be, and how long scars will persist. It is also difficult to predict how successfully scars can be prevented by effective acne treatment.

Nevertheless, the only sure method of preventing or limiting the extent of scars is to treat acne early in its course, and as long as necessary. The more that inflammation can be prevented or moderated, the more likely it is that scars can be prevented. Any person with acne who has a known tendency to scar should be under the care of a dermatologist.

Types Of Acne Scars

There are two general types of acne scars, defined by tissue response to inflammation: scars caused by increased tissue formation, and scars caused by loss of tissue.

Scars Caused By Increased Tissue Formation

The scars caused by increased tissue formation are called keloids, or hypertrophic scars. The word hypertrophy means "enlargement" or "overgrowth." Both hypertrophic and keloid scars are associated with excessive amounts of the cell substance collagen. Overproduction of collagen is a response of skin cells to injury. The excess collagen becomes piled up in fibrous masses, resulting in a characteristic firm, smooth, usually irregularly-shaped scar.

The typical keloid or hypertrophic scar is one to two millimeters in diameter, but some may be one centimeter or larger. Keloid scars tend to "run in families"—that is, abnormal growth of scar tissue is more likely to occur in people who have relatives with similar types of scars.

Hypertrophic and keloid scars persist for years, but may diminish in size over time.

Scars Caused By Loss Of Tissue

Acne scars associated with loss of tissue—similar to scars that result from chickenpox—are more common than keloids and hypertrophic scars. Scars associated with loss of tissue are:

- *Ice-pick scars* usually occur on the cheek. They are typically small, with a somewhat jagged edge and steep sides—like wounds from an ice pick. Ice-pick scars may be shallow or deep, and hard or soft to the touch. Soft scars can be improved by stretching the skin; hard ice-pick scars cannot be stretched out.

- *Depressed fibrotic scars* are usually quite large, with sharp edges and steep sides. The base of these scars is firm to the touch. Ice-pick scars may evolve into depressed fibrotic scars over time.

- *Soft scars*, superficial or deep, are soft to the touch. They have gently sloping rolled edges that merge with normal skin. They are usually small and either circular or linear in shape.

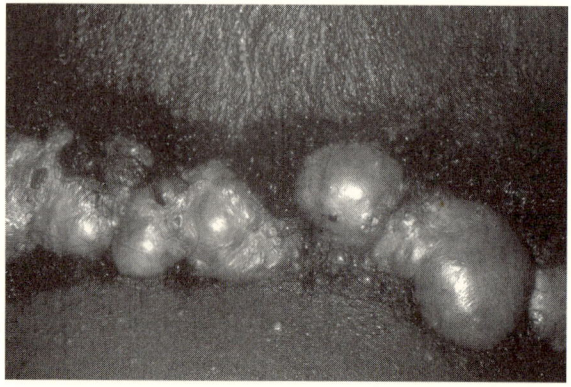

Figure 21.2. A typical severe acne keloid.

Acne Scarring

- *Atrophic macules* are usually fairly small when they occur on the face, but may be a centimeter or larger on the body. They are soft, often with a slightly wrinkled base, and may be bluish in appearance due to blood vessels lying just under the scar. Over time, these scars change from bluish to ivory white in color in white-skinned people and become much less obvious.

> ♣ **It's A Fact!!**
> True acne scars are of two basic types: those that result from an overgrowth (hypertrophy) of the affected tissue, and those that arise from the loss of affected tissue.

- *Follicular macular atrophy* is more likely to occur on the chest or back of a person with acne. These are small, white, soft lesions, often barely raised above the surface of the skin—somewhat like whiteheads that didn't fully develop. This condition is sometimes also called perifollicular elastolysis. The lesions may persist for months to years.

Treatments For Acne Scars

A number of treatments are available for acne scars through dermatologic surgery. The type of treatment selected should be the one that is best for you in terms of your type of skin, the cost, what you want the treatment to accomplish, and the possibility that some types of treatment may result in more scarring if you are very susceptible to scar formation.

A decision to seek dermatologic surgical treatment for acne scars also depends on:

- *The way you feel about scars*. Do acne scars psychologically or emotionally affect your life? Are you willing to "live with your scars" and wait for them to fade over time? These are personal decisions only you can make.

- *The severity of your scars*. Is scarring substantially disfiguring, even by objective assessment?

- *A dermatologist's expert opinion* as to whether scar treatment is justified in your particular case and what scar treatment will be most effective for you.

Before committing to treatment of acne scars, you should have a frank discussion with your dermatologist regarding those questions and any others you feel are important. You need to tell the dermatologist how you feel about your scars. The dermatologist needs to conduct a full examination and determine whether treatment can, or should, be undertaken.

The objective of scar treatment is to give the skin a more acceptable physical appearance. Total restoration of the skin to the way it looked before you had acne is often not possible, but scar treatment does usually improve the appearance of your skin.

The scar treatments that are currently available include:

- *Collagen injection.* Collagen, a normal substance of the body, is injected under the skin to "stretch" and "fill out" certain types of superficial and deep soft scars. Collagen treatment usually does not work as well for ice-pick scars and keloids. Collagen derived from cows or other non-human sources cannot be used in people with autoimmune diseases. Human collagen or fascia is helpful for those allergic to cow-derived collagen. Cosmetic benefit from collagen injection usually lasts three to six months. Additional collagen injections to maintain the cosmetic benefit are done at additional cost.

- *Autologous fat transfer.* Fat is taken from another site on your own body and prepared for injection into your skin. The fat is injected beneath the surface of the skin to elevate depressed scars. This method of autologous (from your own body) fat transfer is usually used to correct deep contour defects caused by scarring from nodulocystic acne. Because the fat is reabsorbed into the skin over a period of 6 to 18 months, the procedure usually must be repeated. Longer-lasting results may be achieved with multiple fat-transfer procedures.

- *Dermabrasion.* This is thought to be the most effective treatment for acne scars. Under local anesthetic, a high-speed brush or fraise used to remove surface skin and alter the contour of scars. Superficial scars may be removed altogether, and deeper scars may be reduced in depth. Dermabrasion does not work for all kinds of scars; for example, it may make ice-pick scars more noticeable if the scars are wider under the

♣ It's A Fact!!
They're Not All Scars

Not every change in the skin following acne is a scar, in the sense that a permanent change has occurred. Still, even though these spots are not true scars and they disappear in time, they are visible and can cause embarrassment.

Macules, or "pseudoscars," are flat, red or reddish spots that are the final stage of most inflamed acne lesions. After an inflamed acne lesion flattens, a macule may remain to "mark the spot" for up to six months. When the macule eventually disappears, no trace of it will remain—unlike a scar.

Postinflammatory pigmentation is discoloration of the skin at the site of a healed or healing inflamed acne lesion. It occurs more frequently in darker-skinned people, but occasionally is seen in people with white skin. Early treatment by a dermatologist may minimize the development of postinflammatory pigmentation. Some postinflammatory pigmentation may persist for up to 18 months, especially with excessive sun exposure. Chemical peeling may hasten the disappearance of postinflammatory pigmentation.

---

skin than at the surface. In darker-skinned people, dermabrasion may cause changes in pigmentation that require additional treatment.

- *Microdermabrasion.* This new technique is a surface form of dermabrasion. Instead of a high-speed brush, microdermabrasion uses aluminum oxide crystals passing through a vacuum tube to remove surface skin. Only the very surface cells of the skin are removed, so no additional wound is created. Multiple procedures are often required, but scars may not be significantly improved.

- *Laser treatment.* Lasers of various wavelength and intensity may be used to recontour scar tissue and reduce the redness of skin around healed acne lesions. The type of laser used is determined by the results that the laser treatment aims to accomplish. Tissue may actually be removed with more powerful instruments such as the carbon dioxide laser. In some cases, a single treatment is all that will be necessary to achieve permanent results. Because the skin absorbs powerful bursts of energy from the laser, there may be posttreatment redness for several months.

- *Skin surgery.* Some ice-pick scars may be removed by "punch" excision of each individual scar. In this procedure each scar is excised down to the layer of subcutaneous fat; the resulting hole in the skin may be repaired with sutures or with a small skin graft. Subcision is a technique in which a surgical probe is used to lift the scar tissue away from unscarred skin, thus elevating a depressed scar.

- *Skin grafting* may be necessary under certain conditions—for example, sometimes dermabrasion unroofs massive and extensive tunnels (also called sinus tracts) caused by inflammatory reaction to sebum and bacteria in sebaceous follicles. Skin grafting may be needed to close the defect of the unroofed sinus tracts.

- *Treatment of keloids*. Surgical removal is seldom if ever used to treat keloids. A person whose skin has a tendency to form keloids from acne damage may also form keloids in response to skin surgery. Sometimes keloids are treated by injecting steroid drugs into the skin around the keloid. Topical retinoic acid may be applied directly on the keloid. In some cases the best treatment for keloids in a highly susceptible person is no treatment at all.

A Final Word

In summary, acne scars are caused by the body's inflammatory response to acne lesions. The best way to prevent scars is to treat acne early and as long as necessary. If scars form, a number of effective treatments are available. Dermatologic surgery treatments should be discussed with a dermatologist.

Chapter 22

Medications That Can Cause Acne

Acne can be caused or aggravated by a number of medications prescribed for other conditions. This is why it is important to tell your dermatologist about all the medications you may be taking. This includes any prescription drugs you may be taking without a prescription—for example, anabolic steroids if you are an athlete attempting to "bulk up."

Hormones

Since sebum production is predominantly under hormonal control—especially in regard to androgenic (male) hormones—it is not surprising that several hormones given as medications can cause or aggravate acne.

- *Testosterone*, a male hormone, can induce acne in females and in preadolescent children.

- *Gonadotropin*, which may be prescribed in certain pituitary disorders, can indirectly induce acne by stimulating testosterone production.

- *Anabolic steroids* are masculinizing hormones that can provoke or aggravate acne. Sometimes anabolic steroids are prescribed for females to treat relatively rare conditions such as familial angioedema. Because

---

About This Chapter: From "Medications That Cause Acne," http://www.derminfonet.com/acnenet/medsthatcause.html. Reprinted with permission from the American Academy of Dermatology, © 2002. All rights reserved.

part of the masculinizing effect of anabolic steroids is "bulking-up" of muscles, these drugs are frequently taken illegally by both male and female athletes. In illegal use, the doses are often large. Androgenic anabolic steroids can increase sebum production and be a direct cause of acne. Self-administered large doses of anabolic steroids are the cause of multiple acne lesions often seen on the faces and bodies of weightlifters, wrestlers, football players, or other athletes whose sports require muscle bulk.

- *Corticosteroids*, taken orally or applied topically to the skin, may cause a degeneration of the epithelial lining of sebaceous follicles, contributing to the plug of dead cellular material that characterizes comedos. The acne precipitated by corticosteroids tends to consist of superficial inflammatory papules and pustules and sometimes occasional comedos. These acne lesions may progress to nodules and cysts if the person has a genetic predisposition to acne. Corticosteroid acne tends to be dose-dependent—that is, higher doses are more likely to precipitate or aggravate acne. Dose-dependent corticosteroid acne rarely occurs in preteen children.

❧ Weird Words

<u>Angioedema</u>: Large recurring areas of redness and swelling in the skin; most common in young women, usually as an allergic reaction to food or medication.

<u>Cyclosporine</u>: A medication that suppresses the immune system and is commonly given after organ transplants.

<u>Gonadotropin</u>: A hormone that stimulates the gonads (sex organs) to grow and function.

<u>Halogenated</u>: A compound that contains iodine or bromine, elements known chemically as halogens.

Source: Adapted from *Stedman's Medical Dictionary, 27th Edition*, © 2000. Lippincott Williams, and Wilkins. All rights reserved. Reprinted with permission.

Antiepileptic Drugs

Individuals with severe epilepsy often have many endocrine (hormonal) problems, including abnormal testosterone secretion. Some studies have shown that in some people with severe epilepsy, acne may persist past age 50 years. There seems to be a complex link between epilepsy and acne that is associated with the endocrine background of each individual. Some antiepilepsy medications may have an effect on the endocrine pattern of some individuals with severe epilepsy. A person with epilepsy and acne should be under the care of a dermatologist.

Antituberculosis Drugs

Isoniazid, the most widely used drug for treating tuberculosis, has been associated with precipitation or aggravation of acne in small numbers of patients. The acne consisted primarily of blackheads and inflammatory papules. Another antituberculosis drug, rifampicin, has been associated with acne-like outbreaks in some patients. The lesions clear up when drug treatment is completed. The appearance of a skin problem such as acne is not a reason to halt treatment with an antituberculosis drug. It is better to treat the acne and complete the tuberculosis treatment. Tuberculosis is a contagious infectious disease that kills millions of people annually worldwide.

Lithium

Acne precipitation or aggravation is one of the dermatologic side effects of lithium, a medication prescribed in the treatment of bipolar disorder. The acne can usually be successfully managed without discontinuing treatment with lithium. A dermatologist should be consulted if acne appears as a side effect of lithium treatment.

Cyclosporine

Dermatologic reactions, including precipitation or aggravation of acne, are frequently seen in posttransplant patients who must take cyclosporine to prevent organ rejection. Since cyclosporine cannot be discontinued in a posttransplant patient, the side effect of acne should be treated by a dermatologist.

Halogenated Drugs

Medications containing iodine or bromine can cause acne-like eruptions. These medications are much less common today than in earlier years, but some are still in use. In the United States today, it is probably more likely to see acne-like outbreaks resulting from heavy consumption of iodine-containing health foods such as kelp.

Iodine-caused acneiform eruptions are not the same as acne vulgaris. The iodine-caused lesions can occur at any age. They occur rapidly after the consumptions of large amounts of iodine and are likely to be widespread on the face and body. Comedos are rare but inflammatory pustules are common.

Chapter 23

Over-The-Counter Acne Treatments

Soap And Water

Gentle cleansing of the skin with soap and water, no more than two or three times a day, removes excess oils (sebum) and may alleviate the "oily skin" appearance often associated with acne. There is no evidence that cleansing with soap and water prevents or clears up acne. Hard scrubbing, excessive cleansing (more than three times a day), or the use of harsh soaps or detergents may injure the skin and cause other skin problems in addition to acne.

Benzoyl Peroxide

A mainstay of over-the-counter acne treatment, and a medication commonly prescribed by physicians to treat mild forms of acne. Benzoyl peroxide has been used in acne treatment for several decades; it was the first agent to be proven effective in the treatment of mild acne.

The anti-acne effects of benzoyl peroxide are believed to be antibacterial with an accompanying decrease in some constituents of sebum. Benzoyl peroxide is available over the counter in a lotion or a gel. Its principal side effect is excessive dryness of the skin.

About This Chapter: From "Over-the-Counter Products," http://www.skincarephysicians.com/acnenet/overthecounter.html. Reprinted with permission from the American Academy of Dermatology, © 2002. All rights reserved.

Salicylic Acid

On the skin, salicylic acid helps to correct the abnormal shedding of cells. For milder acne, salicylic acid helps unclog pores to resolve and prevent lesions. It does not have any effect on sebum production or *Propionibacterium acnes*, the bacterium that causes acne. It must be used continuously, just like benzoyl peroxide, since its effects stop when you stop using it—pores clog up again, and the acne returns. Salicylic acid is available in many acne products, including lotions, creams, and pads.

Sulfur

An acne treatment in use for 50 years or longer. In combination with other agents—for example, alcohol, salicylic acid, and resorcinol—sulfur is still a constituent of some of the most heavily marketed over-the-counter medications. Sulfur is less frequently used by itself as an acne treatment due to its unpleasant odor. Although long used in treatment of acne, it is not known how sulfur acts on the skin to influence the development of acne.

Sulfurated Lime

An older medication for treatment of various skin diseases and scabies. Sulfurated lime probably characterizes the medications that were the best available in past decades.

Resorcinol

Together with sulfur, a constituent of popular over-the-counter acne medications. Resorcinol is less frequently used alone in treatment of acne.

> ♣ **It's A Fact!!**
>
> Benzoyl peroxide can bleach hair and fabric, including sheets, towels, and clothing, so care should be taken when applying it. An old shirt should be worn when benzoyl peroxide is applied to the back or chest overnight.

Alcohol And Acetone

Acetone is a "degreasing" agent, and alcohol has a mild antibacterial activity. The two agents have been sometimes combined in over-the-counter medication. However, when acetone is used alone, it may have no effect in the treatment of acne.

Herbal, Organic, And "Natural" Medications

Over-the-counter products called "herbal," "organic," or "natural" are marketed as acne treatments, but their effectiveness has rarely been tested in clinical trials. The value of such treatments is generally unknown.

Physical Therapies

Comedo Extraction

Extraction of comedones should be performed only by a dermatologist, under sterile conditions, and usually only when comedones have not responded to other treatment. Acne patients should not attempt to extract comedones by squeezing or picking.

Ultraviolet Light Therapy

Ultraviolet light has not been proven effective as an acne treatment. At most, skin tanning may mask acne. However, skin tanning increases risk for other, more serious skin conditions such as melanoma and other skin cancers.

Light Chemical Peels

Glycolic acid and other chemical agents are applied by a dermatologist to loosen blackheads and decrease acne papules.

Chapter 24
Prescription Medications For Acne

The most effective acne medications are available only by physician prescription. As with any potent pharmaceutical agent, they should be used only after examination by a physician and under the supervision of a physician.

The medications physicians prescribe for acne are of two basic types: topical medications, which are applied directly to the acne-affected skin; and oral medications, which are taken by mouth.

Topical Medications
Topical Antibiotics

The antibiotics used topically in treatment of acne are believed to be effective for reasons in addition to antibacterial activity. All antibiotics are powerful drugs that must be used as directed by a physician.

Topical antibiotics alone are not generally recommended. In fact, long-term use may increase risk for antibiotic resistance in skin bacteria. They should be used in combination with other topical agents.

About This Chapter: From "Prescription Medications," http://www.skincarephysicians.com/acnenet/precriptmeds.html. Reviewed by David A. Cooke, M.D., January 1, 2003. Reprinted with permission from the American Academy of Dermatologists, © 2002. All rights reserved.

The most commonly prescribed topical antibiotics include:

- *Azelaic acid*—a naturally occurring acid that has been adapted to use for treating acne. Its anti-acne activities are antimicrobial (reducing populations of *Propionibacterium acnes*), and decrease of hyperkeratinization (may inhibit comedo formation). *P. acnes* is the predominant microbiologic organism in sebaceous follicles. It is generally accepted that *P. acnes* plays a role in acne by releasing metabolic products that contribute to the inflammation of acne. Azelaic acid is applied as a cream. A course of treatment may require several months.

- *Erythromycin*—a member of the macrolide family of antibiotics, erythromycin is active against a broad spectrum of bacteria. Systemically it is used to treat diseases such as pneumonia. Its principal topical use is in treatment of acne vulgaris, for its anti-acne effects are both antimicrobial and anti-inflammatory. A combination erythromycin–benzoyl peroxide agent combines the effects of two antimicrobial agents, and it reduces skin oiliness. A combination erythromycin-zinc acetate is available in some countries but not currently in the United States.

- *Clindamycin*—a semisynthetic antibiotic with antimicrobial activity similar to that of erythromycin. Clindamycin has a long history of use in treatment of acne.

- *Tetracyclines*—broad-spectrum antibiotics, among the first adapted to the topical treatment of acne. Today tetracyclines are used much less frequently in the United States as topical medication. Undesirable side effects of odor and yellow staining of skin limited the acceptance of tetracycline topical agents.

- *Sulfonamide*—among the oldest antibacterial agents, in use since the 1930s. Sodium sulfonamide lotion is available for treatment of acne and reducing inflammatory lesions.

Many other antibiotics are used topically to treat skin infections. The antibiotics discussed above are those in current topical use in the United States to treat acne vulgaris. A dermatologist can determine for each individual patient whether topical antibiotics are appropriate, and which topical antibiotic should be prescribed.

Topical Retinoids

Retinoids are a class of molecules in the vitamin A family of molecules. The retinoids are very potent as anti-acne medications. The retinoid activation of specific retinoid acid receptors (RARs) in the skin normalizes abnormal growth and death of cells in the sebaceous follicle; abnormal follicular cell cycles are believed to play a major role in plugging sebaceous follicles and causing comedones to form.

> ♣ **It's A Fact!!**
>
> Cells in the skin and other tissues contain special receptors called retinoic acid receptors (RARs) that attract and bind retinoic acid, a derivative of vitamin A. The retinoic acid and the RAR form a complex that affects the genetic workings of the cell. One of the effects on the skin cells is a decrease in the output of sebaceous glands, which helps reduce acne.
>
> Reviewed by David A. Cooke, M.D., January 2003.

The most common side effects of topical retinoids are redness, dryness, peeling, and itching of skin in the areas of retinoid application. Risk for birth defects is a major side effect of systemic retinoids; the risk is much lower for topical retinoids but should be discussed with the physician when a female acne patient is pregnant or likely to become pregnant.

The topical natural and synthetic retinoids currently available as acne medications in the United States are:

- *Tretinoin*—also known as vitamin A acid, a natural retinoid. Tretinoin is a molecule in the very large family of vitamin A–type molecules that are important for good vision, good skin quality, and general good health. Tretinoin influences skin cell growth and death cycles by a cascade of events that begins with binding to RARs and ends with both direct and indirect alteration of genes that control follicular cell cycles. Topical tretinoin is available as a cream, gel, or solution; a dermatologist will prescribe the form of application best for each individual patient. The maximum benefit of tretinoin's anti-acne activity may require several weeks of treatment.

- *Adapalene*—a synthetic retinoid applied as a gel or cream, it has potent retinoid and antiinflammatory activity. Side effects are similar to those of tretinoin.

♣ It's A Fact!!

When the U.S. Food and Drug Administration (FDA) approved isotretinoin for acne, the drug was known to able to cause birth defects. It was designated as Category X, meaning that it must be avoided under all circumstances during pregnancy. Nursing mothers also should not use isotretinoin.

Though not every fetus exposed to isotretinoin becomes deformed, the risk of birth defects among pregnant women is extremely high. These defects include hydrocephaly (enlargement of the fluid-filled spaces of the brain) and microcephaly (small head), heart defects, facial deformities such as cleft lip and missing ears, and mental retardation.

Reports in the literature suggest that about 25 to 35 percent of babies will suffer a malformation after exposure. That doesn't account for other defects, such as learning disabilities, that aren't detectable at birth. Miscarriages and premature births have also been reported.

Because the risks of fetal malformations with isotretinoin are so great, special restrictions on its prescribing have been put in place. Only physicians who have been registered with the manufacturer may prescribe it, and prescriptions can only be filled if marked with a special sticker available solely to these doctors. Female patients on isotretinoin therapy are required to use two forms of birth control and have frequent pregnancy tests.

Source: "The Power of Accutane: The Benefits and Risks of a Breakthrough Acne Drug," *FDA Consumer Magazine*, March–April 2001; also available at http://www.fda.gov/fdac/features/2001/201_acne.html.

- *Tazarotene*—a synthetic retinoid applied as a gel or cream, it acts on the follicular cell cycle by a biochemical pathway different from that of tretinoin. Side effects are similar to those of tretinoin.

Oral Medications
Oral Antibiotics

Broad-spectrum antibiotics have been a mainstay of systemic therapy for moderate to severe and persistent acne for many years. Numerous studies have provided evidence supporting the effectiveness of oral broad-spectrum antibiotics. The anti-acne activity of oral antibiotics appears to include physiologic effects in the sebaceous follicle as well as reduction of bacterial populations in the follicle.

Oral tetracycline has a long history in the treatment of acne, and it remains one of the most widely used. A typical tetracycline regimen for treating moderate to severe acne is a starting dose of 500 to 1000 milligrams a day, decreased as improvement is noted. Long-term, low-dose tetracycline therapy may be continued for many months to maintain suppression of acne. Higher doses may be prescribed for very severe acne, with regular monitoring for systemic side effects. Tetracycline may cause staining of teeth in children, and should generally not be taken by children younger than eight years of age. Oral tetracycline may cause permanent teeth staining or skeletal defects in a fetus and therefore should not be taken by a woman who is pregnant.

Oral erythromycin is an alternative to tetracycline that is safe for use in pregnant women and young children.

Oral minocycline and doxycycline are synthetically derived from tetracycline. Some evidence suggests that these antibiotics may be more effective than tetracycline in treating acne. Minocycline has a long history of use in the treatment of acne. Doxycycline may induce sensitivity to sunlight. Neither should be taken by pregnant women.

Hormonal Therapies

Androgenic ("male") hormones are known to have physiologic effects on sebaceous follicles that promote the development of acne. The purpose of hormonal therapy is to block or lessen acne-promoting effects of androgenic hormones.

Estrogen is a "feminine" hormone that counteracts effects of androgenic hormones and decreases sebum secretion in the sebaceous follicles. Estrogen has wide-ranging physiologic effects in the body, and its use must be closely monitored—often by both a gynecologist and a dermatologist. The use of estrogen alone in the treatment of acne may be indicated in carefully selected patients.

Estrogen-containing oral contraceptives are prescribed more frequently than estrogen alone in hormonal therapy of acne in females. The effects of estrogen are balanced by other hormonal constituents of oral contraceptives. While oral contraceptives have a better safety profile than estrogen alone in treating acne, their use must be monitored for side effects of nausea, weight gain, menstrual spotting, and breast tenderness. Hormonal therapy may be a treatment of choice for women whose acne does not respond to other medication.

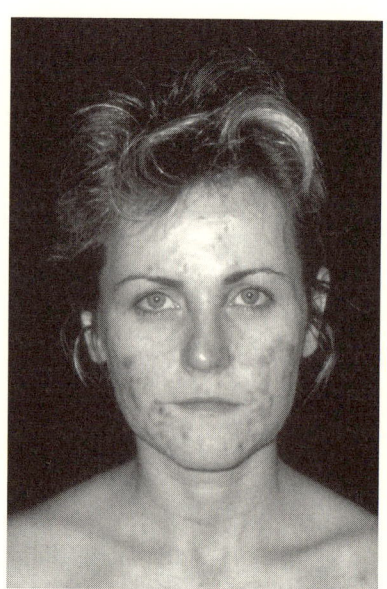

Figure 24.1. A typical case of severe acne before treatment with isotretinoin.

Prescription Medications For Acne

Corticosteroids

These powerful anti-inflammation drugs may be prescribed for short courses to treat very severe acne. Their metabolic effects limit long-term use. Low-dose corticosteroids are helpful in specific instances—for example, to suppress excessive secretion of androgenic hormones. Corticosteroids can induce development of steroid acne with prolonged use.

Other Hormone Therapies

The antiandrogen spironolactone reduces sebum production and improves acne in some patients. Side effects include irregular menstruation in women, breast tenderness, headache, and fatigue. The antiandrogen may be used along with an oral contraceptive to reduce irregular menstrual bleeding.

Flutamide is an antiandrogen sometimes prescribed together with an oral contraceptive to treat acne and hirsutism (excessive growth of facial and body hair) in women. It should not be taken by pregnant women.

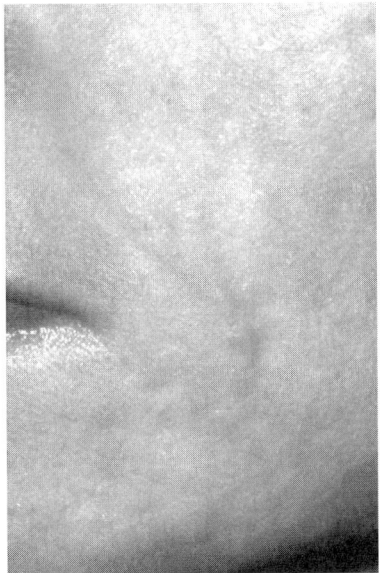

Figure 24.2. A close-up of the same patient after isotretinoin treatment; the acne is much less severe.

Isotretinoin

Isotretinoin, a synthetic retinoid, is the most effective drug available for treatment of severe cystic acne and acne resistant to other medications. Isotretinoin is a potent drug, usually reserved for treatment of very severe cystic acne and acne that is resistant to other medications. It is very effective in treating all forms of acne; the remissions achieved with isotretinoin usually last for many months to many years.

A number of side effects are associated with isotretinoin therapy, the most serious being the potential to cause severe birth defects to a developing fetus. The most common side effect of isotretinoin therapy is dryness of the skin and mucous membranes. Other, less common side effects include nausea and vomiting, bone and joint pain, headache, thinning hair, and changes in blood and enzyme profiles monitored in regular follow-up examinations. Psychological depression, sometimes severe, has been reported to occur in association with isotretinoin therapy. Regularly scheduled monitoring for side effects by the physician is required. For most persons treated with isotretinoin, side effects are tolerable and not a reason to discontinue therapy before remission is achieved.

It is imperative that women of childbearing potential follow the pregnancy prevention program and guidelines. Women who are planning a pregnancy, are pregnant, or are nursing must not use isotretinoin. It is recommended that women planning a pregnancy discontinue the use of isotretinoin for one month.

Chapter 25

Accutane®: The Breakthrough Acne Drug

Acne plagued Julie Harper throughout high school and college. She depended on makeup and wore her hair down over the side of her face. She gave up chocolate and french fries, only to find that neither made a difference. And she went through medicine after medicine, from over-the-counter creams to oral antibiotics.

These were not occasional pimples that vanish after a couple of days. This acne covered her face and left scars on her neck. "I had tried everything and felt frustrated all the time," says Harper, now a physician and assistant professor of dermatology at the University of Alabama-Birmingham—a career she chose due in large part to her struggle with acne.

Harper finally found a successful treatment nine years ago at the age of 22. She took a drug called isotretinoin (trade name Accutane) and watched her skin improve in just a couple of months. By the third month, her acne had disappeared. She says with clearer skin came more self-confidence and higher self-esteem.

About This Chapter: Excerpted from "The Power of Accutane: The Benefits and Risks of a Breakthrough Acne Drug," *FDA Consumer Magazine*, March–April 2001; also available at http://www.fda.gov/fdac/features/2001/201_acne.html. "Why Acne Forms, and How Accutane Knocks It Out" appeared in the original article as a sidebar and is available at http://www.fda.gov/fdac/features/2001/sideacne.html.

Considered the biggest breakthrough in acne drug treatment over the past 20 years, Accutane is the only drug that has the potential to clear severe acne permanently after one course of treatment. One course, which is typically five months, results in prolonged remission of acne in up to 85 percent of patients. A member of a class of drugs known as retinoids, Accutane is highly effective. But it doesn't work for everyone, and some patients need more than one course of treatment. Dr. Harper took a second course of Accutane one year after the first and has been free of severe acne ever since, now only occasionally using a topical medication.

♣ It's A Fact!!

Why Acne Forms And How Accutane Knocks It Out

Acne is the most common skin disorder, and while it usually appears in adolescence, adults can get it too. Acne occurs when hair follicles and the sebaceous glands inside the follicles are inflamed. Sebaceous glands make an oily substance called sebum. Too much sebum can clog the follicles and lead to bacterial growth and inflammation.

According to the American Academy of Dermatology, the four basic mechanisms contributing to acne are hormones, increased sebum production, changes inside hair follicles, and bacteria. Acne usually occurs at age 11 to 14 when the body starts producing male hormones called androgens. Androgens can overstimulate sebaceous glands and make them produce more sebum.

Dead cells inside hair follicles normally are shed and come out onto the surface of the skin. But in people with acne, the cells are shed faster, stick together, mix with sebum, and clog the follicle. Then bacteria contaminate the skin cell and sebum mixture and grow. When the body's immune system tries to destroy the bacteria, inflammation results.

Accutane helps the function of the follicles return to normal, lowers production of sebum, slows the growth of a bacterium called *Propionibacterium acnes* (*P. acnes*), and reduces inflammation and the chance for scarring. The drug is unique in its ability to affect all main underlying causes of acne formation.

No other acne medicine works as well for severe acne. Patients generally have to keep using other medications because they only suppress acne temporarily. But as powerful as Accutane can be in improving patients' lives, its adverse effects can be just as powerful. The drug is known to cause miscarriage and severe birth defects. Patients taking Accutane may develop potentially serious problems affecting a number of organs, including the liver, intestines, eyes, ears, and skeletal system. And some patients taking Accutane have developed serious psychiatric problems, including depression. More rarely, patients have developed suicidal behavior and killed themselves.

Because it is a high-risk drug, Accutane should be reserved for cases of "severe recalcitrant nodular acne," according to the product's labeling. This type of acne is resistant to standard acne treatment, including oral antibiotics, and is characterized by many nodules or cysts—inflammatory lesions filled with pus and lodged deep within the skin. These lesions can cause pain, permanent scarring, and negative psychological effects.

"Sometimes people tend to dismiss the impact of acne because it's not life-threatening, says Kathy O'Connell, M.D., Ph.D., a medical reviewer for Accutane in the U.S. Food and Drug Administration (FDA)'s division of dermatologic and dental drug products, Center for Drug Evaluation and Research (CDER). "But patients with severe acne know all too well the very real suffering caused by this disfiguring disease."

FDA approved Accutane in 1982, and since then, about 5 million people in the United States and 12 million worldwide have been treated with it, according to its manufacturer, Hoffmann-La Roche of Nutley, New Jersey. The number of patients taking the drug has increased, and half are females, most of whom are in their childbearing years (age 15–44). Because of concern about the drug's risks, FDA continues to evaluate Accutane and work with the manufacturer to maximize safe use of the drug.

Warning About Pregnancy Risks

When FDA approved Accutane, the drug was known to be teratogenic—able to cause birth defects. It was designated as Category X, meaning that it must be avoided under all circumstances during pregnancy. Nursing mothers also should not use Accutane.

Though not every fetus exposed to Accutane becomes deformed, the risk of birth defects among pregnant women is extremely high. These defects include hydrocephaly (enlargement of the fluid-filled spaces of the brain) and microcephaly (small head), heart defects, facial deformities such as cleft lip and missing ears, and mental retardation.

Reports in the literature suggest that about 25 to 35 percent of babies will suffer a malformation after exposure, and that doesn't account for other defects, such as learning disabilities, that aren't detectable at birth. Miscarriages and premature births have also been reported.

Though FDA approved labeling in 1982 that warned Accutane should not be used in pregnant women, reports of severe birth defects associated with the drug began to arrive in June 1983. Over the following years, a series of labeling changes and letters to pharmacists and prescribers of the drug stressed pregnancy warnings and sought to increase awareness about reported malformations.

Then, after an FDA review of pregnancy exposures to Accutane, Roche launched the Pregnancy Prevention Program (PPP) in late 1988 to further educate women using Accutane and their physicians about the dangers. The goal was to ensure that prescriptions would only be given to women with severe recalcitrant nodular acne who could comply with contraceptive requirements.

Roche sent PPP kits to physicians and encouraged them to review pregnancy prevention materials with patients before starting the drug. Materials included a contraceptive booklet, checklists to help assess whether patients could adhere to the drug's requirements, and consent forms that patients sign to acknowledge their understanding of the risk of birth defects. Roche also set up a toll-free line, made contraceptive information available in 13 languages, and offered to pay for contraceptive counseling and pregnancy testing by a specialist.

To further reinforce pregnancy prevention, Roche began packaging Accutane in blister packs that include red and black warnings, along with a drawing of a malformed baby and the "Avoid Pregnancy" symbol.

Even though Accutane's labeling recommended use of two reliable forms of contraception, there have been reports of pregnancies occurring in patients who used hormonal contraception, including pills, injectables, and implantables, while taking Accutane. Accutane's labeling was updated in the summer of 2000. One change emphasized the need for two reliable forms of contraception for at least one month before taking Accutane, during treatment, and for one month after discontinuing Accutane, even when one of the forms of contraception is hormonal.

Evaluating Compliance

Yolonda Lawrence of Santa Monica, California, says there was no way she could miss the point about pregnancy prevention before she used Accutane for severe adult-onset acne in 1998. "I got a pamphlet, I signed papers, the doctor told me over and over, and the pictures of what can happen were very clear—babies with no ears" and other deformities, she says.

But reports of Accutane-exposed pregnancies continue, and that's enough to make FDA concerned, says Peter Honig, M.D., director of FDA's office of postmarketing drug risk assessment (OPDRA) in CDER.

Shortly after the Pregnancy Prevention Program began, Roche sponsored a survey of women taking Accutane to assess compliance with the program, and the company encouraged doctors to enroll patients. Run by the Slone Epidemiology Unit at Boston University's School of Public Health, the survey set out to track pregnancy rates and outcomes, patients' awareness of risks, and patient and physician behavior.

Of the 500,000 women enrolled in the Slone survey from 1989 to 1998, there have been 958 pregnancies, 834 of which were terminations (either elective or spontaneous or due to ectopic pregnancies), 110 that resulted in live births, and 14 that had unknown outcomes. Of the 60 infants with available medical records, 8 had congenital abnormalities. Since Accutane's approval, Roche has received close to 2,000 reports of Accutane-exposed pregnancies, 70 percent of which occurred after the PPP began.

According to FDA, exactly how well the PPP has worked is unclear. Experts say the PPP is a significant program that has prevented many pregnancies and is the first of its kind initiated by a pharmaceutical company. Roche has made extraordinary efforts to educate patients that they must not become pregnant while taking Accutane, says a Roche spokesperson.

At a September 2000 meeting of FDA's Dermatologic and Ophthalmic Drugs Advisory Committee, a Roche representative reported that from the company's perspective, pregnancy rates have declined. Amarilys Vega, M.D., an FDA medical officer, agreed. However, because use of the product has increased over the years, the actual number of pregnancies occurring during Accutane use has not declined. One limitation is that the survey is voluntary and only captures about 30 to 40 percent of all patients on Accutane. So there's no way to know exactly how many pregnancy exposures there have been, according to FDA experts. Of serious concern is that women who enroll in the survey may be more likely to comply with the contraceptive requirements than those who don't enroll in the survey. This leaves open critical questions about how representative the PPP group is and about unreported pregnancies among women who don't enroll in the PPP.

> ✔ **Quick Tip**
> **Accutane Resources**
> To learn more, visit FDA's Accutane page on the Internet: www.fda.gov/cder/drug/infopage/accutane. To report adverse events related to Accutane, call Roche Medical Services at 1-800-526-6367 or FDA's MedWatch Program at 1-800-FDA-1088.

Most patients in the Slone survey have reported that they understood Accutane may cause birth defects. And according to Roche, the percentage of female patients who reported they were pregnant when they began Accutane dropped from 30 percent of pregnancies reported in 1989 to 11 percent of pregnancies reported for the period of 1991 to 1997. But substantial noncompliance with the PPP continues to be reported.

For example, a 1997 report on the survey shows that 25 percent of women in the program did not report having a pregnancy test before starting

Accutane, and 33 percent did not report postponing the start of Accutane until a pregnancy test result was known. It is estimated that 40 percent of women taking Accutane are sexually active.

The only patients exempt from Accutane's contraceptive requirements are men, and women who have had a hysterectomy or who say they will abstain from sex during treatment. But the challenge is that going from sexually inactive to active can happen overnight.

Possible Psychiatric Link

Many patients say they feel better about themselves after receiving successful treatment for acne. Evelyn Germanakos, of Los Angeles, California, struggled with acne as an adult, and says she felt like her old self after Accutane cleared up lumpy blemishes in 1997. "I had gotten to the point where I didn't even want to go outside or be with people, let alone look in the mirror," she says. But while Accutane may help lift psychosocial distress such as embarrassment, evidence suggests that it may actually cause serious psychiatric disorders in some people.

Though the drug's label previously listed depression as a possible reaction, FDA strengthened the label warning in 1998 after reviewing cases with serious outcomes reported in the years after the drug was approved. The new labeling states that Accutane may cause depression and psychosis, and that in rare cases it may cause suicidal ideation (thoughts of suicide), suicide attempts, and suicide.

The label also advises providers that simply discontinuing the drug may not remedy any psychiatric problems and that further evaluation may be necessary. "In some cases, stopping Accutane alone may not be enough to relieve the mood changes," says Jonathan Wilkin, M.D., director of CDER's division of dermatologic and dental drug products. "Psychiatric treatment may also be needed."

The relationship between Accutane and depression remains unproven, but some patients have reported that their depression subsided when they stopped the medication and came back when they resumed taking it. And some who have reported problems with depression while taking Accutane had no previous psychiatric history. FDA considers the number of reports of serious depression associated with Accutane high compared to other drugs in its database.

From 1982 to May 2000, FDA received reports of 37 U.S. Accutane patients who committed suicide, 24 while on the drug and 13 after stopping the drug. In addition to suicides, FDA received reports of 110 U.S. Accutane users hospitalized for depression, suicidal ideation, and suicide attempt during the same time period. As of May 2000, FDA had received reports of 284 Accutane users with nonhospitalized depression.

Several factors make it hard to definitively link depression with Accutane. Depression is a common problem, and some patients may be suffering from it before starting Accutane therapy. Additionally, some patients who reported depression with Accutane had previous courses of the drug without depression. Even so, it is recommended that doctors act as if Accutane could have psychiatric effects until there is more information, says FDA's Wilkin.

The Future Of Accutane

Roche does not want to have any Accutane-exposed pregnancies, a company spokesperson says, and plans to continue educational efforts. This year Roche launched a targeted Pregnancy Prevention Program that focuses on women who are at highest risk of becoming pregnant while taking Accutane.

Experts agree that pregnancy prevention education should remain a key part of risk management for Accutane use. But more labeling changes and letters are not likely to make a significant difference, according to FDA's Honig. "During all the time the drug has been on the market and after all of those labeling changes, there are still pregnancies," he says. "It is not expected that another labeling change or 'Dear Doctor' letter will change behavior at this point." Psychiatric adverse events have also continued after labeling changes.

FDA's Dermatologic and Ophthalmic Drugs Advisory Committee met in September 2000 to discuss options for Accutane, and to evaluate whether a framework for safer use of the drug can be developed. One change since then is that all Accutane prescriptions now come with a new Medication

Accutane®: The Breakthrough Acne Drug

Guide that contains warnings about pregnancy and psychiatric issues, plus other important warnings and precautions regarding potentially serious or life-threatening effects.

FDA has also proposed a mandatory registration of patients taking Accutane, prescribers, and pharmacists. "The main reason is to ensure that pregnancy testing is done before the drug is prescribed," says Julie Beitz, M.D., of FDA's office of postmarketing drug risk assessment. The goal would be to have doctors document negative pregnancy tests and to have pharmacies dispense the drug only to women who have had negative pregnancy tests.

The registry for prescribers may involve a continuing education course that doctors would have to take to be able to prescribe Accutane. According to Hoffmann-La Roche, about 85 percent of Accutane prescriptions come from dermatologists and 15 percent come from primary care physicians. The course would be open to all medical doctors. And all Accutane patients would have to sign a mandatory consent form that would address both pregnancy and psychiatric issues, Beitz says.

The American Academy of Dermatology and the Dermatologic Nurses Association were among those who testified at the September 2000 committee meeting in opposition to a mandatory registration, saying that it would be a disservice to patients, making it harder for them to obtain the drug. Others, including the March of Dimes and the Public Citizen's Health Research Group, testified that they want to see stricter measures for Accutane.

FDA's experts say it's a balancing act. The value of Accutane is clear, but when it comes to even one report of death—whether it's suicide, miscarriage, or some other cause—FDA must make choices that will best protect the public's health.

Monthly Accutane Prescriptions Ensure Follow-Up

Evelyn Germanakos of Los Angeles, California, recalls forgetting to have a blood test before returning to her dermatologist for a monthly visit while taking Accutane. "He sent me right away to get it, and said he wouldn't renew the prescription without it," she says.

Experts say that kind of follow-up is critical. Doctors should only give one-month prescriptions for Accutane and should conduct urine or blood pregnancy testing and contraceptive counseling each month of treatment.

Monthly blood tests also allow doctors to monitor patients for other adverse effects. Elevated triglyceride levels, which can be associated with pancreatitis, have occurred in about 25 percent of patients in clinical trials for Accutane, and about 7 percent of patients showed an increase in cholesterol levels.

Alan N. Moshell, MD, director of the skin diseases branch at the National Institute of Arthritis and Musculoskeletal and Skin Diseases, says he's heard about severe adverse effects such as liver damage in cases where a full dose of Accutane has been prescribed with inadequate follow-up. "It has usually been a situation in which the full five-month course has been prescribed at the first visit and then the patient was not brought back, or simply failed to follow instructions about follow-up visits and blood tests." In such cases, patients may keep taking the drug and only return to the doctor when it's too late and they've experienced an adverse effect.

More common side effects of Accutane include lip inflammation and drying of the skin and mucous membranes. Germanakos says her mouth was incredibly dry. "I drank about 15 to 16 glasses of water a day, and I was still thirsty," she says. She also experienced skin peeling on her eyelids and dry nasal passages, and she says her acne got worse before it got better.

—by Michelle Meadows

Chapter 26

Chemical Peeling For Acne Scars

Chemical peeling is a technique used to improve the appearance of the skin which is typically performed on the face, neck, or hands. In this treatment, a chemical solution is applied to the skin that causes it to "blister" and eventually peel off. The new, regenerated skin is usually smoother and less wrinkled than the old skin. The new skin is also temporarily more sensitive to the sun.

Dermatologic surgeons have used various peeling agents for the last 50 years and are experts in performing multiple types of chemical peels. A thorough evaluation by your dermatologic surgeon is imperative before embarking upon a chemical peel.

What Can A Chemical Peel Do?

Chemical peeling is often used to treat fine lines under the eyes and around the mouth. Wrinkles caused by sun damage, aging, and hereditary factors can often be reduced or even eliminated with this procedure. However, sags, bulges, and more severe wrinkles do not respond well to peeling and may require other kinds of cosmetic surgical procedures, such as a face lift, brow lift, eye lift, or soft-tissue filler.

About This Chapter: Adapted from "Chemical Peeling," © 2002 American Society for Dermatological Surgery (ASDS), http://www.asds-net.org/FactSheets/chemical_peeling.html. Reprinted with permission.

Mild scarring and certain types of acne can also be treated with chemical peels. In addition, pigmentation of the skin in the form of sun spots, age spots, liver spots, freckles, splotching due to taking birth control pills, and skin that is dull in texture and color may be improved with chemical peeling.

Chemical peeling may be combined with laser resurfacing, dermabrasion, or soft-tissue fillers to achieve cost-effective skin rejuvenation customized to the needs of the individual patient. Areas of sun-damaged, precancerous keratoses or scaling patches may improve after chemical peeling. Following treatment, new lesions or patches are less likely to appear.

Generally, fair-skinned and light-haired patients are ideal candidates for chemical peels. Darker skin types may also experience good results, depending upon the type of skin problem encountered.

How Are Chemical Peels Performed?

Prior to surgery, instructions may include the elimination of certain drugs and the preparation of the skin with topical preconditioning medications. The patient may be advised to clean the area with an antiseptic soap the day before surgery.

A chemical peel can be performed in a doctor's office or in a surgery center as an outpatient procedure. At the time of treatment, the skin is thoroughly cleansed with an agent that removes excess oils, and the eyes and hair are protected. One or more chemical solutions—an alpha hydroxy acid, such

---

✎ Weird Words

Keratosis (keratoses, plural): Any area on the surface of the skin covered with an unusual growth of the outer, horny layers.

Source: Adapted from *Stedman's Medical Dictionary, 27th Edition,* © 2000. Lippincott Williams, and Wilkins. All rights reserved. Reprinted with permission.

as glycolic acid, salicylic acid, or lactic acid; trichloroacetic acid (TCA); or carbolic acid (phenol)—are used. Dermatologic surgeons are well qualified to select the proper peeling agent based upon the type of skin damage. During a chemical peel, the physician applies the solution to small areas on the skin. These applications produce a controlled wound, enabling new, refreshed skin to appear. Most patients experience a warm to somewhat hot sensation that lasts about 5 to 10 minutes, followed by a stinging sensation. A deeper peel may require pain medication during or after the procedure.

What Should Be Expected After Treatment?

Depending upon the type of peel, a reaction similar to a sunburn occurs following a chemical peel. Superficial peeling usually involves redness, followed by scaling that ends within three to seven days. Medium-depth and deep peeling may result in swelling and the presence of water blisters that may break, crust, turn brown, and peel off over a period of 7 to 14 days. Some peels may require bandages to be placed on part or all of the treated skin. Bandages are usually removed in several days and may improve the effectiveness of the treatment. It is important to avoid overexposure to the sun after a chemical peel, since the new skin is fragile and more susceptible to complications. The dermatologic surgeon will prescribe the proper follow-up care to reduce the tendency to develop abnormal skin color after peeling.

What Are The Possible Complications?

In certain skin types, there is a risk of developing a temporary or permanent color change in the skin. Taking birth control pills, pregnancy, or a family history of brownish discoloration on the face may increase the possibility of developing abnormal pigmentation. Although low, there is a risk of scarring in certain areas of the face, and certain individuals may be more prone to scarring. There is a small incidence of the reactivation of cold sores in patients with *Herpes* infection. This problem is treated with medication prescribed by the dermatologic surgeon. Prior to treatment, it is important for a patient to inform the physician of any history of keloids, unusual scarring tendencies, extensive x-rays on the face, or recurring cold sores.

Part 4

Understanding And Preventing Skin Cancer

Chapter 27

Everything You Need To Know About Sun And Skin

The Burden Of Skin Cancer

Skin cancer is the most common form of cancer in the United States. More than one million new cases of skin cancer will be diagnosed in 2002. The three major types of skin cancer are basal cell carcinoma, squamous cell carcinoma, and melanoma. Although basal cell and squamous cell carcinomas can be cured if detected and treated early, these cancers can cause considerable damage and disfigurement. Melanoma is the deadliest form of skin cancer, causing more than 75 percent of all skin cancer deaths. About 53,600 people in the United States will be diagnosed with a melanoma skin cancer in 2002, and approximately 7,400 will die.

Exposure to the sun's ultraviolet (UV) rays appears to be the most important environmental factor in the development of skin cancer. Skin cancer can be prevented when sun-protective practices are used consistently. UV rays from artificial sources of light, such as tanning beds and sun lamps, are just

---

About This Chapter: Adapted from "Skin Cancer: Preventing America's Most Common Cancer," National Center for Chronic Disease Prevention and Health Promotion, Centers for Disease Control, August 8, 2002, available at http://www.cdc.gov/cancer/nscpep/skin.htm; and from "Choose Your Cover Skin Cancer Prevention Campaign: Questions and Answers," National Center for Chronic Disease Prevention and Health Promotion, Centers for Disease Control, November 15, 2001, available at http://www.cdc.gov/chooseyourcover/qanda.htm.

as dangerous as those from the sun, and should also be avoided. Although both tanning and burning can increase a person's risk for skin cancer, most Americans do not consistently protect themselves from UV rays.

Sun Exposure

When do I need to protect myself from sun exposure?

Protection from sun exposure is important all year round, not just during the summer or at the beach. Any time the sun's ultraviolet (UV) rays are able to reach the earth, you need to protect yourself from excessive sun exposure. UV rays can cause skin damage during any season or temperature.

Relatively speaking, the hours between 10 a.m. and 4 p.m. during daylight savings time (9 a.m.–3 p.m. during standard time) are the most hazardous for UV exposure in the continental United States. UV radiation is the greatest during the late spring and early summer in North America.

UV Rays

What exactly are "ultraviolet rays"?

Ultraviolet (UV) rays are a part of sunlight that is an invisible form of radiation. UV rays can penetrate and change the structure of skin cells.

> **Remember!!**
> UV rays reach you on cloudy and hazy days, as well as on bright and sunny days. UV rays will also reflect off any surface like water, cement, sand, and snow.

There are three types of UV rays: ultraviolet A (UVA), ultraviolet B (UVB), and ultraviolet C (UVC). UVA is the most abundant source of solar radiation at the earth's surface and penetrates beyond the top layer of human skin. Scientists believe that UVA radiation can cause damage to connective tissue and increase a person's risk for developing skin cancer.

UVB rays are less abundant at the earth's surface than UVA because a significant portion of UVB rays is absorbed by the ozone layer. UVB rays penetrate less deeply into the skin than do UVA rays, but also can be damaging.

UVC radiation is extremely hazardous to skin, but it is completely absorbed by the stratospheric ozone layer and does not reach the surface of the earth.

How can I protect myself from the sun's UV rays?

When possible, avoid outdoor activities during midday, when the sun's rays are strongest. This usually means the hours between 10 a.m. and 4 p.m. You can also wear protective clothing, such as a wide-brimmed hat, long-sleeved shirt, and long pants.

For eye protection, wear wraparound sunglasses that provide 100 percent UV ray protection. And always wear a broad-spectrum (protection against both UVA and UVB rays) sunscreen and lipscreen with at least SPF 15. Remember to reapply as indicated by the manufacturer's directions.

Also, check the sunscreen's expiration date. Sunscreen without an expiration date has a shelf life of no more than three years. Exposure to extreme temperatures can shorten the expiration date or shelf life of sunscreen.

What can excessive exposure to UV rays do to my health?

UV exposure appears to be the most important environmental factor in the development of skin cancer and a primary factor in the development of lip cancer.

Although getting some sun exposure can yield a few positive benefits, excessive and unprotected exposure to the sun can result in premature aging and undesirable changes in skin texture. Such exposure has been associated with various types of skin cancer, including melanoma, one of the most serious and deadly forms.

UV rays also have been found to be associated with various eye conditions, such as cataracts.

UV Index

What is the UV Index?

The UV Index was developed by the National Weather Service and the Environmental Protection Agency. It provides a forecast of the expected risk of overexposure to UV rays and indicates the degree of caution you should take when working, playing, or exercising outdoors.

The UV Index predicts exposure levels on a 0–10+ scale, where 0 indicates a low risk of overexposure and 10+ means a very high risk of overexposure. Calculated on a next-day basis for dozens of cities across the U.S., the UV Index takes into account clouds and other local conditions that affect the amount of UV radiation reaching the ground.

The level of danger calculated for the basic categories of the index are for a person with Type II skin (see Table 27.1). For a person with type II skin, for example, an index value of 5 or 6 represents a moderate possibility of UV overexposure.

Tanning And Burning

What does a suntan indicate? Why does the skin tan when exposed to the sun?

The penetration of UV rays to the skin's inner layer results in the production of more melanin. That melanin eventually moves toward the outer layers of the skin and becomes visible as a tan.

♣ **It's A Fact!!**

Table 27.1. Sunburn And Skin Type

Skin Type	Tanning and Sunburning History
I	Always burns, never tans, sensitive to sun exposure
II	Burns easily, tans minimally
III	Burns moderately, tans gradually to light brown
IV	Burns minimally, always tans well to moderately brown
V	Rarely burns, tans profusely to dark
VI	Never burns, deeply pigmented, least sensitive

Though everyone is at risk for damage as a result of excessive sun exposure, people with skin types I and II are at the highest risk.

A suntan is not an indicator of good health. Some physicians consider the skin's tanning a response to injury because it appears after the sun's UV rays have killed some cells and damaged others.

Not everyone burns or tans in the same manner. Are there ways to classify different skin types?

Whether individuals burn or tan depends on a number of factors, including their skin type, the time of year, and the amount of sun exposure they have received recently. The skin's susceptibility to burning can be classified on the five-point scale outlined in the Table 27.1.

Rub It On

Does it matter what kind of sunscreen I use?

Sunscreens come in a variety of forms such as lotions, gels, and sprays, so there are plenty of different options. There are also sunscreens made for specific purposes, such as the scalp, sensitive skin, and use on babies. Regardless of the type of sunscreen you choose, be sure that you use one that blocks both UVA and UVB rays and that it offers at least SPF 15.

What does a sunscreen's SPF rating mean?

Sunscreens are assigned a sun protection factor (SPF) number according to their effectiveness in offering protection from UV rays. Higher numbers indicate more protection. As a rule of thumb, you should always use a sunscreen with at least SPF 15.

Do sunscreens need to be reapplied during the course of a day?

You should follow the manufacturer's directions regarding reapplication, or you risk not getting the protection that you might think you are getting. Though recently developed sunscreens are more resistant to loss through sweating and getting wet than previous sunscreens were, you should still reapply frequently, especially during peak sun hours or after swimming or sweating.

How do sunscreens work?

Most sun protection products work by absorbing, reflecting, or scattering the sun's rays. Such products contain chemicals that interact with the skin to protect it from UV rays. Sunscreens help prevent problems related to sun exposure, such as aging skin and precancerous growths.

Keep in mind that sunscreen is not meant to allow you to spend more time in the sun than you would otherwise. That's why it is important to complement sunscreen use with other sun protection options: cover up, wear a hat and sunglasses, and seek shade.

Some cosmetic products claim to protect you from UV rays. Can they?

There are cosmetics and lip protectors that contain some of the same protective chemicals used by sunscreens on the market. However, not all of these products meet the standard of having at least SPF 15, and therefore do not offer sufficient protection by themselves.

Cover Up

What kinds of clothing best protect my skin from UV rays?

Clothing that covers your skin protects against the sun's UV rays. Loose-fitting long-sleeved shirts and long pants made from tightly woven fabric offer the best protection. A wet T-shirt offers you much less UV protection than does a dry one.

If wearing this type of clothing isn't practical, at least try to wear a T-shirt or a beach cover-up. Keep in mind, however, that a typical T-shirt actually has an SPF rating substantially lower than the recommended SPF 15, so double up on protection by using sunscreen with at least SPF 15 (and UVA and UVB protection) and staying in the shade when you can.

Does protective clothing have to be a certain color?

Wearing clothing made of tightly woven fabric is best for protecting your skin, regardless of the color. Darker colors, though, may offer more protection than lighter colors.

It gets so hot here in the summer, there's no way I could be comfortable in long pants and a long-sleeved shirt. So, what else can I do to protect my skin?

Protecting yourself from the sun's UV rays doesn't have to be a major chore; it's just a matter of knowing your options and using them. Wearing a

Everything You Need To Know About Sun And Skin

dry T-shirt is a good start, but it is not enough if you are going to be outside for more than a few minutes.

If you can't wear long pants and a long-sleeved shirt, you can boost your protection by seeking shade whenever possible and by always wearing sunscreen with at least SPF 15.

Get A Hat

Will a hat help protect my skin? Are there recommended styles for the best protection?

Hats can help shield your skin from the sun's UV rays. Choose a hat that provides shade for all of your head and neck. For the most protection, wear a hat with a brim all the way around that shades your face, ears, and the back of your neck.

If you choose to wear a baseball cap, you should also protect your ears and the back of your neck by wearing clothing that covers those areas, using sunscreen with at least SPF 15, or staying in the shade.

For the best protection, what material should I look for in a hat?

A tightly woven fabric, such as canvas, works best to protect your skin from UV rays. When possible, avoid straw hats with holes that let sunlight through.

Does the color of my hat matter?

The amount of shade offered by a particular hat appears to be its most important prevention characteristic. If a darker hat is an option, though, it may offer even more UV protection.

Grab Shades

Are sunglasses an important part of my sun protection plan?

Yes. Sunglasses protect your eyes from UV rays and reduce the risk of cataracts. They also protect the tender skin around your eyes from sun exposure.

What type of sunglasses best protects my eyes from UV rays?

Sunglasses that block both UVA and UVB rays offer the best protection. The majority of sunglasses sold in the United States, regardless of cost, meet this standard. Wrap-around sunglasses work best because they block UV rays from sneaking in from the side.

Seek Shade

Is there any particular time I should try to stay in the shade?

The sun's UV rays are strongest and do the most damage during midday, so it's best to avoid direct exposure between 10:00 a.m. and 4:00 p.m. You can reduce your risk of skin damage and skin cancer by seeking shade under an umbrella, tree, or other shelter before you need relief from the sun.

I work outdoors all summer and can't stay in the shade. What can I do to protect my skin?

If you can't avoid the sun, you can protect your skin by wearing a wide-brimmed hat, wraparound sunglasses that block both UVA and UVB rays, long-sleeved shirt, and long pants. You can also wear a sunscreen and lipscreen with at least SPF 15 and UVA and UVB protection and reapply according to the manufacturer's directions. When you can, take your breaks and your lunch in the shade.

If I stay in the shade, should I still use sunscreen and wear a hat?

UV rays can reflect off virtually any surface (including sand, snow and concrete) and can reach you in the shade. Your best bet to protect your skin and lips is to use sunscreen or wear protective clothing when you're outside—even when you're in the shade.

Chapter 28

Seven Steps To Safer Sunning

Put away the baby oil. Toss out that old metal sun reflector. Cancel your next appointment to the local tanning salon.

These are new days with new ways of sunning, and the practices that traditionally have gone into obtaining the so-called "healthy tanned" look are on the verge of fading into history.

In their place: safer sun practices that preserve people's natural skin color and condition.

That's what health experts are hoping for as the evidence against exposure to the sun and sunlamps continues to mount. Both emit harmful ultraviolet (UV) radiation that in the short term can cause painful sunburn and in the long term may lead to unsightly skin blemishes, premature aging of the skin, cataracts and other eye problems, skin cancer, and a weakened immune system.

The problems may become more prevalent, too, if, as some scientists predict, the earth's ozone layer continues to be depleted. According to the Environmental Protection Agency, scientists began accumulating evidence in

---

About This Chapter: Originally appeared in *FDA Consumer* in 1996; revised in 1997 and available at http://www.fda.gov/fdac/features/596_7sun.html. Reviewed by David A. Cooke, M.D., on October 8, 2002.

the 1980s that the ozone layer—a thin shield in the stratosphere that protects life from UV radiation—is being depleted by certain widely used chemicals. According to the most recent estimates from the National Aeronautics and Space Administration, the ozone layer is being depleted at a rate of 4 to 6 percent each decade. This means additional UV radiation reaching the earth's surface—and our bodies.

Although people with light skin are more susceptible to sun damage, darker-skinned people, including African Americans and Hispanic Americans, also can be affected.

You may have already started to take precautions. But are you doing all you can?

The following recommendations come from various expert organizations, including the American Academy of Dermatology, American Cancer Society, American Academy of Ophthalmology, Skin Cancer Foundation, American Academy of Pediatrics, National Cancer Institute, National Weather Service, and Food and Drug Administration. FDA regulates many items related to sun safety, including sunscreens and sunblocks, sunglasses, and sun-protective clothing that makes medical claims. The agency also sets performance standards for sunlamps.

Here are seven steps to safer sunning.

1. Avoid The Sun

This is especially important between 10 a.m. and 3 p.m., when the sun's rays are strongest. Also avoid the sun when the UV Index is high in your area.

> ✔ **Quick Tip**
> The National Weather Service forecasts the UV Index daily in 58 U.S. cities. You can learn the UV Index in your area by checking the National Weather Service Climate Prediction Center's website. Go to (http://www.cpc.ncep.noaa.gov/products/stratosphere/uv_index/uv_current.htm).

The UV Index is a number from 0 to 10+ that indicates the amount of UV radiation reaching the earth's surface during the hour around noon. The higher the number, the greater your exposure to UV radiation if you go outdoors.

Seven Steps To Safer Sunning

Don't be fooled by cloudy skies. Clouds block only as much as 20 percent of UV radiation. UV radiation also can pass through water, so don't assume you're safe from UV radiation if you're in the water and feeling cool. Also, be especially careful on the beach and in the snow because sand and snow reflect sunlight and increase the amount of UV radiation you receive.

People with darker skin will resist the sun's rays by tanning, which is actually an indication that the skin has been injured. Tanning occurs when ultraviolet radiation is absorbed by the skin, causing an increase in the activity and number of melanocytes, the cells that produce the pigment melanin. Melanin helps to block out damaging rays up to a point.

Those with lighter skin are more likely to burn. Too much sun exposure in a short period results in sunburn. A sunburn causes skin redness, tenderness, pain, swelling, and blistering. Although there is no quick cure, the American Academy of Dermatology recommends using wet compresses, cool baths, bland moisturizers, and over-the-counter hydrocortisone creams.

Sunburn becomes a more serious problem with fever, chills, upset stomach, and confusion. If these symptoms develop, see a doctor.

2. Use Sunscreen

With labels stating "sunscreen" or "sunblock," these lotions, creams, ointments, gels, or wax sticks, when applied to the skin, absorb, reflect, or scatter some or all of the sun's rays.

Some sunscreen products, labeled "broad-spectrum," protect against two types of radiation: UVA and UVB. Scientists now believe that both UVA and UVB can damage the skin and lead to skin cancer.

Other products protect only against UVB, previously thought to be the only damaging type.

Some cosmetics, such as some lipsticks, also are considered sunscreen products if they contain sunscreen and their labels state they do.

Sunblock products block a large percentage of UV radiation.

FDA requires the labels of all sunscreen and sunblock products to state the product's sun protection factor, or SPF, from 2 on up. The higher the number, the longer a person can stay in the sun before burning.

Experts recommend broad-spectrum products with SPFs of at least 15. They also suggest applying the product liberally—about 30 milliliters (1 ounce) per application for the average-size person, according to The Skin Cancer Foundation—15 to 30 minutes every time before going outdoors. It should be applied evenly on all exposed skin, including lips, nose, ears, neck, scalp (if hair is thinning), hands, feet, and eyelids, although care should be taken not to get it in the eyes because it can irritate them. If contact occurs, rinse eyes thoroughly with water.

Sunscreens should not be used on babies younger than six months because their bodies may not be developed enough to handle sunscreen chemicals. Instead, use hats, clothing, and shading to protect small babies from the sun. If you think your baby may need a sunscreen, check with your pediatrician.

For children six months to two years, use a sunscreen with at least an SPF of 4, although 15 or higher is best.

Use sunscreen products regularly on children, advises Stephen Katz, M.D., Ph.D., director of the National Institute of Arthritis and Musculoskeletal and Skin Diseases and chief of the National Cancer Institute's dermatology branch. "Get them used to it, so they can use it regularly like toothpaste," Katz says.

3. Wear A Hat

A hat with at least a 3-inch brim all around is ideal because it can protect areas often exposed to the sun, such as the neck, ears, eyes, and scalp. A shade cap (which looks like a baseball cap with about 7 inches of material draping down the sides and back) also is good. These are often sold in sports and outdoor clothing and supply stores.

A baseball cap or visor provides only limited protection but is better than nothing.

4. Wear Sunglasses

Sunglasses can help protect your eyes from sun damage.

The ideal sunglasses don't have to be expensive, but they should block 99 to 100 percent of UVA and UVB radiation. Check the label to see that they do. If there's no label, don't buy the glasses. And, don't go by how dark the glasses are because UV protection comes from an invisible chemical applied to the lenses, not from the color or darkness of the lenses.

Large-framed wraparound sunglasses are best because they can protect your eyes from all angles.

Children should wear sunglasses, too, starting as young as one, advises Gerhard Cibis, a pediatric ophthalmologist in Kansas City, Missouri. They need smaller versions of real, protective adult sunglasses—not toy sunglasses. Kids' sunglasses are available at many optical stores, Cibis says.

Ideally, says the American Academy of Ophthalmology, all types of eyewear, including prescription glasses, contact lenses, and intraocular lens implants used in cataract surgery, should absorb the entire UV spectrum.

You may want to put sunscreen on the eyelids and around the eyes, too, even if you're wearing sunglasses. According to Cibis, sunglasses prevent UV rays from getting into the eyes; they won't help protect the skin around them.

5. Cover Up

Wear lightweight, loose-fitting, long-sleeved shirts, pants, or long skirts as much as possible when in the sun. Most materials and colors absorb or reflect UV rays. Tightly weaved cloth is best.

> ♣ **It's A Fact!!**
>
> You can get a nasty sunburn even on a cloudy day. Clouds block only 20 percent of UV radiation.

Avoid wearing wet clothes, such as a wet T-shirt, because when clothes get wet, the sun's rays can more easily pass through. If you see light through a fabric, UV rays can get through, too.

FDA's policy is that so-called "sun-protective" clothing will be regulated by the agency only if the clothing's label makes a medical claim, such as that it prevents skin cancer.

6. Avoid Artificial Tanning

Many people believe that the UV rays of tanning beds are harmless because sunlamps in tanning beds emit primarily UVA and little, if any, UVB, the rays once thought to be the most hazardous. However, UVA can cause serious skin damage, too. According to some scientists, UVA may be linked to the most serious form of skin cancer, melanoma. A 1996 unpublished risk analysis by FDA scientists Sharon Miller, Scott Hamilton, and Howard Cyr, Ph.D., concluded that people who use sunlamps about 100 times a year may be increasing their exposure to "melanoma-inducing" radiation by up to 24 times compared with the amount they would receive from the sun. This would depend on the type of sunlamp used and whether sunscreen is used regularly. The authors note that home users are a major concern because they may use their sunlamps as often as every day. But, Miller said, "This analysis was based on data from a nonmammalian animal model and the assumption that cumulative UV exposure—not just exposure that resulted in sunburns—contributes to the development of melanoma. The dose-response behavior of melanoma is not well understood, so our results must be regarded with caution."

Because of sunlamps' dangers, health experts advise people to avoid them for tanning.

Sunlamps remain on the market because, according to George Jan, Ph.D., a physicist in FDA's Center for Devices and Radiological Health, they represent an alternative to the sun, and unlike the sun, can be regulated to promote greater safety.

Under FDA regulations, sunlamp products must:

- Have a timer to limit the amount of exposure a person can receive in one session

- Have a label with recommended exposure position or distance from the sunlamp to reduce the risk of overexposure, even when the timer is set at its maximum limit

- Limit the amount of short-wave UV radiation emitted from the product
- Come with UV-blocking goggles, which the user should always wear
- Carry a prominent warning about the dangers of overexposure, especially to those who are sensitive to UV radiation
- Provide information on proper use

Several products that claim to give a tan without UV radiation carry safety risks, too. These include so-called "tanning pills" containing carotenoid color additives derived from substances similar to beta-carotene, which gives carrots their orange color. The additives are distributed throughout the body, especially in skin, making it orange. Although FDA has approved some of these additives for coloring food, it has not approved them for use in tanning agents. And, at the high levels that are consumed in tanning pills, they may be harmful. According to John Bailey, Ph.D., acting director of FDA's Office of Cosmetics and Colors, the main ingredient in tanning pills, canthaxanthin, can deposit in the eyes as crystals, which may cause injury and impaired vision. There also has been one reported case of a woman who died from aplastic anemia that her doctor attributed to her use of tanning pills.

Tanning accelerators, such as those formulated with the amino acid tyrosine or tyrosine derivatives, are ineffective and also may be dangerous. Marketers promote these products as substances that stimulate the body's own tanning process, although the evidence suggests they don't work, Bailey says. FDA considers them unapproved new drugs that have not been proved safe and effective.

Two other tanning products, bronzers and extenders, are considered cosmetics for external use. Bronzers, made from color additives approved by FDA for cosmetic use, stain the skin when applied and can be washed off with soap and water. Extenders, when applied to the skin, interact with protein on the surface of the skin to produce color. The color tends to wear off after a few days. The only color additive approved for extenders is dihydroxyacetone.

Although they give skin a golden color, these products do not offer sunscreen protection. Also, the chemicals in bronzers may react differently on various areas of your body, producing a tan of many shades.

7. Check Skin Regularly

You can improve your chances of finding precancerous skin conditions, such as actinic keratosis—a dry, scaly, reddish, and slightly raised lesion—and skin cancer by performing simple skin self-exams regularly. The earlier you identify signs and see a doctor, the greater the chances for successful treatment.

The best time to do skin exams is after a shower or bath. Get used to your birthmarks, moles, and blemishes so that you know what they usually look like and then can easily identify any changes they undergo. Signs to look for are changes in size, texture, shape, and color of blemishes or a sore that does not heal.

If you find any changes, see your doctor. Also, during regular checkups, ask your doctor to check your skin.

The more of these practices you can incorporate into your life, the greater your chances of reducing the damage sun can cause. And by teaching these same practices to your children, you can help them get off to a lifetime of safer sun practices.

Who's Most At Risk?

Take extra care to protect babies and children from the sun. Studies show that one or more severe, blistering sunburns as a child or teenager could increase the risk for melanoma, an often fatal form of skin cancer.

You need to be especially careful to play it safe in the sun if you:

- Have fair skin; blond, red, or light brown hair; and blue, green, or gray eyes
- Have freckles and burn before tanning
- Spend a lot of time outdoors
- Were previously treated for skin cancer
- Have a family history of skin cancer, especially melanoma
- Work indoors all week and then try to catch up on your tan on weekends

Seven Steps To Safer Sunning

- Live or vacation at high altitudes (ultraviolet radiation from the sun increases 4 to 5 percent for every 1,000 feet above sea level)
- Live or vacation close to the equator
- Have certain diseases, such as lupus erythematosus
- Take certain medicines, including:
  - ◊ Acne medicines
  - ◊ Antibiotics, such as tetracyclines
  - ◊ Antihistamines
  - ◊ Oral contraceptives containing estrogen
  - ◊ Nonsteroidal anti-inflammatory drugs, such as naproxen sodium
  - ◊ Phenothiazines (major tranquilizers and anti-nausea drugs)
  - ◊ Sulfa drugs
  - ◊ Tricyclic antidepressants
  - ◊ Thiazide diuretics
  - ◊ Sulfonylureas, such as oral anti-diabetics

Ask your doctor about the risk of any medicines you may be taking that could be harmful to you when you are in the sun.

—by Paula Kurtzweil

☞ Remember!!

The seven steps to safer sunning are:

1. Avoid the sun.
2. Use sunscreen.
3. Wear a hat.
4. Wear sunglasses.
5. Cover up.
6. Avoid artificial tanning.
7. Check skin regularly.

Chapter 29

Sunscreens And Sun Safety

You would think that all the questions about sunscreens have been answered by now. You slather it on before you go to the beach. It keeps you from being fried to a crisp. And, if you use enough, it helps prevent your skin from taking on that wrinkled, leathery look of photoaged skin. Best of all, it protects you from the harmful ultraviolet rays that cause skin cancer.

If that's your perception, you're mostly right, but that view is not complete. While all the basic information remains true—sunscreens do protect skin from sunburn—a scientific debate simmers about the importance of lower-energy ultraviolet light to skin damage and whether current sunscreens provide adequate protection.

Sunburns And Suntans

Sunburn, which is caused by a type of ultraviolet (UV) light known as UVB, has served as a surrogate for more serious skin disorders, such as melanoma and basal and squamous cell carcinoma, three forms of skin cancer. Basically, the thinking was if you prevent sunburn, you'd prevent skin cancer.

> About This Chapter: Main text adapted from "Trying to Look SUNsational? Complexity Persists in Using SUNSCREENS," *FDA Consumer Magazine*, July–August 2000, available at http://www.fda.gov/fdac/features/2000/400_sun.html. Additional material from "Sunscreens, Tanning Products, and Sun Safety," Office of Cosmetics and Colors Fact Sheet, Center for Food Safety and Applied Nutrition, U. S. Food and Drug Administration; available at http://vm.cfsan.fda.gov/~dms/cos-220.html, June 27, 2000.

In recent years, however, scientists have come to appreciate that a different form of ultraviolet light, called UVA, may be just as, or even more, important in causing some skin disorders. Although experts still believe that UVB is responsible for much of the skin damage caused by sunlight—especially sunburn—UVA may be an important factor in other types of sun damage, including photoaging and the development of skin cancers. Most sunscreens do a good job blocking UVB, but fewer filter out most of the UVA.

"Both laboratory and epidemiological studies indicate that sunscreens may not block the initiation or promotion of melanoma formation," says Ronald D. Ley, Ph.D., at the University of New Mexico School of Medicine's Steve Schiff Center for Skin Cancer in Albuquerque, New Mexico. Studies using a fish model of melanoma induction "suggest that the action spectrum [the defined wavelength of ultraviolet light that damages skin] for erythema induction is different than the action spectrum for the induction of melanoma." Erythema means red skin; that is, sunburn.

"There are a lot of data on both sides of the question about the tanning link to melanoma," says John Lipnicki of the U.S. Food and Drug Administration (FDA)'s Center for Drug Evaluation and Research (CDER).

Risks And Reality

The death rate from melanoma in the United States has been going up about 4 percent a year since 1973, according to the Centers for Disease Control and Prevention in Atlanta. Although melanoma represents only about 47,000 of the nearly 1.8 million cases of skin cancer diagnosed each year, according to the American Cancer Society, it will cause 79 percent of skin cancer deaths. While cancer treatments continue to improve, melanoma recovery rates remain disappointing. Prevention is the better solution.

As prevention, however, sunscreens alone appear to be imperfect. In the first study to test the protective effect of sunscreens on people—not just the hairless mice or other models used in laboratory studies—researchers at the Queensland Institute for Medical Research in Brisbane, Australia, reported in September 1999 that sunscreen use reduces the risk of developing squamous cell carcinoma by 40 percent. But using sunscreen did not reduce the risk of developing melanoma or basal cell carcinoma. The Australian study followed 1,383 adults for five years.

The U.S. Food and Drug Administration (FDA) believes that sunscreens are an important part of a person's total sun protection strategy, but sunscreen use alone will not prevent all of the possible harmful effects due to sun exposure, according to agency statements. Borrowing the "Slip, Slop, Slap" slogan from an Australian skin cancer prevention campaign, the American Cancer Society recommends that anyone out in the sun slip on a shirt, slop on sunscreen, and slap on a hat.

The education campaign's benefits in Australia have been promising, says Robin Marks, M.B., of the University of Melbourne. "Suntans are out of fashion, especially deep tans. We can measure sunburn rates, and they have gone down." Most importantly, the epidemiological studies show the rates of skin cancer, including melanoma, are going down in the younger groups, says Marks, but not in the older groups whose skin already has been damaged by prior exposure to the sun.

UVA Versus UVB

The complexities of light quickly overwhelm freshmen physics students, but some basic principles can be readily understood. In one model of how light works, the electromagnetic radiation can be thought of as a series of waves, like ocean waves at the beach, steadily marching toward shore. At the beach, the wind makes the waves by transferring kinetic or mechanical energy into the water. The harder the wind blows, the more energy in the water and the higher and closer together the ocean waves. On a calm summer day, widely spaced waves lap mildly against the shore. During a hurricane, the wave action intensifies, pounding the sand with closely packed wave after wave of crashing white foam strong enough to wipe away the beach.

The electromagnetic energy in sunlight works much the same way: The higher the energy of the light, the closer together its waves. Some types of light have waves that are far apart—like ocean waves on a calm day. Other types of light have waves that are packed closely together, like ocean waves on a windy day.

This difference in closeness of a light's waves, its wavelength, gives different parts of the electromagnetic spectrum its characteristics, such as the colors of visible light and the destructive capabilities of x-rays and ultraviolet light.

Physicists classify ultraviolet light into three types, by its wavelengths: UVA, UVB, and UVC. The dimensions of their wavelengths are roughly 400 to 320 nanometers (nm) for UVA, 320 to 290 nm for UVB, and 290 to 200 nm for UVC. Although it may seem backwards, the shorter the wavelength and the lower the number, the greater the energy level of the light and the more damage it can do. For example, direct exposure to UVC for a length of time would destroy the skin. Fortunately, UVC is completely absorbed by gases in the atmosphere before it reaches the ground.

The longer wavelengths of UVB and UVA, however, pass right through the atmosphere, even on a cloudy day. That's why you can still get sunburned on a cloudy or hazy day. The

♣ It's A Fact!!
Teens And Sunscreen

Although industry studies show that consumer use of sunscreen products continues to improve—up 13 percent in 1999—the American Academy of Dermatology (AAD) says that consumers still do not apply the correct amounts of sunscreen to achieve the full benefit.

A study sponsored by Seventeen Magazine, Beiersdorf Inc.'s Nivea brand, and the AAD found an increase in the use of sunscreen by teens, but also found problems: Eighty-eight percent of teens spend a significant amount of time in the sun, but only 72 percent say they use sunscreen at least some of the time. Only about 40 percent of the teens say they use sunscreen often or all of the time. Young women use sunscreen more than young men (46.2 percent compared to 30.5 percent), and the reasons given for not using it include the belief that they never burn (30 percent), inconvenience (17 percent), and the desire for a dark tan (6 percent).

The difficulty, of course, is that teenagers won't see the effects of sun damage until they reach their forties and fifties or later. By then, however, the damage already is done.

Sunscreens And Sun Safety

molecules in sunscreens absorb most UVB and prevent it from reaching the skin, just as the molecules of the atmosphere absorb UVC and prevent it from reaching the ground.

UVA, however, is another story.

According to a 1998 review article, most sunscreens do not protect the skin from the longer UVA wavelengths. And that may be critical to the creation of skin cancer. Approximately 65 percent of melanomas and 90 percent of basal and squamous cell skin cancers are attributed to UV exposure.

The precise wavelengths of ultraviolet that contribute to the formation of skin cancer still need to be sorted out. And scientists must still figure out how best to formulate sunscreens to provide effective protection against these wavelengths.

Scientists use a number of techniques to measure the UV-blocking ability of a sunscreen. Some rely on electronic laboratory equipment, some on living tissue or live animals. Some testing procedures even use human volunteers.

"We have a good way of measuring UVB protection with a sunburn or erythema test in humans," says Sharon Miller, an optical engineer in FDA's Center for Devices and Radiological Health. But scientists lack a simple measure of UVA's impact on the skin, she says. That makes it difficult to determine how much UVA protection a sunscreen provides.

That leaves FDA with an unresolved technical dilemma that it is trying to resolve through additional research. "We are trying to determine a testing method that will demonstrate that a sunscreen is providing UVA protection," Lipnicki says. A claim such as "broad spectrum" on a sunscreen label needs to be supported by evidence that the product provides significant and meaningful protection across the entire UVB/UVA spectrum.

To Australia's Robin Marks, however, the issue is not UVA versus UVB or even UVA combined with UVB. "The most common skin cancers seen in humans are related to sunlight, not to a limited band of the solar spectrum," Marks says. "It is the whole of all light coming from the sun. Don't concentrate on one band, but the entire spectrum. Keep it off the skin."

☞ Remember!!

Different Sun Products, And What They Do

Sunscreens

Sunscreens play an important role in a total program to reduce the harmful effects of the sun, along with limiting sun exposure and wearing protective clothing. FDA regulates sunscreens as over-the-counter (OTC) drugs. Cosmetic products that are marketed with sun-protection claims are regulated as both drugs and cosmetics.

To help consumers select products that best suit their needs, sunscreens are labeled with SPF numbers. SPF stands for "sun protection factor." The higher the SPF number, the more sunburn protection the product provides. Remember, sunscreen use alone will not prevent all of the possible harmful effects of the sun.

The effectiveness of a sunscreen is reduced if it is not applied in adequate amounts or it is washed off, rubbed off, sweated off, or otherwise removed. For maximum effectiveness, apply a sunscreen liberally and reapply it frequently.

Tanning Accelerators

Lotions and pills marketed as "tanning accelerators" generally contain tyrosine (an amino acid), often in combination with other substances. Tanning accelerators are marketed with the claim that they enhance tanning by stimulating and increasing melanin formation. FDA has concluded that these "tanning accelerators" are actually unapproved drugs, and the agency has issued warning letters to several manufacturers of these products. There are no scientific data showing that they work; in fact, at least one study has found them ineffective.

Tanning Pills

Pills that contain large doses of canthaxanthin are sometimes marketed as "tanning pills." Although FDA has approved canthaxanthin for use as a color additive in foods, where it is used in small amounts, its use as a tanning agent is not approved. Imported tanning pills containing canthaxanthin are subject to import detention as products containing nonpermitted color additives.

When a person ingests canthaxanthin in large quantities, the substance is deposited in various parts of the body, including the skin, where it imparts a color ranging from orange to brownish. Tanning pills have been associated with side effects, particularly a condition called canthaxanthin retinopathy, the formation of yellow deposits in the retina of the eye.

Sunless Tanners And Bronzers

Sunless tanners, sometimes referred to as self-tanners or tanning extenders, are promoted as a way to get tan without the sun. They produce a tanned appearance by interacting with amino acids on the skin's surface. The only color additive currently approved by FDA for this purpose is dihydroxyacetone (DHA). These products can be difficult to apply, and the chemicals may react differently on various areas of your body, resulting in uneven coloring.

The term "bronzer" refers to a variety of products used to achieve a temporary tanned appearance. Some are applied topically to stain the skin temporarily. Usually, soap and water will remove them. They may streak after application and, when wet, some may stain clothing.

Among other products marketed as bronzers are tinted moisturizers and brush-on powders. These also produce a temporary effect, similar to other types of makeup. Still others are combination products that also contain DHA.

Sunless tanners and bronzers may or may not contain sunscreen ingredients or be labeled with SPF numbers. Consumers are advised to read the labeling carefully to determine whether or not these products provide protection from the sun.

The SPF Debate

To figure out how much protection a sunscreen provides, most consumers turn to a simple number: the SPF, or sun protection factor, listed on the label. Studies show that most consumers understand that the higher the number, the more the product protects the skin.

Unfortunately, studies also show that people often have the mistaken notion that the higher the SPF number of the sunscreen they use, the longer they can stay—and will stay—in the sun. In August 1999, the *Journal of the National Cancer Institute* published a study showing that use of higher-SPF sunscreens led to increased sun exposure. Two groups of French and Swiss volunteers used unlabeled sunscreen during their vacations. One group used SPF 10 and the other group used SPF 30. The group using the higher-SPF sunscreen spent 20 percent more time in the sun (72.6 hours versus 58.2 hours) than the group using the lower-SPF sunscreen.

"Because of variations between individuals, products, exposures, and conditions of use, there is no really easy way to explain SPF in a few words," says FDA's Lipnicki. "In the past, it was explained in terms of the amount of time you could stay in the sun longer with sunscreen than without it before getting 'burned.' We have gotten away from that. Sunscreen should not be used to prolong time spent in the sun. Even with a sunscreen, you are not going to prevent all the possible damage from the sun. Some of the newer research in the last several years shows that the suberythemal doses [exposure to the sun that does not cause reddening of the skin], as little as one-tenth the energy needed to get a sunburn, start the process of skin damage of one sort or another."

In the final monograph completed last year, FDA proposed limiting SPF values on a sunscreen label to 30. Products with higher SPFs would be labeled "30+" (or "30 plus"). The agency took this action for two reasons: inadequacies in the testing methodologies for higher-level SPF formulations, and concern that the high SPF labeling may lead consumers to spend more time in the sun than they should.

The SPF portion of FDA's monograph immediately produced opposition from both industry groups and consumer organizations. The National

Coalition for Sun Safety, an organization supported by the American Academy of Dermatology, advocated "a floor rather than a cap on SPF," wrote coalition co-chairmen Rex Arnonette, M.D., and Roger Ceilley, M.D. The organization wants a minimum level of SPF to ensure that all products provide some protection.

Industry, primarily represented by the Cosmetic, Toiletry, and Fragrance Association (CTFA), opposed the 30-plus cap for several reasons, including consumer confusion, fear that manufacturers would remove effective sunscreen protection in their products to avoid misbranding, and unresolved scientific issues about UVA. With the deferral of the monograph's implementation, the industry, along with the agency, will have additional time to resolve the issues.

The Labeling Controversy

The questions surrounding labeling, which may have less to do with science and more to do with motivating human behavior, may prove to be the thorniest of all. Everyone agrees on the goal: Create a simple label that consumers can easily understand.

In addition to recommending the SPF limit on labels, FDA has proposed further label changes to help clarify the risks and benefits of sunscreen use and how to use the products properly. For example, FDA wants the label to avoid unsupported, misleading or, confusing terms such as "sunblock," "waterproof," "all-day protection," and "visible and/or infrared light protection." And when the label says the product is "water resistant," or "very water resistant," it must mean that the product provides the stated SPF level after water resistance testing for a specified length of time. FDA and the industry also are wrestling with what it means to claim that a sunscreen is "broad-spectrum"; that is, protective against both UVA and UVB.

Complexity is the problem because consumers want simplicity. Industry already has conducted studies that test the effectiveness of different ways to present information on the label. For example, Schering-Plough Health Care Products of Berkeley Heights, New Jersey, tested a label that contained another number in addition to the SPF to indicate the degree to which the product protected against UVA. "The second protection number created unnecessary complications and confusion for the consumer," says Patricia Agin, Ph.D., Schering-Plough's photobiology research director. "UVA should complement and not distract from SPF on the label. A descriptive approach better conveyed to consumers the added benefit of UVA protection and did not distract from the SPF number."

"SPF should remain the primary index of efficacy," agrees Jay Nash, Ph.D., of Proctor & Gamble Pharmaceuticals, Inc., of Mason, Ohio, "and any additional descriptor should be independent and commensurate with this information. Simplicity is the key to public policy."

Simple or not, the labeling issue is not trivial because studies already show that consumers may not use sunscreens correctly. The public under-applies sunscreens by as much as half of the recommended amount, concluded a study published in the *Archives of Dermatology*. Consequently, the study argued, consumers are receiving only half of the SPF protection they believe the product provides.

Couple that with prolonged periods of baking in the sun and you have a recipe for future disease.

✔ **Quick Tip**

A Label Caution

One new requirement for over-the-counter sunscreen products went into effect on May 22, 2000. The new regulation requires all tanning products that do not contain sunscreen to bear the following warning statement on the label:

"Warning—This product does not contain a sunscreen and does not protect against sunburn. Repeated exposure of unprotected skin while tanning may increase the risk of skin aging, skin cancer, and other harmful effects to the skin even if you do not burn."

Tanning products that do not contain sunscreens and do not protect against the harmful effects of UV light are regulated as cosmetics. FDA requires this warning statement so that consumers are fully informed that such products do not provide protection from the sun.

How Sunlight Ages Skin

Take a look at a long-haul trucker sometime, a guy who's been driving for decades. Look closely at his face. One side will have more wrinkles than the other. Guess which one? The left side, the side of his face most exposed to the open window. Do you know why it has more wrinkles? Because it absorbs more direct sunlight than the right side of his face that's shaded inside the truck cab.

Look at the face of a long-haul trucker from a country like Great Britain, where people drive on the left side of the road. The right side of his face has more wrinkles because that's the side that faces the open window.

We're not talking lying in the sun here. We're not talking sunburn. We're talking chronic, long-term exposure to microdoses of ultraviolet light that never overtly damages the skin, but over the years causes a collection of microscars that leaves a telling impression: wrinkles.

The epidermis, the outer layer of skin, "is as thin as a sheet of paper," says John J. Voorhees, M.D., chairman of dermatology at the University of Michigan Medical School. "Ninety percent of the mass of the skin is collagen," a large protein composed of three intertwined chains of amino acids that contributes to the form, function, and strength of the skin. That also makes collagen the principal recipient of ultraviolet light damage.

But the pathway to aged skin is not straightforward. Sunlight itself does little direct damage to the collagen protein. A growing body of research shows, instead, that ultraviolet light turns genes "on" and "off"—and which genes get turned on can make all the difference.

Normal skin maintains a dynamic collagen exchange. A common type of skin cell called a fibroblast exudes new layers of collagen when collagen genes are turned on. When collagen is damaged, skin cells produce enzymes that digest and liquefy the large collagen proteins into gelatin for disposal.

Voorhees's group discovered a complex genetic pathway through which sunlight can suppress collagen production by turning off the collagen-producing genes. At the same time sunlight activates collagen digestion by stimulating production of the destructive enzymes.

Damaged skin results. The skin now carries a wound, and it needs to heal. "Anytime you cut yourself more than superficially, there is always a little bit of a scar," Voorhees says. "Our claim is that wound healing is never perfect. It could be 99.9 percent perfect, but never perfect. And that 99.9 percent [healing after sun damage] is going to lead to the slightest imperfection that is not visible to the human eye, but after thousands of these over a lifetime, the microscars become macroscars. This is the UV-induced aging we call photoaging, and it is piled on top of natural aging that has nothing to do with the sun."

Prematurely wrinkled skin results. Although FDA has approved retinoic acid to treat chronic photoaging, prevention remains the more effective approach.

Here's the really tricky part: Most of the genetic changes and resulting photoaging appear to come from so-called UVA, the wavelengths of ultraviolet light in the A band of the spectrum. Most sunscreens currently on the market provide excellent protection against UVB, but not all provide equally good protection against UVA. "If you put on gobs of sunscreen, it blocks" the damage, Voorhees says. "But if you don't use much, it does not block [the damage] at all."

Moreover, sunlight turns on the genetic destruction quickly, but it also stops quickly when you get out of the sun. The level of collagen production is completely back to normal in two days.

"The average person thinks, 'I didn't get pink so I have no photoaging,'" Voorhees says. "Our data suggest that is not true. You are going to be getting the photoaged [signals that turn genes on and off] and develop the microscars without getting any pinkness at all. You can get photoaged damage long before you get pink or sunburned."

—by Larry Thompson

Chapter 30

Indoor Tanning Increases The Risk Of Skin Cancer

"Tan indoors with absolutely no harmful side effects."

"No burning, no drying, and no sun damage."

"Unlike the sun, indoor tanning will not cause skin cancer or skin aging."

Beware of claims like these. Ads that claim indoor tanning devices are a safe alternative to outdoor tanning may be false.

Tanning indoors damages your skin. That's because indoor tanning devices emit ultraviolet rays. Tanning occurs when the skin produces additional pigment (coloring) to protect itself against burn from ultraviolet rays. Overexposure to these rays can cause eye injury, premature wrinkling of the skin, and light-induced skin rashes, and it can increase your chances of developing skin cancer.

The most popular device used in tanning salons is a clamshell-like tanning bed. The customer lies down on a Plexiglas® surface as lights from above and below reach the body.

About This Chapter: Text compiled from the fact sheet "Indoor Tanning," Federal Trade Commission, http://www.ftc.gov/bcp/conline/pubs/health/indootan.htm, 1997; and from information provided by The Skin Cancer Foundation, New York, New York, www.skincancer.org © 2000; reprinted with permission. Reviewed by David A. Cooke, M.D., December 13, 2002.

Many older tanning devices used light sources that emitted shortwave ultraviolet rays (UVB) that actually caused burning. Aware of the harmful effects of UVB radiation, salon owners began using tanning beds that emit mostly longwave (UVA) light sources. Some salons claim this is safe. While UVA rays are less likely to cause burning than UVB rays, they are suspected to have links to malignant melanoma and immune system damage.

Advertising Claims

Here are some claims commonly made about indoor tanning—and the facts.

"You can achieve a deep year-round tan with gentle, comfortable, and safe UVA light."

Ultraviolet light is divided into two wavelength bands. Shortwave ultraviolet rays called UVB can burn the outer layer of skin. Longwave ultraviolet rays called UVA penetrate more deeply and can weaken the skin's inner connective tissue.

Long-term exposure to the sun and to artificial sources of ultraviolet light contributes to the risk of developing skin cancer. Two types of skin cancer, basal cell and squamous cell, are treatable if detected early. Melanoma, another type of skin cancer, can be fatal.

> ♣ **It's A Fact!!**
> Despite claims to the contrary, the bulbs used in cosmetic tanning devices typically emit 5 percent UVB. Some go as high as 10 percent. UVB is the portion of the light spectrum that causes sunburn and increases the chance of contracting skin cancer, including the fatal form known as melanoma.

"No harsh glare, so no goggles or eye shades are necessary."

Studies show that too much exposure to ultraviolet rays, including UVA rays, can damage the retina. Overexposure can burn the cornea, and repeated exposure over many years can change the structure of the lens so that it begins to cloud, forming a cataract. Left untreated, cataracts can cause blindness.

The United States Food and Drug Administration (FDA) requires tanning salons to direct all customers to wear protective eye goggles. Closing

Indoor Tanning Increases The Risk Of Skin Cancer

your eyes, wearing ordinary sunglasses, and using cotton wads do not protect the cornea from the intensity of UV radiation in tanning devices.

Long-term exposure to natural sunlight also can result in eye damage, but in the sun, people generally are more aware that their eyelids are burning. Under indoor UV lights, exposed skin remains cool to the touch. In addition, the intensity of lights used in tanning devices is much greater—and potentially more damaging to the eyes—than the intensity of UV rays in natural sunlight.

"Tan year-round without the harmful side effects often associated with natural sunlight."

Exposure to tanning salon rays increases the damage caused by sunlight. This occurs because ultraviolet light actually thins the skin, making it less able to heal.

Unprotected exposure to ultraviolet rays also results in premature skin aging. A tan is damaged skin that is more likely to wrinkle and sag than skin that hasn't been tanned. Over time, you may notice certain undesirable changes in the way your skin looks and heals. According to some skin specialists, skin that has a dry, wrinkled, leathery appearance early in middle age is a result of UV exposure that occurred in youth.

"No danger in exposure or burning."

Whether you tan indoors or out, studies show the combination of ultraviolet rays and some medicines, birth control pills, cosmetics, and soaps may accelerate skin burns or produce painful adverse skin reactions, such as rashes. In addition, tanning devices may induce common light-sensitive skin ailments like cold sores.

Who's In Charge?

While the FDA regulates tanning machine quality and labeling, it does not have sufficient resources to oversee how the machines are used in each tanning salon around the country. In great part, it falls to individual states or municipalities to monitor salons in their own jurisdictions. However, only

27 states have passed any state legislation governing tanning parlors, and only about half a dozen have shown much commitment to enforcing either federal or state legislation. Elsewhere, the FDA's labeling and exposure standards are not being routinely followed by tanning parlors or strictly enforced. Therefore, the practices of individual tanning salons nationwide vary drastically.

The FDA has established 4 MEDs (minimal erythemal doses) as the maximum single-session exposure for a skin type II individual. This may range from 10 to 30 minutes depending upon the amount of UV emitted. In the first week of tanning, sessions are actually supposed to be limited to no more than 0.75 MEDs per exposure, with a gradual increase in exposure thereafter up to 4 MEDs. However, some salons fail to increase MEDs gradually, and some sell additional minutes of tanning beyond the 4-MED maximum. Some have even installed hotter bulbs than the systems are labeled for, making the posted maximum time limit inappropriate.

✔ **Quick Tip**

Protecting Yourself

If you do tan indoors, here's what you can do to lessen the risk of damage:

- *Limit your exposure to avoid sunburn.* If you tan with a device, ask whether the manufacturer or the salon staff recommends, exposure limits for your skin type. Set a timer on the tanning device that automatically shuts off the lights or somehow signals that you've reached your exposure time. Remember that exposure time affects burning and that your age at the time of exposure is important relative to burning. Studies suggest that children and adolescents are harmed more by equivalent amounts of UVB rays than adults. The earlier you start tanning, the earlier skin injury may occur.

Indoor Tanning Increases The Risk Of Skin Cancer

Making matters worse, many salons sell unlimited tanning, meaning that they will allow someone to tan once a day. This defies the FDA's exposure schedule (meant to be posted clearly on the machines' labels), which indicates that individuals should tan no more than three times a week, with at least a 48-hour rest period between exposures, for a total of no more than 12 MEDs of UV a week. With daily tanning, users may accumulate 28 MEDs of exposure weekly—more than twice as much as legally allowed.

Staggering Numbers

There are more than 18,000 tanning salons, with more than one million people using them each day. The majority of these people consider themselves "serious" tanners who have been tanning more than three times a week for longer than four years. Considering that most cosmetic tanners are young, and that UV exposure in youth is believed to play a major role in the etiology of most melanomas, such an exposure regimen could have an immense

---

- *Use goggles to protect your eyes.* Ask whether safety goggles are provided and if their use is mandatory. Make sure the goggles fit snugly. Check to see that the salon sterilizes the goggles after each use to prevent the spread of eye infections.

- *Consider your medical history.* If you are undergoing treatment for lupus or diabetes or are susceptible to cold sores, be aware that these conditions can be aggravated through exposure to ultraviolet radiation from tanning devices, sunlamps, or natural sunlight. In addition, your skin may be more sensitive to artificial light or sunlight if you use certain medications—for example, antihistamines, tranquilizers, or birth control pills. Your tanning salon may keep a file with information on your medical history, medications, and treatments. Make sure you update it as necessary.

impact. By the turn of the century—15 years after tanning machines were first approved for marketing by the FDA—the effect on the melanoma rate could be substantial.

Conclusions

In our opinion, the massive, inadequately controlled experiment being conducted each day on millions of Americans in tanning salons represents a great danger to public health. Those who voluntarily seek an indoor tan do so for cosmetic reasons only. In their case, can the heightened risk of melanoma ever be justified?

Health professionals should steer patients—especially young ones—away from cosmetic tanning devices and tanning salons, and should provide them with educational materials about their dangers. They should also lobby for stronger regulatory action at all levels. Tanning units must be systematically labeled or relabeled to reflect appropriate exposure schedules based on their UV output, and warnings should be included that the machines may cause skin cancer. Unlimited tanning memberships should be outlawed, and all salon owners and operators should go through a rigorous certification program. The promotion of tanning salons should be scrupulously monitored for misleading statements. And tanning accelerators, many of which contain unapproved and untested ingredients, should be held to the same standards of safety and efficacy as other drugs.

Chapter 31

Treating Skin Cancer

Skin cancer is the uncontrollable growth of abnormal cells in a layer of the skin. It attacks one out of every seven Americans each year, making it the most prevalent form of cancer. However, the majority of all skin cancers can be cured if detected and treated in time.

Types of Skin Cancer

There are several different kinds of skin cancers, distinguished by the types of cells affected. The three most common forms of skin cancer are:

- *Basal cell carcinoma.* Basal cell carcinomas usually appear as raised, translucent lumps. This cancer develops in 300,000 to 400,000 Americans each year. Although the disease does not usually spread to other parts of the body through the bloodstream, it may cause considerable damage by direct growth and invasion.

- *Squamous cell carcinoma.* This type of skin cancer is usually distinguished by raised reddish lumps or growths. This form of cancer develops in 80,000 to 100,000 Americans per year. The disease can spread to other parts of the body. Approximately 2,000 deaths occur each year from this form of cancer.

About This Chapter: Adapted from "Skin Cancer," American Society for Dermatological Surgery (ASDS), http://www.asds-net.org/FactSheets/skin_cancer.html, 2002. Reprinted with permission.

- *Malignant melanoma.* Malignant melanoma typically first appears as a light brown to black, irregularly shaped blemish. This serious form of cancer results in death if undetected and untreated. It can spread to other parts of the body through the bloodstream and the lymph drainage system.

Skin Cancer Treatments

Your dermatologic surgeon will select the most appropriate treatment for a particular skin cancer or precancerous condition from among the following procedures and techniques:

- *Curettage.* Malignant tissue is scraped away with a sharp instrument. This method is most effective for small, superficial cancers that have not been treated previously. Curettage is often followed by destruction of the cancerous tissue with an electric needle.

- *Surgical excision.* This technique involves cutting into the skin and removing the growth. The skin is then closed with stitches.

- *Cryosurgery.* Liquid nitrogen is applied directly to the skin to freeze cancerous tissue.

- *Topical chemotherapy.* The application to the skin surface of chemicals capable of destroying precancerous growths.

- *MOHS micrographic surgery.* Excision of a tumor and its surrounding skin with the aid of a microscope. This method allows the dermatologic surgeon to trace the outline of a cancerous growth, layer by layer, with exceptional accuracy.

- *Laser surgery.* Intense waves of light are beamed at cancerous skin to cut away or vaporize the tissue.

> ♣ **It's A Fact!!**
> Melanoma is by far the most dangerous form of skin cancer. Although it is almost completely curable when discovered early, the cancer spreads if untreated and eventually results in death. Over the past 10 years, the incidence of melanoma has been increasing faster than any other type of cancer. Currently, about 51,000 cases are reported to the American Cancer Society each year.
>
> Source:
>
> Information provided by The Skin Cancer Foundation, New York, New York, © 2000; http://www.skincancer.org/melanoma/index.html; reprinted with permission.

Chapter 32

Moles And Cancer

Moles

Moles are growths on the skin. Doctors call moles nevi (one mole is a nevus). These growths occur when cells in the skin, called melanocytes, grow in a cluster with tissue surrounding them. Moles are usually pink, tan, brown, or flesh-colored. Melanocytes are also spread evenly throughout the skin and produce the pigment that gives skin its natural color. When skin is exposed to the sun, melanocytes produce more pigment, causing the skin to tan, or darken.

Moles are very common. Most people have between 10 and 40 moles. A person may develop new moles from time to time, usually until about age 40. Moles can be flat or raised. They are usually round or oval and no larger than a pencil eraser. Many moles begin as a small, flat spot and slowly become larger in diameter and raised. Over many years, they may flatten again, become flesh-colored, and go away.

Dysplastic Nevi

About one out of every ten people has at least one unusual (or atypical) mole that looks different from an ordinary mole (see Table 32.1). The medical term for these unusual moles is dysplastic nevi.

About This Chapter: Excerpted from "What You Need To Know About™ Moles and Dysplastic Nevi," NIH Publication No. 99-3133, updated January 22, 2002; available online at http://www.cancer.gov.

Doctors believe that dysplastic nevi are more likely than ordinary moles to develop into a type of skin cancer called melanoma. Because of this, moles should be checked regularly by a doctor or nurse specialist, especially if they look unusual; grow larger; or change in color, outline, or any other way.

Melanoma

Melanoma is a type of skin cancer—one of the most serious types because advanced melanomas have the ability to spread to other parts of the body. (Melanoma can also develop in the eye, called intraocular melanoma, or rarely in other parts of the body where pigment cells are found.) Melanoma begins when melanocytes (pigment cells) gradually become more abnormal and divide without control or order. These cells can invade and destroy the normal cells around them. The abnormal cells form a growth of malignant tissue (a cancerous tumor) on the surface of the skin. Melanoma can begin either in an existing mole or as a new growth on the skin. A doctor or nurse specialist can tell whether an abnormal-looking

> ### ✎ Weird Words
>
> <u>Dermatologist</u>: A doctor who specializes in the diagnosis and treatment of skin problems.
>
> <u>Dysplastic nevi</u>: Atypical moles; moles whose appearance is different from that of common moles. Dysplastic nevi are generally larger than ordinary moles and have irregular and indistinct borders. Their color frequently is not uniform and ranges from pink to dark brown; they usually are flat, but parts may be raised above the skin surface.
>
> <u>Excisional biopsy</u>: A surgical procedure in which an entire lump or suspicious area is removed for diagnosis. The tissue is then examined under a microscope.
>
> <u>Melanocytes</u>: Cells in the skin that produce and contain the pigment called melanin.
>
> <u>Melanoma</u>: A form of skin cancer that arises in melanocytes, the cells that produce pigment. Melanoma usually begins in a mole.
>
> <u>Metastasis</u>: The spread of cancer cells from their site of origin to other parts of the body.
>
> <u>Nevus</u>: Medical term for a mole; the plural of nevus is nevi.
>
> <u>Shave biopsy</u>: A procedure in which the parts of a mole that are above and just below the surface of the skin are removed with a small blade. There is no need for stitches with this procedure.

mole should be closely watched or should be removed and checked for melanoma cells. The purpose of routine skin exams is to identify and follow abnormal moles.

The removal of the entire mole or a sample of tissue for examination under a microscope is called a biopsy. If possible, it is best to remove moles by an excisional biopsy rather than a shave biopsy.

If the biopsy results in a diagnosis of melanoma, the patient and the doctor should work together to make treatment decisions. In many cases, melanoma can be cured by minimal surgery if the tumor is discovered when it is thin (before it has grown downward from the skin surface) and before the cancer cells have begun to spread to other places in the body. However, if melanoma is not found early, the cancer cells can spread through the bloodstream and lymphatic system to form tumors in other parts of the body. Melanoma is much harder to control when it has spread. The spread of cancer is called metastasis.

Doctors and scientists believe that it is possible to prevent many melanomas and to detect most others early, when the disease is more likely to be cured with minimal surgery. In the past several decades, an increasing percentage of melanomas have been diagnosed at very early stages, when they are quite thin and unlikely to have spread. Learning about prevention and early detection, while important for everyone, is especially important for people who have an increased risk for melanoma. People who are at an increased risk include those who have dysplastic nevi or a very large number of ordinary moles.

Risk Factors For Melanoma

The odds for getting melanoma are higher in people with one or more of the following characteristics:

- Family history of melanoma
- Dysplastic nevi
- History of melanoma
- Weakened immune system
- Many ordinary moles (more than 50)
- Exposure to ultraviolet (UV) radiation, particularly sunlight
- Severe, blistering sunburns
- Freckles
- Fair skin

✔ **Quick Tip**

Table 32.1 Telling Ordinary Moles And Dysplastic Nevi Apart

Characteristic	Ordinary Moles	Dysplastic Nevi
Color	Evenly tan or brown; all typical moles on one person tend to look similar.	Mixture of tan, brown, and red or pink. A person's moles often look quite different from one another.
Shape	Round or oval, with a distinct edge that separates the mole from the rest of the skin.	Have irregular, sometimes notched edges. May fade into the skin around it. The flat portion of the mole may be level with the skin.
Surface	Begin as flat, smooth spots on skin; may rise and form a smooth bump.	May have a smooth, slightly scaly, or rough, irregular, "pebbly" appearance.
Size	Usually less than 5 millimeters (about 1/4 inch) across (size of a pencil eraser).	Often larger than 5 millimeters (about 1/4 inch) across and sometimes larger than 10 millimeters (about 1/2 inch).
Number	Between 10 and 40 typical moles may be present on an adult's body.	May be present in large numbers (more than 100 on the same person). However, some people have only a few dysplastic nevi.
Location	Usually found above the waist on sun-exposed surfaces of the body. Scalp, breasts, and buttocks rarely have normal moles.	May occur anywhere on the body but most frequently on the back and areas exposed to the sun. May also appear below the waist and on the scalp, breasts, and buttocks.

It is important to remember that not everyone who has dysplastic nevi or other risk factors for melanoma gets the disease. In fact, most do not. Also, about half the people who develop melanoma do not have dysplastic nevi, and they may not have any other known risk factor for the disease. At this time, no one can explain why one person gets melanoma while another does not. Research has shown that sun exposure, especially excessive exposure that leads to bad, blistering sunburns, is an important and avoidable risk factor. Scientists are continuing their studies of risk factors for melanoma.

Prevention Of Melanoma

The number of people in the world who develop melanoma is increasing each year. In the United States, the number has more than doubled in the past 20 years. Experts believe that much of the worldwide increase in melanoma is related to an increase in the amount of time people spend in the sun.

Ultraviolet (UV) radiation from the sun and from sunlamps and tanning booths damages the skin and can lead to melanoma and other types of skin cancer. Everyone, especially those who have dysplastic nevi or other risk factors, should try to reduce the risk of developing melanoma by protecting the skin from UV radiation. The intensity of UV radiation from the sun is greatest in the summer, particularly during midday hours. A simple rule is to avoid the sun or protect your skin whenever your shadow is shorter than you are.

People who work or play in the sun should wear protective clothing, such as a hat and long sleeves. Also, lotion, cream, or gel that contains sunscreen can help protect the skin. Many doctors believe sunscreens may help prevent melanoma, especially those that reflect, absorb, and/or scatter both types of ultraviolet radiation.

Sunscreens are rated in strength according to a sun protection factor (SPF). The higher the SPF, the more sunburn protection is provided. Sunscreens with an SPF value of 2 to 11 provide minimal protection against sunburns. Sunscreens with an SPF of 12 to 29 provide moderate protection. Those with an SPF of 30 or higher provide high protection against sunburn.

Sunglasses that have UV-absorbing lenses should also be worn. The label should specify that the lenses block at least 99 percent of UVA and UVB radiation.

Early Detection Of Melanoma

Because melanoma usually begins on the surface of the skin, it often can be detected at an early stage with a total skin examination by a trained health care worker. Checking the skin regularly for any signs of the disease increases the chance of finding melanoma early. A monthly skin self-exam is very important for people who have any of the known risk factors, but doing skin self-exams routinely is a good idea for everyone.

Here is how to do a skin self-exam:

- After a bath or shower, stand in front of a full-length mirror in a well-lighted room. Use a hand-held mirror to look at hard-to-see areas.

- Begin with the face and scalp and work downward, checking the head, neck, shoulders, back, chest, and so on. Be sure to check the front, back, and sides of the arms and legs. Also, check the groin, the palms, the fingernails, the soles of the feet, the toenails, and the area between the toes.

> ♣ **It's A Fact!!**
> In the United States in just the past 20 years, melanoma has become twice as common. The reason? Most likely it's the greater amount of time we spend in the sun.

- Be sure to check the hard-to-see areas of the body, such as the scalp and neck. A friend or relative may be able to help inspect these areas. Use a comb or a blow dryer to help move hair so you can see the scalp and neck better.

- Be aware of where your moles are and how they look. By checking your skin regularly, you will become familiar with what your moles look like. Look for any signs of change, particularly a new black mole or a change in outline, shape, size, color (especially a new black area), or feel of an existing mole. Also, note any new, unusual, or "ugly-looking" moles. If your doctor has taken photos of your skin, compare these pictures with the way your skin looks on self-examination.

- Check moles carefully during times of hormone changes, such as adolescence, pregnancy, and menopause. As hormone levels change, moles may change.

It may be helpful to record the dates of your skin exams and to write notes about the way your skin looks. If you find anything unusual, see your doctor right away.

In addition to doing routine skin self-exams, people should have their skin checked regularly by a doctor or nurse specialist. A doctor can do a skin exam during visits for regular checkups. People who think they have dysplastic nevi should point them out to the doctor. It is also important to tell the doctor about any new, changing, or "ugly-looking" moles.

Sometimes it is necessary to see a specialist. A dermatologist (skin doctor) is likely to have the most training in diseases of the skin. Some plastic surgeons, general surgeons, oncologists, internists, and family doctors also have a special interest and training in moles and melanoma.

Melanoma may run in families, and members of these families are at high risk for the disease. In some of these families, certain members also have a large number (usually over 100) of dysplastic nevi. These people have an especially high risk of developing melanoma. When two or more family members develop melanoma, it is important for all of the patients' close relatives (parents, brothers, sisters, and children above the age of 10) to see a doctor and be examined carefully for dysplastic nevi or any signs of melanoma. The doctor can then decide how often each person needs to be seen. (Doctors may recommend that these family members have checkups every six months.) Anyone who has a large number of dysplastic nevi also should be examined regularly.

A doctor may want to watch a slightly abnormal mole closely to see whether it changes over time. Pictures taken at one visit may be compared with the appearance of the mole at the next visit. Sometimes a doctor decides that a mole should be removed so that the tissue can be examined under a microscope. The removal of a mole, called a biopsy, is usually done in the doctor's office with a local anesthetic. It generally takes only a few minutes. The patient may require stitches, and a small scar will remain after healing. A pathologist examines the tissue under a microscope to see whether the melanocytes are normal, dysplastic, or cancerous.

Because most moles, including most dysplastic nevi, do not develop into melanoma, removing all of them is not necessary. A doctor can recommend when and when not to remove moles. Usually, only moles that look like melanoma, those that change, or those that are both new and look abnormal need to be removed.

Distinguishing Characteristics Of Melanoma

- *Large size.* Most melanomas are at least 5 millimeters (about 1/4 inch) across when they are found; many are much larger. An unusually large mole may be melanoma.

- *Many colors.* A mixture of tan, brown, white, pink, red, gray, blue, and especially black in a mole suggests melanoma.

- *Irregular border.* If a mole has an edge that is irregular or notched, it may be melanoma.

- *Abnormal surface.* If a mole is scaly, flaky, oozing, or bleeding, has an open sore that does not heal, or has a hard lump in it, it may be melanoma.

- *Unusual sensation.* If a mole itches or is painful or tender, melanoma may be present.

- *Abnormal skin around mole.* If color from the mole spreads into the skin around it or if this skin becomes red or loses its color (becomes white or gray), melanoma may be present.

☞ **Remember!!**
The earlier a melanoma is found, the better the chance for a cure.

Chapter 33

All About Melanoma

Melanoma is the most serious form of skin cancer. Even so, if diagnosed and removed while it is still thin and limited to the outermost skin layer, it is almost 100 percent curable. Once the cancer advances and metastasizes (spreads) to other parts of the body, it is hard to treat and can be deadly. During the past 10 years, the number of cases of melanoma has increased more rapidly than that of any other cancer. Over 51,000 new cases are reported to the American Cancer Society each year, and it is probable that a great many more occur and are not reported.

What Is Melanoma?

Melanoma is a malignant tumor that originates in melanocytes, the cells which produce the pigment melanin that colors our skin, hair, and eyes and is heavily concentrated in most moles. The majority of melanomas, therefore, are black or brown. However, melanomas occasionally stop producing pigment. When that happens, the melanomas may no longer be dark, but are skin-colored, pink, red, or purple.

Some Are More Dangerous

The physician will tell you whether the melanoma is early or advanced by describing it as either *in situ* or invasive. "In situ" is Latin and means "in one

---

About This Chapter: Information provided by The Skin Cancer Foundation, New York, New York, www.skincancer.org. © 2000; reprinted with permission.

site" or "localized." Melanomas *in situ* occupy only the uppermost part of the epidermis, the top layers of the skin.

Invasive melanomas are the more serious, as they have penetrated more deeply into the skin and may have traveled from the original tumor through the body.

The Four Basic Types

Melanomas fall into four basic categories. Three of them begin *in situ* and sometimes become invasive; the fourth is invasive from the start. It is helpful to recognize the names and be able to define the characteristics of each type.

Superficial Spreading Melanoma

Superficial spreading melanoma is by far the most common type, accounting for about 70 percent of all cases. As you might expect, this melanoma travels along the top layer of the skin for a fairly long time before penetrating more deeply.

The first sign is the appearance of a flat or slightly raised discolored patch that has irregular borders and is somewhat geometrical in form. The color varies, and you may see areas of tan, brown, black, red, blue, or white. Sometimes an older mole will change in these ways, or a new one will arise. The melanoma can be seen almost anywhere on the body, but is most likely to occur on the trunk in men, the legs in women, and the upper back in both. Most melanomas found in the young are of the superficial spreading type.

Lentigo Maligna

Lentigo maligna is similar to the superficial spreading type, as it also remains close to the skin surface for quite a while, and usually appears as a flat or mildly elevated mottled tan, brown, or dark brown discoloration.

This type of *in situ* melanoma is found most often in the elderly, arising on chronically sun-exposed, damaged skin on the face, ears, arms, and upper trunk. Lentigo maligna is the most common form of melanoma in Hawaii.

Lentigo maligna melanoma is the invasive form.

Acral Lentiginous Melanoma

The third type of melanoma, acral lentiginous melanoma, also spreads superficially before penetrating more deeply. It is quite different from the others, though, as it usually appears as a black or brown discoloration under the nails or on the soles of the feet or palms of the hands. This type of melanoma is sometimes found in dark-skinned people.

It is the most common melanoma in African Americans and Asians, and the least common among Caucasians.

Nodular Melanoma

Unlike the other three types, nodular melanoma, is usually invasive at the time it is first diagnosed. The malignancy is recognized when it becomes a bump. The color is most often black, but occasionally is blue, gray, white, brown, tan, red, or skin tone.

✔ **Quick Tip**

How To Spot Skin Cancer

Coupled with a yearly skin exam by a doctor, self-examination of your skin at least every three months is the best way to detect the early warning signs of basal cell carcinoma, squamous cell carcinoma, and malignant melanoma, the three main types of skin cancer. Look for a new growth or any skin change.

What you'll need: a bright light, a full-length mirror, a hand mirror, two chairs or stools, and a blow-dryer.

- Examine head and face, using one or both mirrors. Use blow-dryer to inspect scalp.
- Check hands, including nails. In full-length mirror, examine elbows, arms, underarms.
- Focus on neck, chest, torso. Women: Check under breasts.
- With back to the mirror, use hand mirror to inspect back of neck, shoulders, upper arms, back, buttocks, legs.
- Sitting down, check legs and feet, including soles, heels, and nails. Use hand mirror to examine genitals.

The most frequent locations are the trunk, legs, and arms, mainly of elderly people, as well as the scalp in men. This is the most aggressive of the melanomas, and is found in 10 to 15 percent of cases.

The ABCD's Of Moles And Melanoma

When a melanoma is detected at an early stage and treated, it is usually curable. Some melanomas are hidden in everyday life—by inconspicuous locations on the body, by clothing, even by hair on our heads. But many, if not most, melanomas can be spotted as soon as they arise—if you know what to look for and check for these signs. The ABCD's of melanoma are asymmetry, border irregularity, color variability, and diameter larger than a pencil eraser.

Most people have a number of brownish spots on their skin—freckles, birthmarks, moles. Almost all such spots are normal, but some may be skin cancers. Be alert to irregularities in shape, edges, color, and size.

Asymmetry

Most early melanomas are asymmetrical: a line through the middle would not create matching halves. Common moles are round and symmetrical.

Border

The borders of early melanomas are often uneven and may have scalloped or notched edges. Common moles have smoother, more even borders.

Color

Common moles usually are a single shade of brown. Varied shades of brown, tan, or black are often the first sign of melanoma. As melanomas progress, the colors red, white, and blue may appear.

Diameter

Early melanomas tend to grow larger than common moles—generally to at least the size of a pencil eraser (about 6 millimeters, or 1/4 inch, in diameter).

All About Melanoma

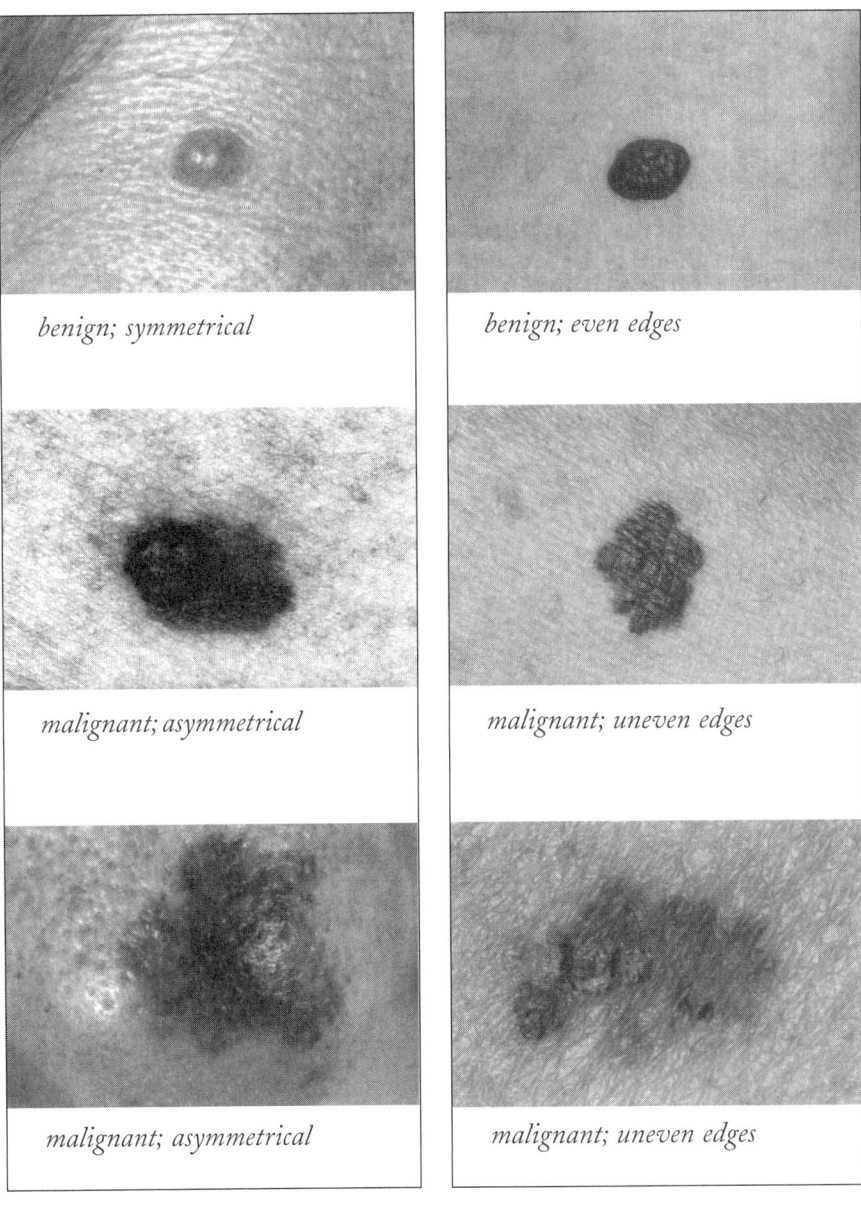

Figure 33.1. Some forms of early malignant melanoma are asymmetrical, meaning a line drawn through the middle will not create matching halves. Common moles are round and symmetrical.

Figure 33.2. The borders of early melanomas are frequently uneven, often containing scalloped or notched edges. Common moles have smooth, even borders.

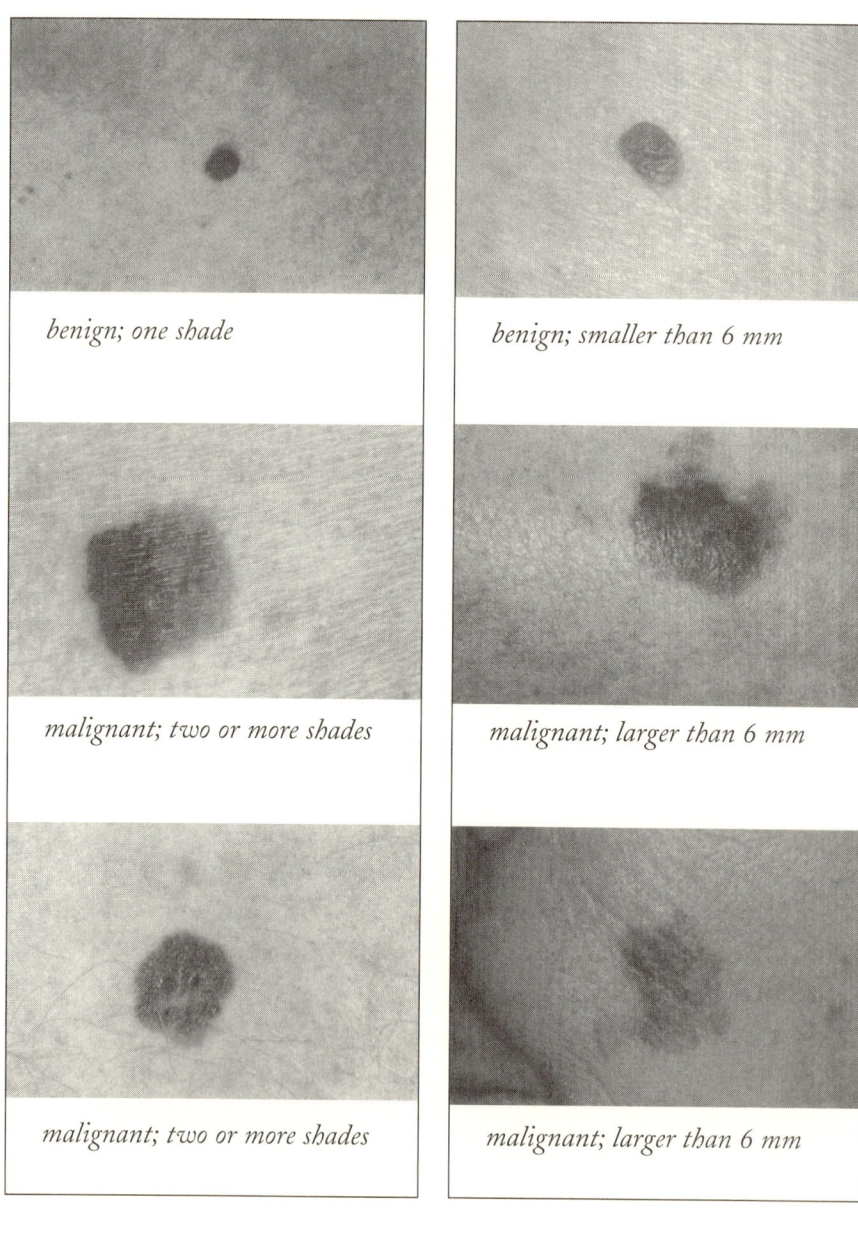

Figure 33.3. Different shades of brown or black are often the first sign of a malignant melanoma. Common moles usually have a single shade of brown.

Figure 33.4. Common moles are usually less than 6 mm in diameter (¼"), the size of a pencil eraser. Early melanomas tend to be larger than 6 mm.

☞ Remember!!

In addition to being aware of the ABCD's of melanoma, know these warning signs of change in a mole. If one of them should appear, contact your physician.

- **Size.** The mole suddenly or continuously gets larger.

- **Color.** A wide variety of colors or color combinations appear. Color might spread from the edge into the surrounding tissue.

- **Elevation.** A mole that was flat or slightly elevated increases in height rapidly.

- **Surrounding skin.** The skin around a mole becomes red or develops colored blemishes or swellings.

- **Surface.** A smooth mole develops scaliness, erosion, oozing. Crusting, ulceration, or bleeding are signs of more advanced disease.

- **Sensation.** Itching is the most common early symptom, and there may also be feelings of tenderness or pain. Nonetheless, remember that skin cancers are usually painless.

Part 5

Other Diseases and Conditions That Affect The Skin, Nails, And Scalp

Chapter 34
Eczema

Atopic dermatitis is often referred to as "eczema," which is a general term for the many types of dermatitis. Atopic dermatitis is the most common of the many types of eczema; several have very similar symptoms.

Atopic dermatitis is a chronic (long-lasting) disease that affects the skin. The word "dermatitis" means inflammation of the skin. "Atopic" refers to a group of diseases that are hereditary (that is, run in families) and often occur together, including asthma, allergies such as hay fever, and atopic dermatitis. In atopic dermatitis, the skin becomes extremely itchy and inflamed, causing redness, swelling, cracking, weeping, crusting, and scaling. Atopic dermatitis most often affects infants and young children, but it can continue into adulthood or first show up later in life. In most cases, there are periods of time when the disease is worse, called exacerbations or flares, followed by periods when the skin improves or clears up entirely, called remissions. Many children with atopic dermatitis will experience a permanent remission of the disease when they get older, although their skin often remains dry and easily irritated. Environmental factors can bring on symptoms of atopic dermatitis at any time in the lives of individuals who have inherited the atopic disease trait.

About This Chapter: Taken from "Handout on Health: Atopic Dermatitis," January 1999; available electronically at http://www.niams.nih.gov/hi/topics/dermatitis/index.html and in printed form from National Arthritis and Musculoskeletal and Skin Diseases Information Clearinghouse, NIAMS, National Institutes of Health, 1 AMS Circle, Bethesda, Maryland 20892-3675.

Atopic dermatitis is very common. It affects males and females equally and accounts for 10 to 20 percent of all referrals to dermatologists (doctors who specialize in the care and treatment of skin diseases). Atopic dermatitis occurs most often in infants and children, and its onset decreases substantially with age. Scientists estimate that 65 percent of patients develop symptoms in the first year of life, and 90 percent develop symptoms before the age of five. Onset after age 30 is less common and often occurs after exposure of skin to harsh conditions. People who live in urban areas and in climates with low humidity seem to be at an increased risk for developing atopic dermatitis.

Although it is difficult to identify exactly how many people are affected by atopic dermatitis, an estimated 10 percent of infants and young children experience symptoms of the disease. Roughly 60 percent of these infants continue to have one or more symptoms of atopic dermatitis into adulthood. This means that more than 15 million people in the United States have symptoms of the disease.

✎ Weird Words

<u>Dermatitis</u>: Inflammation of the skin from any cause.

<u>Atopic</u>: Pertaining to an inherited state of extreme sensitivity to allergy-causing substances.

<u>Eczema</u>: A common term for any inflammatory reaction or disease of the skin.

<u>Allergen</u>: A substance that causes an extreme, or allergic, response from the body's immune system.

<u>Phototherapy</u>: Treatment of a disease with light rays.

<u>Immunosuppressive drug</u>: A medication that inhibits or slows the body's immune response.

<u>Immunoglobulin E (IgE)</u>: A special protein produced by the body's immune system that recognizes and helps fight and destroy viruses, bacteria, and other foreign substances that invade the body.

The cause of atopic dermatitis is not known, but the disease seems to result from a combination of genetic (hereditary) and environmental factors. Evidence suggests the disease is associated with other so-called atopic disorders such as hay fever and asthma, which many people with atopic dermatitis also have. In addition, many children who outgrow the symptoms of atopic dermatitis go on to develop hay fever or asthma. Although one disorder does not cause another, they may be related, thereby giving researchers clues to understanding atopic dermatitis.

In the past, doctors thought that atopic dermatitis was caused by an emotional disorder. We now know that emotional factors, such as stress, can make the condition worse, but they do not cause the disease. Also, atopic dermatitis is not contagious; it cannot be passed from one person to another.

Symptoms Of Atopic Dermatitis

Symptoms vary from person to person. The most common symptoms are dry, itchy skin; cracks behind the ears; and rashes on the cheeks, arms, and legs. The itchy feeling is an important factor in atopic dermatitis, because scratching and rubbing in response to itching worsen the skin inflammation characteristic of this disease. People with atopic dermatitis seem to be more sensitive to itching and feel the need to scratch longer in response. They develop what is referred to as "the itch-scratch cycle": The extreme itchiness of the skin causes the person to scratch, which in turn worsens the itch, and so on. Itching is particularly a problem during sleep, when conscious control of scratching decreases and the absence of other outside stimuli makes the itchiness more noticeable.

The way the skin is affected by atopic dermatitis can be changed by patterns of scratching and resulting skin infections. Some people with the disease develop red, scaling skin where the immune system in the skin is becoming very activated. Others develop thick and leathery skin as a result of constant scratching and rubbing. This condition is called lichenification. Still others develop papules, or small raised bumps, on their skin. When the papules are scratched, they may open (excoriations) and become crusty and infected. These conditions can also be found in people without atopic dermatitis or with other types of skin disorders.

Atopic dermatitis may also affect the skin around the eyes, the eyelids, and the eyebrows and lashes. Scratching and rubbing the eye area can cause the skin to change in appearance. Some people with atopic dermatitis develop an extra fold of skin under their eyes, called an atopic pleat or Dennie-Morgan fold. Other people may have hyperpigmented eyelids, meaning that the skin on their eyelids darkens from inflammation or hay fever (allergic shiners). Patchy eyebrows and eyelashes may also result from scratching or rubbing.

Researchers have noted differences in the skin of people with atopic dermatitis that may contribute to the symptoms of the disease. The epidermis, which is the outermost layer of skin, is divided into two parts: The inner part contains moist, living cells, and the outer part, known as the horny layer or stratum corneum, contains dry, flattened, dead cells. Under

> ♣ **It's A Fact!!**
>
> There are many different types of dermatitis. Here are the most common ones:
>
> - *Atopic dermatitis*: a chronic skin disease characterized by itchy, inflamed skin
> - *Contact eczema*: a localized reaction that includes redness, itching, and burning where the skin has come into contact with an allergen (an allergy-causing substance) or with an irritant such as an acid, a cleaning agent, or other chemical
> - *Allergic contact eczema (dermatitis)*: a red, itchy, weepy reaction where the skin has come into contact with a substance that the immune system recognizes as foreign, such as poison ivy or certain preservatives in creams and lotions
> - *Seborrheic eczema*: yellowish, oily, scaly patches of skin on the scalp, face, and occasionally other parts of the body
> - *Nummular eczema*: coin-shaped patches of irritated skin—most common on the arms, back, buttocks, and lower legs—that may be crusted, scaling, and extremely itchy
> - *Neurodermatitis*: scaly patches of skin on the head, lower legs, wrists, or forearms caused by a localized itch (such as an insect bite) that becomes intensely irritated when scratched
> - *Stasis dermatitis*: a skin irritation on the lower legs, generally related to circulatory problems
> - *Dyshidrotic eczema*: irritation of the skin on the palms of hands and soles of the feet characterized by clear, deep blisters that itch and burn

Eczema

normal conditions the stratum corneum acts as a barrier, keeping the rest of the skin from drying out and protecting other layers of skin from damage caused by irritants and infections. When this barrier is damaged, irritants act more intensely on the skin.

The skin of a person with atopic dermatitis loses too much moisture from the epidermal layer, allowing the skin to become very dry and reducing its protective abilities. In addition, the patient's skin is very susceptible to recurring infections, such as staphylococcal and streptococcal bacterial skin infections and warts, herpes simplex, and molluscum contagiosum (skin disorders caused by a virus).

Skin Features Of Atopic Dermatitis

- Lichenification: thick, leathery skin resulting from constant scratching and rubbing
- Papules: small raised bumps that may open when scratched, becoming crusty and infected
- Ichthyosis: dry, rectangular scales on the skin
- Keratosis pilaris: small, rough bumps, generally on the face, upper arms, and thighs
- Hyperlinear palms: increased number of skin creases on the palms
- Urticaria: hives (red, raised bumps), often after exposure to an allergen, at the beginning of flares, or after exercise or a hot bath
- Cheilitis: inflammation of the skin on and around the lips
- Atopic pleat (Dennie-Morgan fold): an extra fold of skin that develops under the eye
- Hyperpigmented eyelids: eyelids that have become darker in color from inflammation or hay fever

Stages Of Atopic Dermatitis

Atopic dermatitis is more common in infancy and childhood. It affects each child differently, in terms of both onset and severity of symptoms. In infants, atopic dermatitis typically begins around 6 to 12 weeks of age. It may first appear around the cheeks and chin as a patchy facial rash, which can progress to red, scaling, oozing skin. The skin may become infected. Once the infant becomes more mobile and begins crawling, exposed areas such as knees and elbows may also be affected. An infant with atopic dermatitis may be restless and irritable because of the itching and discomfort of the disease. Many infants get better by 18 months of age, although they remain at greater than normal risk for dry skin or hand eczema later in life.

In childhood, the rash tends to occur behind the knees and inside the elbows; on the sides of the neck; and on the wrists, ankles, and hands. Often, the rash begins with papules that become hard and scaly when scratched. The skin around the lips may be inflamed, and constant licking of the area may lead to small, painful cracks in the skin around the mouth. Severe cases of atopic dermatitis may affect growth, and the child may be shorter than average.

The disease may go into remission. The length of a remission varies, and it may last months or even years. In some children, the disease gets better for a long time only to come back at the onset of puberty when hormones, stress, and the use of irritating skin care products or cosmetics may cause the disease to flare.

Although a number of people who developed atopic dermatitis as children also experience symptoms as adults, it is unusual (but possible) for the disease to show up first in adulthood. The pattern in adults is similar to that seen in children; that is, the disease may be widespread or limited to a more restricted form. In some adults, only the hands or feet may be affected and become dry, itchy, red, and cracked. Sleep patterns and work performance may be affected, and long-term use of medications to treat the atopic dermatitis may cause complications. Adults with atopic dermatitis also have a predisposition toward irritant contact dermatitis, especially if they are in occupations involving frequent hand wetting or hand washing or exposure to chemicals. Some people develop a rash around their nipples. These localized symptoms are difficult to treat, and people often do not tell their doctor because of modesty or embarrassment. Adults may also develop cataracts that are difficult to detect because they cause no symptoms. Therefore, the doctor may recommend regular eye exams.

Eczema

Diagnosing Atopic Dermatitis

Currently, there is no test to diagnose atopic dermatitis and no single symptom or feature used to identify the disease. Each patient experiences a unique combination of symptoms, and the symptoms and severity of the disease may vary over time. The doctor will base his or her diagnosis on the symptoms the patient experiences and may need to see the patient several times to make an accurate diagnosis. It is important for the doctor to rule out other diseases and conditions that might cause skin irritation. In some cases, the family doctor or pediatrician may refer the patient to a dermatologist or allergist (allergy specialist) for further evaluation.

Several tools help the doctor better understand a patient's symptoms and their possible causes. The most valuable diagnostic tool is a thorough medical history, which provides important clues. The doctor may ask about family history of allergic disease; whether the patient also has diseases such as hay fever or asthma; and about exposure to irritants, sleep disturbances, any foods that seem to be related to skin flares, previous treatments for skin-related symptoms, use of steroids, and the effect of symptoms on schoolwork, career, or social life. Sometimes it is necessary to do a biopsy of the skin or patch testing to see if the skin immune system overreacts to certain chemicals or preservatives in skin creams. A preliminary diagnosis of atopic dermatitis can be made if the patient has three or more features from each of two categories: major features and minor features.

Skin scratch/prick tests (scratching or pricking the skin with a needle that contains a small amount of a suspected allergen) and blood tests for airborne allergens generally are not as useful in the diagnosis of atopic dermatitis as a medical history and careful observation of symptoms. However, they may occasionally help the doctor rule out or confirm a specific allergen that might be considered important in diagnosis. Although negative results on skin tests are reliable and may help rule out the possibility that certain substances cause skin inflammation in the patient, positive skin scratch/prick test results are difficult to interpret in people with atopic dermatitis and are often inaccurate. Blood tests, including measurements of certain antibodies to allergens, are not recommended in most cases because they have a high rate of false positives and are expensive. In some cases, where the type of dermatitis is unclear, blood tests to check the level of eosinophils (a type of white blood cell) or IgE (an antibody whose levels are often high in atopic dermatitis) are helpful.

Exacerbating Factors

Many factors or conditions can make symptoms of atopic dermatitis worse, further triggering the already overactive immune system in the skin, aggravating the itch-scratch cycle, and increasing damage to the skin. These exacerbating factors can be broken down into two main categories: irritants and allergens. Emotional factors and some infections can also influence atopic dermatitis.

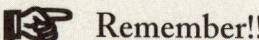 **Remember!!**

Major And Minor Features Of Atopic Dermatitis

Major features

- Intense itching
- Characteristic rash in locations typical of the disease
- Chronic or repeatedly occurring symptoms
- Personal or family history of atopic disorders (eczema, hay fever, asthma)

Minor features

- Early age of onset
- Dry, rough skin
- High levels of immunoglobulin E (IgE), an antibody, in the blood
- Ichthyosis
- Hyperlinear palms
- Keratosis pilaris
- Hand or foot dermatitis
- Cheilitis
- Nipple eczema
- Susceptibility to skin infection
- Positive allergy skin tests

Irritants are substances that directly affect the skin and, when used in high enough concentrations with long enough contact, cause the skin to become red and itchy or to burn. Specific irritants affect people with atopic dermatitis to different degrees. Over time, many patients and their families learn to identify the irritants most troublesome to them. For example, wool or synthetic fibers may affect some patients. Also, rough or poorly fitting clothing can rub the skin, trigger inflammation, and cause the itch-scratch cycle to begin. Soaps and detergents may have a drying effect and worsen itching, and some perfumes and cosmetics may irritate the skin. Exposure to certain substances, such as chlorine, mineral oil, or solvents, or to irritants, such as dust or sand, may also make the condition worse. Cigarette smoke may irritate the eyelids. Because irritants vary from one person to another, each person has to determine for himself or herself what substances or circumstances cause the disease to flare.

Allergens are substances from foods, plants, or animals that inflame the skin because the immune system overreacts to the substance. Inflammation occurs even when the person is exposed to small amounts of the substance for a limited time. Some examples of allergens are pollen and dog or cat dander (tiny particles from the animal's skin or hair). When people with atopic dermatitis come into contact with an irritant or allergen they are sensitive to, inflammation-producing cells come into the skin from elsewhere in the body. These cells release chemicals that cause itching and redness. As the person scratches and rubs the skin in response, further damage occurs.

Some doctors and scientists believe that certain foods act as allergens and may trigger atopic dermatitis or cause it to become worse. Other researchers think that food allergens play a role in only a limited number of cases of atopic dermatitis, primarily in infants and children. An allergic reaction to food can cause skin inflammation (generally hives), gastrointestinal symptoms (vomiting, diarrhea), upper respiratory tract symptoms (congestion, sneezing), and wheezing. The most common allergenic (allergy-causing) foods are eggs, peanuts, milk, fish, soy products, and wheat. Although the data remain inconclusive, some studies suggest that mothers of children with a family history of atopic diseases should avoid eating commonly allergenic foods themselves during late pregnancy and (if breast-feeding) while they are breast-feeding the baby. Although not all researchers agree, some think that breast feeding the infant for at least four months may have a protective effect for the child.

Currently, no reliable laboratory test identifies a food allergy, including skin or blood tests. If a food allergy is suspected, it may be helpful to keep a careful diary of everything the patient eats, noting any reactions. Identifying the food allergen may be difficult if the patient is also being exposed to other allergens, and may require supervision by an allergist. One helpful way to explore the possibility of a food allergy is to eliminate the suspected food and then, if improvement is noticed, reintroduce it into the diet under carefully controlled conditions. If this causes no symptoms or if there has been no improvement in two weeks of eliminating that food, other foods may be eliminated in turn.

> ♣ **It's A Fact!!**
>
> A number of common irritants can make atopic dermatitis worse. They include:
> - Wool or synthetic fibers
> - Soaps and detergents
> - Some perfumes and cosmetics
> - Substances such as chlorine, mineral oil, or solvents
> - Dust or sand
> - Cigarette smoke

Changing the diet of a person who has atopic dermatitis may not always relieve symptoms. A change may be helpful, however, when a patient's medical history and specific symptoms strongly suggest a food allergy. It is up to the patient and his or her family and physician to judge whether the dietary restrictions outweigh the impact of the disease itself. Restricted diets often are emotionally and financially difficult for patients and their families to follow. Unless properly monitored, diets with many restrictions can also contribute to nutritional problems in children.

Other types of allergens called aeroallergens (because they are present in the air) may also play a role in atopic dermatitis. Common aeroallergens are dust mites, pollens, molds, and dander from animal hair or skin. These aeroallergens, particularly the house dust mite, may worsen the symptoms of atopic dermatitis in some people. Although some researchers think that aeroallergens are an important contributing factor to atopic dermatitis, others do not think that they are significant. Scientists also don't understand the way aeroallergens affect the skin—whether the aeroallergen is inhaled by the patient or the aeroallergen actually penetrates the patient's skin.

No reliable test is available that determines whether a specific aeroallergen is an exacerbating factor in any given individual. If the doctor suspects that an aeroallergen is contributing to the symptoms a person is experiencing, the doctor may recommend ways to reduce exposure to the aeroallergen. For example, the presence of the house dust mite can be limited by encasing mattresses and pillows in special dust-proof covers, frequently washing bedding in hot water, and removing carpeting. However, there is no way to completely rid the environment of aeroallergens.

In addition to irritants and allergens, other factors—such as emotional issues, temperature and climate, and skin infections—play a role in atopic dermatitis. Although the disease itself is not caused by emotional factors or personality, it can be made worse by stress, anger, and frustration. Interpersonal problems or major life changes, such as divorce, job changes, or the death of a loved one, can also make the disease worse. Often, emotional stress seems to trigger a flare of the disease.

Bathing without proper moisturizing afterward is a common factor that triggers a flare of atopic dermatitis. The low humidity of winter or the dry year-round climate of some geographic areas can make the disease worse, as can overheated indoor areas and long or hot baths and showers. Alternately sweating and chilling can trigger a flare in some people. Bacterial infections can also trigger or increase the severity of atopic dermatitis. If a patient experiences a sudden flare of illness, the doctor may check for a viral infection (such as herpes simplex) or fungal infection (such as ringworm or athlete's foot).

Treating Atopic Dermatitis

Treatment involves a partnership among the patient, family members, and doctor. The doctor will suggest a treatment plan based on the patient's age, symptoms, and general health. The patient and the patient's family play a large role in the success of the treatment plan by carefully following the doctor's instructions. Some of the primary components of treatment programs are described below. Most patients can be successfully treated with proper skin care and lifestyle changes and do not require the more intensive treatments discussed.

The doctor has three main goals in treating atopic dermatitis: healing the skin and keeping it healthy, preventing flares, and treating symptoms when they do occur. Much of caring for the skin and preventing flares has to do with developing skin care routines, identifying exacerbating factors, and avoiding circumstances that trigger the skin's immune system and the itch-scratch cycle. It is important for the patient and his or her family to note any changes in skin condition in response to treatment, and to be persistent in identifying the most effective treatment strategy.

Skin Care

Healing the skin and keeping it healthy are of primary importance as part of both preventing further damage and enhancing quality of life. Developing and sticking with a daily skin care routine is critical to preventing flares. Key factors are proper bathing and the application of lubricants, such as creams or ointments, within three minutes of bathing. People with atopic dermatitis should avoid hot or long (more than 10 to 15 minutes) baths and showers. A lukewarm bath helps to cleanse and moisturize the skin without drying it excessively. Because soaps can be drying to the skin, the doctor may recommend limited use of a mild bar soap or nonsoap cleanser. Bath oils are not usually helpful.

Once the bath is finished, the patient should air-dry the skin or pat it dry gently (avoiding rubbing or brisk drying) and apply a lubricant immediately. Lubrication restores the skin's moisture, increases the rate of healing, and establishes a barrier against further drying and irritation. Several kinds of lubricants can be used. Lotions have a high water or alcohol content and evaporate more quickly, so they generally are not the best choice. Creams and ointments work better at healing the skin. Tar preparations can be very helpful in healing very dry, lichenified areas. Whatever preparation is chosen, it should be as free of fragrances and chemicals as possible.

Another key to protecting and restoring the skin is taking steps to avoid repeated skin infections. Although it may not be possible to avoid infection

Eczema

altogether, the effect of an infection may be minimized if it is identified and treated early. People with atopic dermatitis and their families should learn to recognize signs of skin infections, including tiny pustules (pus-filled bumps) on arms and legs, appearance of oozing areas, or crusty yellow blisters. If symptoms of a skin infection develop, the doctor should be consulted and treatment should begin as soon as possible.

Medications And Phototherapy

If a flare of atopic dermatitis does occur, several methods can be used to treat the symptoms. The doctor will select a treatment according to the age of the patient and the severity of the symptoms. With proper treatment, most symptoms can be brought under control within three weeks. If symptoms fail to respond, this may be due to a flare that is stronger than the medication can handle, a treatment program that is not fully effective for a particular individual, or the presence of trigger factors that were not addressed in the initial treatment program. These factors can include a reaction to a medication, infection, or emotional stress. Continued symptoms may also occur because the patient is not following the treatment program instructions.

Corticosteroid creams and ointments are the most frequently used treatment. Sometimes over-the-counter preparations are used, but in many cases the doctor will prescribe a stronger corticosteroid cream or ointment. The doctor will take into account the patient's age, location of the skin to be treated, severity of the symptoms, and type of preparation (cream or ointment) when prescribing a medication. Sometimes the base used in certain brands of corticosteroid creams and ointments is irritating for a particular patient. Side effects of repeated or long-term use of topical corticosteroids can include thinning of the skin, infections, growth suppression (in children), and stretch marks on the skin.

Some treatments reduce specific symptoms of the disease. Antibiotics to treat skin infections may be applied directly to the skin in an ointment, but are usually more effective when taken by mouth. Certain antihistamines that cause drowsiness can reduce nighttime scratching and allow more restful sleep when taken at bedtime. This effect can be particularly helpful for patients whose nighttime scratching makes the disease worse. If viral or fungal infections are present, the doctor may also prescribe medications to treat those infections.

Phototherapy (treatment with light) that uses ultraviolet A or B light waves, or both together, can be an effective treatment for mild to moderate dermatitis in older children (over 12 years old) and adults. Photochemotherapy, a combination of ultraviolet light therapy and a drug called psoralen, can also be used in cases that are resistant to phototherapy alone. Possible long-term side effects of this treatment include premature skin aging and skin cancer. If the doctor thinks that phototherapy may be useful to treat the symptoms of atopic dermatitis, he or she will use the minimum exposure necessary and monitor the skin carefully.

When other treatments are not effective, the doctor may prescribe systemic corticosteroids: drugs that are taken by mouth or injected into muscle instead of being applied directly to the skin. An example of a commonly prescribed corticosteroid is prednisone. Typically, these medications are used only in resistant cases and only given for short periods. The side effects of systemic corticosteroids can include skin damage, thinned or weakened bones, high blood pressure, high blood sugar, infections, and cataracts. It can be dangerous to suddenly stop taking corticosteroids, so it is very important that the doctor and patient work together in changing the corticosteroid dose.

In adults, immunosuppressive drugs, such as cyclosporine, are also used to treat severe cases of atopic dermatitis that have failed to respond to any other forms of therapy. Immunosuppressive drugs restrain the overactive immune system by blocking the production of some immune cells and curbing the action of others. The side effects of cyclosporine can include high blood pressure, nausea, vomiting, kidney problems, headaches, tingling or numbness, and a possible increased risk of cancer and infections. There is a risk of relapse after the drug is stopped. Because of their toxic side effects, systemic corticosteroids and immunosuppressive drugs are used only in severe cases and then for as short a time as possible. Patients requiring systemic corticosteroids should be referred to dermatologists or allergists specializing in the care of atopic dermatitis to help identify trigger factors and alternative therapies.

In rare cases, when no other treatments have been successful, the patient may have to be hospitalized. A five- to seven-day stay in the hospital allows intensive skin care and reduces the patient's exposure to irritants and allergens and the stresses of day-to-day life. Under these conditions, the symptoms usually clear quickly if environmental factors play a role or if the patient is not able to carry out adequate skin care at home.

A number of promising experimental medications are being tested for atopic dermatitis. These medications affect the immune system and offer additional options for patients with difficult-to-treat symptoms. Researchers are also actively pursuing the development of alternative treatments for atopic dermatitis.

> ✔ **Quick Tip**
> **Working With Your Doctor**
>
> - Provide complete, accurate medical information about yourself.
> - Make a list of your questions and concerns in advance.
> - Be honest and share your point of view with the doctor.
> - Ask for clarification or further explanation if you need it.
> - Talk to other members of the health care team, such as nurses, therapists, or pharmacists.
> - Don't hesitate to discuss sensitive subjects with your doctor.
> - Discuss changes to any medical treatment or medications with your doctor before making them.

Atopic Dermatitis And Quality of Life

Despite the symptoms caused by atopic dermatitis, it is possible for people with the disorder to maintain a high quality of life. The key to quality of life lies in education, awareness, and developing a partnership among patient, family, and doctor. Good communication is essential, both within the family and among the patient, the family, and the doctor. It is important that the doctor provide understandable information about the disease and its symptoms to the patient and family and demonstrate any treatment measures recommended to ensure that they will be properly carried out.

> ♣ **It's A Fact!!**
>
> Here are the best ways to control atopic dermatitis and its symptoms:
> - Prevent scratching or rubbing whenever possible.
> - Protect skin from excessive moisture, irritants, and rough clothing.
> - Maintain a cool, stable temperature and consistent humidity levels.
> - Limit exposure to dust, cigarette smoke, pollens, and animal dander.
> - Recognize and limit emotional stress.

When a child has atopic dermatitis, the entire family may be affected. It is important that families have additional support to help them cope with the stress and frustration associated with the disease. The child may be fussy and difficult, and often is unable to keep from scratching and rubbing the skin. Distracting the child and providing as many activities that keep the hands busy is key, but it requires much effort and work on the part of parents or caregivers. Another issue families face is the social and emotional stress associated with disfigurement caused by atopic dermatitis. The child may face difficulty in school or other social relationships and may need additional support and encouragement from family members.

Adults with atopic dermatitis can enhance their quality of life by caring regularly for their skin and being mindful of other effects of the disease and how to treat them. Adults should develop a skin care regimen as part of their daily routine, which can be adapted as circumstances and skin conditions change. Stress management and relaxation techniques may help decrease the likelihood of flares due to emotional stress. Developing a network of support that includes family, friends, health professionals, and support groups or organizations can be beneficial. Chronic anxiety and depression may be relieved by short-term psychological therapy.

Recognizing the situations when scratching is most likely to occur may also help. For example, many patients find that they scratch more when they are idle, so structured activity that keeps the hands occupied may prevent further damage to the skin. Occupational counseling also may be helpful to identify or change career goals if a job involves contact with irritants or involves frequent hand washing, such as kitchen work or auto mechanics.

Eczema

Current Research

Research on atopic dermatitis is active. Scientists, including some supported by the National Institute of Arthritis and Musculoskeletal and Skin Diseases and other institutes of the National Institutes of Health, are working to better understand what causes the disease and how it can be managed, treated, and, ultimately, prevented. Several avenues of research offer promise.

Genetics

Although atopic dermatitis runs in families, the role of genetics remains unclear. It does appear that more than one gene is involved in the development of the disease. Researchers suspect that atopic dermatitis may be caused by environmental factors acting in people who are genetically predisposed to the disease.

Research has helped shed light on the patterns of inheritance of atopic dermatitis. Studies show that children are at increased risk for developing the disorder if there is a family history of other atopic disease, such as hay fever or asthma. The risk is significantly higher if both parents have an atopic disease. In addition, studies of identical twins, who have the exact same genes, show that in an estimated 80 to 90 percent of cases, if one twin has an atopic disease, the other does also. Fraternal (nonidentical) twins, who have only some genes in common, are no more likely than two other people in the general population to both have an atopic disease. These findings suggest that genes play an important role in determining who gets the disease.

Biochemical Abnormalities

Scientists suspect that changes in the skin's protective barrier make people with atopic dermatitis more sensitive to irritants. Such people have lower levels of fatty acids (substances that provide moisture and elasticity) in their skin, which causes dryness and reduces the skin's ability to control inflammation.

Other research evidence points to a possible defect in a type of white blood cell called a monocyte. In people with atopic dermatitis, monocytes appear to play a role in the decreased production of an immune system hormone called interferon gamma (IFN-), which helps regulate allergic reactions. This defect may cause exaggerated immune and inflammatory responses in the blood and tissues of people with atopic dermatitis.

Faulty Regulation Of Immunoglobulin E (IgE)

IgE is a type of antibody that controls the immune system's allergic response. An antibody is a special protein produced by the immune system that recognizes and helps fight and destroy viruses, bacteria, and other foreign substances that invade the body. Normally, IgE is present in very small amounts, but levels are high in 80 to 90 percent of people with atopic dermatitis. Researchers suspect that IgE may play a role in the disease.

In allergic diseases, IgE antibodies are produced in response to different allergens. When an allergen comes into contact with IgE on specialized immune cells, the cells release various chemicals, including histamine. These chemicals cause the symptoms of an allergic reaction, such as wheezing, sneezing, runny eyes, and itching. Scientists originally thought the release of histamine played an important role in the development of atopic dermatitis. However, the release of histamine and other chemicals alone cannot explain the typical longer-term symptoms of the disease. Research is underway to identify factors that may explain why too much IgE is produced and how it plays a role in the disease.

Immune System Imbalance

Researchers also think that an imbalance in the immune system may contribute to the development of atopic dermatitis. It appears that the part of the immune system responsible for stimulating IgE is overactive, and the part that makes IFN-g and handles skin viral and fungal infections is underactive. Indeed, the skin of people with atopic dermatitis shows increased susceptibility to skin infections. This imbalance appears to result in the skin's inability to prevent dermatitis, or inflammation, even in areas of skin that appear normal.

Hyperactivity of one type of immune cell in the skin, called a Langerhans cell, may be involved in atopic dermatitis. Langerhans cells are responsible for picking up viruses, bacteria, allergens, and other foreign substances that

Eczema

invade the body and delivering them to other cells in the immune defense system. Langerhans cells appear to be hyperactive in the skin of people with atopic diseases. In atopic skin certain Langerhans cells are particularly potent at activating white blood cells called T cells, which produce proteins that promote allergic response. This function results in an exaggerated response of the skin to tiny amounts of allergens.

Treatments

Scientists are also focusing on identifying new treatments for atopic dermatitis, including biologic agents, fatty acid supplements, and new forms of phototherapy. Researchers are working to understand how ultraviolet light affects the immune system in healthy and diseased skin. They are also investigating biologic agents, including several aimed at modifying the response of the immune system. A biologic agent is a new type of drug based on molecules that occur naturally in the body. One promising treatment is the use of the proteins IFN and thymopentin (and similar agents) to reestablish balance in the immune system.

Researchers also continue to look for immunosuppressive drugs that may help treat severe atopic dermatitis. Clinical trials are underway with a drug called FK506, which is applied to the skin rather than taken orally. Two anti-inflammatory drugs called phosphodiesterase inhibitors, currently in clinical trials, also appear promising as treatments for atopic dermatitis. These drugs affect multiple cells and cell functions and may prove to be an effective alternative to corticosteroids in the treatment of atopic dermatitis.

Several experimental treatments are being evaluated that attempt to replace substances that are deficient in people with atopic dermatitis. Evening primrose oil is a substance rich in gamma-linolenic acid, one of the fatty acids that is decreased in the skin of people with atopic dermatitis. Studies to date using evening primrose oil have yielded contradictory results. Clinical trials with another substance, a dietary fatty acid supplement called eicosapentaenoic acid, have resulted in only slight improvement. There is also a great deal of interest in the use of Chinese herbs and herbal teas to treat the disease. Studies to date do show some benefit, but concerns remain about toxicity and the risks of suppression of the immune system.

Hope For The Future

Although the symptoms of atopic dermatitis can be difficult and uncomfortable, the disease can be successfully managed. People with atopic dermatitis, as well as their families, can lead healthy, normal lives. As scientists learn more about atopic dermatitis and what causes it, they continue to move closer to effective treatments and perhaps, ultimately, a cure.

Chapter 35
Psoriasis

What Is Psoriasis?

Psoriasis is a chronic (long-lasting) skin disease characterized by scaling and inflammation. Scaling occurs when cells in the outer layer of the skin reproduce faster than normal and pile up on the skin's surface.

Psoriasis affects between 1 and 2 percent of the United States population, or about 5.5 million people. Although the disease occurs in all age groups and about equally in men and women, it primarily affects adults. People with psoriasis may suffer discomfort, including pain and itching, restricted motion in their joints, and emotional distress.

In its most typical form, psoriasis results in patches of thick, red skin covered with silvery scales. These patches, which are sometimes referred to as plaques, usually itch and may burn. The skin at the joints may crack. Psoriasis most often occurs on the elbows, knees, scalp, lower back, face, palms, and soles of the feet, but it can affect any skin site. The disease may also affect the fingernails, the toenails, and the soft tissues inside the mouth and genitalia. About 15 percent of people with psoriasis have joint inflammation that produces arthritis symptoms. This condition is called psoriatic arthritis.

About This Chapter: Adapted from "Questions and Answers About Psoriasis," the National Institute of Arthritis and Musculoskeletal and Skin Diseases, http://www.niams.nih.gov/hi/topics/psoriasis/psoriafs.htm, published September 1999 and updated January 2002.

What Causes Psoriasis?

Recent research indicates that psoriasis is likely a disorder of the immune system (autoimmune disease). This system includes a type of white blood cell, called a T-cell, that normally helps protect the body against infection and disease. Scientists now think that, in psoriasis, an abnormal immune system causes activity by T-cells in the skin. These T-cells trigger the inflammation and excessive skin cell reproduction seen in people with psoriasis.

> **Weird Words**
>
> <u>Autoimmune disease</u>: A disease in which the immune system destroys or attacks a person's own tissues.
>
> <u>Plaques</u>: Patches of thickened and reddened skin that are covered by silvery scales.
>
> <u>Toxic</u>: Pertaining to a drug's ability to cause harmful or unpleasant side effects.

In about one-third of the cases, psoriasis is inherited. Researchers are studying large families affected by psoriasis to identify a gene or genes that cause the disease. (Genes govern every bodily function and determine the inherited traits passed from parent to child.)

People with psoriasis may notice that there are times when their skin worsens, then improves. Conditions that may cause flare-ups include changes in climate, infections, stress, and dry skin. Also, certain medicines—most notably beta-blockers, which are used to treat high blood pressure; lithium; and drugs used to treat depression—may trigger an outbreak or worsen the disease.

How Is Psoriasis Diagnosed?

Doctors usually diagnose psoriasis after a careful examination of the skin. However, diagnosis may be difficult because psoriasis can look like other skin diseases. A pathologist may assist with diagnosis by examining a small skin sample (biopsy) under a microscope.

There are several forms of psoriasis. The most common form is plaque psoriasis (its scientific name is psoriasis vulgaris). In plaque psoriasis, lesions have a reddened base covered by silvery scales. Other forms of psoriasis include:

- *Guttate psoriasis.* Small, drop-like lesions appear on the trunk, limbs, and scalp. Guttate psoriasis is most often triggered by bacterial infections (for example, *Streptococcus*).
- *Pustular psoriasis.* Blisters of noninfectious pus appear on the skin. Attacks of pustular psoriasis may be triggered by medications, infections, emotional stress, or exposure to certain chemicals. Pustular psoriasis may affect either small or large areas of the body.
- *Inverse psoriasis.* Large, dry, smooth, vividly red plaques occur in the folds of the skin near the genitals, under the breasts, or in the armpits. Inverse psoriasis is related to increased sensitivity to friction and sweating and may be painful or itchy.
- *Erythrodermic psoriasis.* Widespread reddening and scaling of the skin is often accompanied by itching or pain. Erythrodermic psoriasis may be precipitated by severe sunburn, use of oral steroids (such as cortisone), or a drug-related rash.

What Treatments Are Available For Psoriasis?

Doctors generally treat psoriasis in steps based on the severity of the disease, the extent of the areas involved, the type of psoriasis, or the patient's responsiveness to initial treatments. This is sometimes called the "1-2-3" approach. In step 1, medicines are applied to the skin (topical treatment). Step 2 focuses on light treatments (phototherapy). Step 3 involves taking medicines internally, usually by mouth (systemic treatment).

Over time, affected skin can become resistant to treatment, especially when topical corticosteroids are used. Also, a treatment that works very well in one person may have little effect in another. Thus, doctors commonly use a trial-and-error approach to find a treatment that works, and they may switch treatments periodically (for example, every 12 to 24 months) if resistance or adverse reactions occur. Treatment depends on the location of lesions, their size, the amount of skin affected, previous response to treatment, and patients' perceptions about their skin condition and preferences for treatment. In addition, treatment is often tailored to the specific form of the disorder.

Topical Treatment

Treatments applied directly to the skin are sometimes effective in clearing psoriasis. Doctors find that some patients respond well to sunlight, corticosteroid ointments, medicines derived from vitamin D_3, vitamin A (retinoids), coal tar, or anthralin. Other topical measures, such as bath solutions and moisturizers, may be soothing but are seldom strong enough to clear lesions over the long term and may need to be combined with more potent remedies.

- *Sunlight.* Daily, regular, short doses of sunlight that do not produce a sunburn clear psoriasis in many people.

- *Corticosteroids.* Available in different strengths, corticosteroids (cortisone) are usually applied twice a day. Short-term treatment is often effective in improving but not completely clearing psoriasis. If less than 10 percent of the skin is involved, some doctors will begin treatment with a high-potency corticosteroid ointment (for example, Diprolene®, Temovate®, Ultravate®, or Psorcon®). High-potency steroids may also be used for treatment-resistant plaques, particularly those on the hands or feet. Long-term use or overuse of high-potency steroids can lead to worsening of the psoriasis, thinning of the skin, internal side effects, and resistance to the treatment's benefits. Medium-potency corticosteroids may be used on the torso or limbs; low-potency preparations are used on delicate skin areas.

- *Calcipotriene.* This drug is a synthetic form of vitamin D_3. (It is not the same as vitamin D supplements.) Applying calcipotriene ointment (for example, Dovonex®) twice a day controls excessive production of skin cells. Because calcipotriene can irritate the skin, however, it is not recommended for the face or genitals. After four months of treatment, about 60 percent of patients have a good to excellent response. The safety of using the drug for cases affecting more than 20 percent of the skin is unknown, and using it on widespread areas of the skin may raise the amount of calcium in the body to unhealthy levels.

- *Coal tar.* Coal tar may be applied directly to the skin, used in a bath solution, or used on the scalp as a shampoo. It is available in different strengths, but the most potent form may be irritating. It is sometimes combined with ultraviolet B (UVB) phototherapy. Compared with steroids, coal tar has fewer side effects, but it is messy and less effective and thus is not popular with many patients. Other drawbacks include its failure to provide long-term help for most patients, its strong odor, and its tendency to stain skin or clothing.

- *Anthralin.* Doctors sometimes use a 15- to 30-minute application of anthralin ointment, cream, or paste to treat chronic psoriasis lesions. However, this treatment often fails to adequately clear lesions, may irritate the skin, and stains skin and clothing brown or purple. In addition, anthralin is unsuitable for acute or actively inflamed eruptions.
- *Topical retinoid.* The retinoid tazarotene (Tazorac®) is a fast-drying, clear gel that is applied to the surface of the skin. Although this preparation does not act as quickly as topical corticosteroids, it has fewer side effects. Because it is irritating to normal skin, it should be used with caution in skin folds. Women of childbearing age should use birth control when using tazarotene.
- *Salicylic acid.* Salicylic acid is used to remove scales, and is most effective when combined with topical steroids, anthralin, or coal tar.
- *Bath solutions.* People with psoriasis may find that bathing in water with an oil added, then applying a moisturizer, can soothe their skin. Scales can be removed and itching reduced by soaking for 15 minutes in water containing a tar solution, oiled oatmeal, Epsom salts, or Dead Sea salts.
- *Moisturizers.* When applied regularly over a long period, moisturizers have a cosmetic and soothing effect. Preparations that are thick and greasy usually work best because they hold water in the skin, reducing the scales and the itching.

Phototherapy

Ultraviolet (UV) light from the sun causes the activated T-cells in the skin to die, a process called apoptosis. Apoptosis reduces inflammation and slows the overproduction of skin cells that causes scaling. Daily, short, nonburning exposure to sunlight clears or improves psoriasis in many people.

Therefore, sunlight may be included among initial treatments for the disease. A more controlled form of artificial light treatment may be used in mild psoriasis (UVB phototherapy) or in more severe or extensive psoriasis (psoralen and ultraviolet A [PUVA] therapy).

UVB Phototherapy

Some artificial sources of UVB light are similar to sunlight. Newer sources, called narrow-band UVB, emit the part of the ultraviolet spectrum band that is most helpful for psoriasis. Some physicians will start with UVB treatments instead of topical agents. UVB phototherapy is also used to treat widespread psoriasis and lesions that resist topical treatment. This type of phototherapy is normally administered in a doctor's office by using a light panel or light box, although some patients can use UVB light boxes at home with a doctor's guidance. Generally at least three treatments a week for two or three months are needed. UVB phototherapy may be combined with other treatments as well. One combined therapy program, referred to as the Ingram regime, involves a coal tar bath, UVB phototherapy, and application of an anthralin-salicylic acid paste, which is left on the skin for 6 to 24 hours. A similar regime, the Goeckerman treatment, involves application of coal tar ointment and UVB phototherapy.

PUVA

This treatment combines oral or topical administration of a medicine called psoralen with exposure to ultraviolet A (UVA) light. Psoralen makes the body more sensitive to this light. PUVA is normally used when more than 10 percent of the skin is affected or when rapid clearing is required because the disease interferes with a person's occupation (for example, when a model's face or a carpenter's hands are involved). Compared with UVB treatment, PUVA treatment taken two to three times a week clears psoriasis more consistently and in fewer treatments. However, it is associated with more short-term side effects, including nausea, headache, fatigue, burning, and itching. Long-term treatment is associated with an increased risk of squamous cell and melanoma skin cancers. PUVA can be combined with some oral medications (retinoids and hydroxyurea) to increase its effectiveness. Simultaneous use of drugs that suppress the immune system, such as cyclosporine, have little beneficial effect and increase the risk of cancer. In very rare cases, patients who must travel long distances for PUVA treatments may, with a physician's close supervision, be taught to administer this treatment at home.

Systemic Treatment

For more severe forms of psoriasis, doctors sometimes prescribe medicines that are taken internally:

- *Methotrexate.* This treatment, which can be taken by pill or injection, slows cell production by suppressing the immune system. Patients taking methotrexate must be closely monitored because it can cause liver damage and/or decrease the production of oxygen-carrying red blood cells, infection-fighting white blood cells, and clot-enhancing platelets. As a precaution, doctors do not prescribe the drug for people with long-term liver disease or anemia. Methotrexate should not be used by pregnant women, by women who are planning to get pregnant, or by their male partners.

- *Cyclosporine.* Taken orally, cyclosporine (Neoral®) acts by suppressing the immune system in a way that slows the rapid turnover of skin cells. It may provide quick relief of symptoms, but it is usually effective only during the course of treatment. The best candidates for this therapy are those with severe psoriasis who have not responded to or cannot tolerate other systemic therapies. Cyclosporine may impair kidney function or cause high blood pressure (hypertension), so patients must be carefully monitored by a doctor. Also, cyclosporine is not recommended for patients who have a weak immune system, those who have had substantial exposure to UVB or PUVA in the past, or those who are pregnant or breast-feeding.

- *Hydroxyurea (Hydrea®).* Compared with methotrexate and cyclosporine, hydroxyurea is less toxic but also less effective. It is sometimes combined with PUVA or UVB. Possible side effects include anemia and a decrease in white blood cells and platelets. Like methotrexate and cyclosporine, hydroxyurea must be avoided by pregnant women or those who are planning to become pregnant.

- *Retinoids*. A retinoid, such as acitretin (Soriatane®), is a compound with vitamin A-like properties that may be prescribed for severe cases of psoriasis that do not respond to other therapies. Because this treatment also may cause birth defects, women must protect themselves from pregnancy beginning one month before through three years after treatment. Most patients experience a recurrence of psoriasis after acitretin is discontinued.

- Antibiotics. Although not indicated in routine treatment, antibiotics may be employed when an infection, such as *Streptococcus*, triggers the outbreak of psoriasis, as in certain cases of guttate psoriasis.

What Are Some Promising Areas Of Psoriasis Research?

Researchers continue to search for genes that contribute to the inherited and other causes of psoriasis. Scientists are also working to improve our understanding of what happens in the body to trigger this disease. In addition, much research is focused on developing new and better treatments. Some of these experimental treatments, such as agents directed at the specific types of T-cells involved, work to improve the disease with less overall suppression of the immune system.

The National Psoriasis Tissue Bank, which is supported by the National Psoriasis Foundation, is helping researchers worldwide study the inherited tendency toward psoriasis. The tissue bank has DNA from the white blood cells of more than 250 families affected by the disease. There is particular interest in large families in which psoriasis is both common and spans two or more generations. More recently, the tissue bank has begun research involving families having at least two siblings with psoriasis. People seeking more information or families interested in participating in a study should contact

National Psoriasis Foundation Tissue Bank
6600 SW 92nd Avenue, Suite 300
Portland, OR 97223-7195
(503) 244-7404
(800) 723-9166
Fax: (503) 245-0626
http://www.psoriasis.org

Chapter 36
Cellulitis

What Is Cellulitis?

Cellulitis is a spreading infection of the skin that usually begins as a small area of tenderness, swelling, and redness on the skin. As this red area begins to spread, the person may develop a fever, sometimes with chills and sweats, and swollen lymph nodes ("swollen glands") near the area of infected skin.

Unlike impetigo, which is a very superficial skin infection, cellulitis refers to an infection involving the skin's deeper layers; the dermis and subcutaneous tissue. The main pathogen involved in cellulitis is *Staphylococcus* ("staph"), the same bacterium that causes many cases of impetigo. Occasionally, other bacteria may cause cellulitis as well.

Where Does Cellulitis Occur?

Some cases of cellulitis appear on areas of trauma, where the skin has broken open, such as the skin near ulcers or surgical wounds. Many times, however, cellulitis occurs where there has been no break in the skin at all. In such cases, it is anyone's guess where the bacteria came from. Patients who have diabetes or impairment of the immune system (for example, from HIV/AIDS or from drugs that depress the immune system) are particularly prone to developing cellulitis.

About This Chapter: Source: MedicineNet, Inc. (www.medicinenet.com). © 2002; reprinted with permission.

What Does Cellulitis Look Like?

The signs of cellulitis are those of any inflammation: redness, warmth, swelling, and pain. Any skin wound or ulcer that exhibits these signs may be developing cellulitis.

Other forms of uninfected inflammation may mimic cellulitis. People with poor leg circulation, for instance, often develop scaly redness on the shins and ankles; this is called "stasis dermatitis" and is often mistaken for the bacterial infection of cellulitis.

What Causes Cellulitis?

Staph (*Staphylococcus aureus*) is the most common bacterium that causes cellulitis.

Strep (Group A *Streptococcus*) is next most common bacterium that causes cellulitis. A form of rather superficial cellulitis caused by strep is called erysipelas; it is characterized by the spreading of a hot, bright-red, circumscribed area on the skin with a sharp, raised border. The so-called "flesh-eating bacteria" are, in fact, also a strain of strep that can in severe cases destroy tissue almost as fast as surgeons can cut it out.

Cellulitis can be caused by many other types of bacteria. In children under six, *Haemophilus influenzae* bacteria can cause cellulitis, especially on the face, arms, and upper torso. Cellulitis from a dog or cat bite or scratch may be caused by the *Pasteurella multocida* bacterium, which has a very short incubation period of only 4 to 24 hours. Cellulitis after an injury from a saltwater fish or shellfish (like a fish bite, a puncture from a fish spine, or a crab pinch) can be due to *Erysipelothrix rhusiopathiae* bacteria. These same bacteria can also cause cellulitis after a skin injury on the farm, especially if it happened while working with pigs or poultry.

Is Cellulitis Contagious?

Cellulitis is not contagious because it is an infection of the skin's deeper layers, the dermis and subcutaneous tissue, and the skin's top layer (the epidermis) provides a cover over the infection. In this regard, cellulitis is different

Cellulitis

from impetigo, in which there is a very superficial skin infection that can be contagious.

How Is Cellulitis Treated?

First, it is crucial for the doctor to distinguish whether or not the inflammation is due to an infection. The history and physical exam can provide clues in this regard, as sometimes the white blood cell count can. A culture for bacteria may also be of value.

When it is difficult or impossible to distinguish whether or not the inflammation is due to an infection, doctors sometimes treat with antibiotics just to be sure. If the condition does not respond, it may need to be addressed by different methods dealing with types of inflammation that are not infected. For example, if the inflammation is thought to be due to an autoimmune disorder, treatment may be with a corticosteroid.

Antibiotics such as derivatives of penicillin or other types of antibiotics that are effective against the staph germ are used to treat cellulitis. If other bacteria, as determined by culture tests, turn out to be the cause, or if patients are allergic to penicillin, other appropriate antibiotics can be substituted.

Chapter 37

Lichen Sclerosis

What Is Lichen Sclerosis?

Lichen sclerosis (pronounced LIKE-in skler-O-sus) is a skin disorder that can affect men, women, or children, but is most common in women. It usually occurs on the vulva (the outer genitalia or sex organs) in women, but sometimes develops on the head of the penis in men. Occasionally, lichen sclerosis is seen on other parts of the body, especially the upper body, breasts, and upper arms.

The symptoms are the same in children and adults. Early in the disease, small, subtle white spots appear. These areas are usually slightly shiny and smooth. As time goes on, the spots develop into bigger patches, and the skin surface becomes thinned and crinkled. As a result, the skin tears easily, and bright red or purple discoloration from bleeding inside the skin is common. More severe cases of lichen sclerosis produce scarring that may cause the inner lips of the vulva to shrink and disappear, the clitoris to become covered with scar tissue, and the opening of the vagina to narrow.

Lichen sclerosis of the penis occurs almost exclusively in uncircumcised men (those who have not had the foreskin removed). The foreskin

About This Chapter: Adapted from "Questions and Answers About Lichen Sclerosis," National Institute of Arthritis and Musculoskeletal and Skin Diseases, http://www.niams.nih.gov/hi/topics/lichen/lichen.htm, March 2000.

can scar, tighten, and shrink over the head of the penis. Skin on other areas of the body affected by lichen sclerosis usually does not experience scarring.

How Common Is It?

Although definitive data are not available, lichen sclerosis is considered a rare disorder that can develop in people of all ages. It primarily affects the vulva. Fewer than one in 20 women who have vulvar lichen sclerosis have the disease on other skin surfaces. The disease is much less common in childhood. In boys, it is a major cause of tightening of the foreskin, which requires circumcision. Otherwise, it is very uncommon in men.

What Are The Symptoms?

Symptoms vary depending on the area affected. Patients experience very different degrees of discomfort. When lichen sclerosis occurs on parts of the body other than the genital area, most often there are no symptoms other than itching. If the disease is severe, bleeding, tearing, and blistering caused by rubbing or bumping the skin can cause pain.

Very mild lichen sclerosis of the genital area may cause itching, but often causes no symptoms at all. If the disease worsens, itching is the most common symptom. Rarely, lichen sclerosis of the vulva may cause extreme itching that interferes with sleep and daily activities. Rubbing or scratching to relieve the itching can create painful sores and bruising, so that many women must avoid sexual intercourse, tight clothing, tampons, riding bicycles, and other common activities that involve pressure or friction. Urination can be accompanied by burning or pain, and bleeding can occur, especially during intercourse. When lichen sclerosis develops around the anus, the discomfort can lead to constipation. This is particularly common in children.

Most men with genital lichen sclerosis have not been circumcised. They sometimes experience difficulty pulling back the foreskin and have decreased sensation in the tip of the penis. Occasionally, erections are painful, and the urethra (the tube through which urine flows) can become narrow or obstructed.

Lichen Sclerosis

What Causes Lichen Sclerosis?

The cause is unknown, although an overactive immune system may play a role. Some people may have a genetic tendency toward the disease, and studies suggest that abnormal hormone levels may also play a role. Some scientists believe that an infectious bacterium, called a spirochete, may cause the changes in the immune system that lead to lichen sclerosis.

Is It Contagious?

No, lichen sclerosis is not contagious.

How Is It Diagnosed?

Doctors can diagnose an advanced case by looking at the skin. However, early or mild disease often requires a biopsy (removal and examination of a small sample of affected skin). Because other diseases of the genitalia can look like lichen sclerosis, a biopsy is advised whenever the appearance of the skin is not typical of lichen sclerosis.

How Is It Treated?

Patients with lichen sclerosis of nongenital skin often do not need treatment because the symptoms are very mild and usually go away over time. (The amount of time varies from patient to patient.)

However, lichen sclerosis of the genital skin should be treated, even when it is not causing itching or pain, because it can lead to scarring that may narrow openings in the genital area and interfere with either urination or sexual intercourse or both. There is also a very small chance that cancer may develop.

In uncircumcised men, circumcision is the most widely used therapy for lichen sclerosis. This procedure removes the affected skin, and the disease usually does not recur.

Prescription medications are required to treat vulvar lichen sclerosis, nongenital lichen sclerosis that is causing symptoms, and lichen sclerosis of the penis that is not cured by circumcision. The treatment of choice is an ultrapotent topical corticosteroid. Daily use of these creams or ointments can stop itching within a few days and restore the skin's normal texture and strength after several months. However, treatment does not reverse the scarring that may have already occurred.

Because ultrapotent corticosteroid creams and ointments are very strong, frequent evaluation by a doctor is necessary to check the skin for side effects when the medication is used every day. Once the symptoms are gone and the skin has regained its strength, medication can be used less frequently, although use must continue indefinitely, several times a week, to keep vulvar lichen sclerosis in remission.

> ♣ **It's A Fact!!**
> Here is a list of the ultrapotent corticosteroids available by prescription in the United States:
> - Betamethasone dipropionate
> - Clobetasol propionate
> - Diflorasone diacetate
> - Halobetasol propionate

Young girls may not require lifelong treatment, since lichen sclerosis can sometimes, but not always, disappear permanently at puberty. Scarring and changes in skin color, however, may remain even after the symptoms have disappeared.

Because ultrapotent topical corticosteroids are so effective, other therapies are rarely prescribed. The previous standard therapy was testosterone ointment or cream, but this has recently been proven to produce no more benefit than a placebo (inactive) cream. Another hormone cream, progesterone, was previously used to treat the disease, but also has little beneficial effect. Retinoids, or vitamin A–like medications, may be helpful for patients who cannot tolerate or are not helped by ultrapotent topical corticosteroids.

Patients who need medication should ask their doctor how it works, what side effects it might have, and why it is the best treatment for lichen sclerosis.

For women and girls, surgery to remove the affected skin is not an acceptable option. Surgery may be useful for scarring, but only after lichen sclerosis is controlled with medication.

Sometimes, people do not respond to the ultrapotent topical corticosteroid. Other factors, such as low estrogen levels that cause vaginal dryness and soreness, a skin infection, or irritation or allergy to the medication, can keep symptoms from clearing up. Your doctor may need to treat these factors as well. If you feel that you are not improving as you would expect, talk to your doctor.

Can People With Lichen Sclerosis Have Sexual Intercourse?

Women with severe lichen sclerosis may not be able to have sexual intercourse because of pain or scarring that narrows the entrance to the vagina. However, proper treatment with an ultrapotent topical corticosteroid should restore normal sexual ability, unless severe scarring has already narrowed the vaginal opening. In this case, surgery may be needed to correct the problem, but only after the disease has been controlled.

Is Lichen Sclerosis Related To Cancer?

Lichen sclerosis does not cause skin cancer. However, skin that is scarred by lichen sclerosis is more likely to develop skin cancer. About one in 20 women with untreated vulvar lichen sclerosis develops skin cancer. The frequency of skin cancer in men with lichen sclerosis is not known. It is important for people who have the disease to receive proper treatment and to see their doctor every 6 to 12 months, so that he or she can monitor and treat any changes that might signal skin cancer.

What Kind Of Doctor Treats Lichen Sclerosis?

Lichen sclerosis is treated by dermatologists (skin doctors) and by gynecologists if the female genitalia are involved. Urologists and primary care health providers with a special interest in genital diseases also treat this disease. To find a doctor who treats lichen sclerosis, ask your family doctor for a referral, call a local or state department of health, look in the local telephone directory, or contact a local medical center. The American Academy of Dermatology also provides referrals to dermatologists in your area, and the American College of Obstetricians and Gynecologists can refer you to a gynecologist. The *Directory of Medical Specialists*, available at most public libraries, lists dermatologists, gynecologists, and urologists in your area.

Chapter 38

Vitiligo

What Is Vitiligo?

Vitiligo (pronounced vit-ill-EYE-go) is a pigmentation disorder in which melanocytes (the cells that make pigment) in the skin, the mucous membranes (tissues that line the inside of the mouth and nose and genital and rectal areas), and the retina (inner layer of the eyeball) are destroyed. As a result, white patches of skin appear on different parts of the body. The hair that grows in areas affected by vitiligo usually turns white.

The cause of vitiligo is not known, but doctors and researchers have several different theories. One theory is that people develop antibodies that destroy the melanocytes in their own bodies. Another theory is that melanocytes destroy themselves. Finally, some people have reported that a single event such as sunburn or emotional distress triggered vitiligo; however, these events have not been scientifically proven to cause vitiligo.

Who Is Affected by Vitiligo?

About 1 to 2 percent of the world's population, or 40 to 50 million people, have vitiligo. In the United States, 2 to 5 million people have the

About This Chapter: Adapted from "Questions and Answers About Vitiligo," March 2001; available electronically at http://www.niams.nih.gov/hi/topics/vitiligo/vitiligo.htm and in printed form as NIH Publication No. 01-4909, National Arthritis and Musculoskeletal and Skin Diseases Information Clearinghouse, NIAMS, National Institutes of Health, 1 AMS Circle, Bethesda, Maryland 20892-3675.

disorder. Ninety-five percent of people who have vitiligo develop it before their fortieth birthday. The disorder affects all races and both sexes equally.

Vitiligo seems to be more common in people with certain autoimmune diseases (diseases in which a person's immune system reacts against the body's own organs or tissues). These autoimmune diseases include hyperthyroidism (an overactive thyroid gland), adrenocortical insufficiency (the adrenal gland does not produce enough of the hormone called corticosteroid), alopecia areata (patches of baldness), and pernicious anemia (a low level of red blood cells caused by failure of the body to absorb vitamin B_{12}). Scientists do not know the reason for the association between vitiligo and these autoimmune diseases. However, most people with vitiligo have no other autoimmune disease.

Vitiligo may also be hereditary; that is, it can run in families. Children whose parents have the disorder are more likely to develop vitiligo. However, most children will not get vitiligo even if a parent has it, and most people with vitiligo do not have a family history of the disorder.

What Are The Symptoms Of Vitiligo?

People who develop vitiligo usually first notice white patches (depigmentation) on their skin. These patches are more common in sun-exposed areas, including the hands, feet, arms, face, and lips. Other common areas for white

> ### 🕮 Weird Words
>
> <u>Antibodies</u>: Protective proteins produced by the body's immune system to fight infectious agents (such as bacteria or viruses) or other "foreign" substances. Occasionally, antibodies develop that can attack a part of the body and cause an "autoimmune" disease. These antibodies are called autoantibodies.
>
> <u>Pigmentation</u>: Coloring of the skin, hair, mucous membranes, and retina of the eye.
>
> <u>Depigmentation</u>: Loss of color in the skin, hair, mucous membranes, or retina of the eye.
>
> <u>Melanin</u>: A yellow, brown, or black pigment that determines skin color. Melanin also acts as a sunscreen and protects the skin from ultraviolet light.

patches to appear are the armpits and groin and around the mouth, eyes, nostrils, navel, and genitals.

Vitiligo generally appears in one of three patterns. In one pattern (focal pattern), the depigmentation is limited to one or only a few areas. Some people develop depigmented patches on only one side of their bodies (segmental pattern). But for most people who have vitiligo, depigmentation occurs on different parts of the body (generalized pattern). In addition to white patches on the skin, people with vitiligo may have premature graying of the scalp hair, eyelashes, eyebrows, and beard. People with dark skin may notice a loss of color inside their mouths.

Will The Depigmented Patches Spread?

There is no way to predict if vitiligo will spread. For some people, the depigmented patches do not spread. The disorder is usually progressive, however, and over time the white patches will spread to other areas of the body. For some people, vitiligo spreads slowly, over many years. For other people, spreading occurs rapidly. Some people have reported additional depigmentation following periods of physical or emotional stress.

How Is Vitiligo Diagnosed?

If a doctor suspects that a person has vitiligo, he or she usually begins by asking the person about his or her medical history. Important factors in a person's medical history are a family history of vitiligo; a rash, sunburn, or other skin trauma at the site of vitiligo two to three months before depigmentation started; stress or physical illness; and premature (before age 35) graying of the hair. In addition, the doctor will need to know whether the patient or anyone in the patient's family has had any autoimmune diseases and whether the patient is very sensitive to the sun. The doctor will then examine the patient to rule out other medical problems. The doctor may take a small sample (biopsy) of the affected skin. He or she may also take a blood sample to check the blood-cell count and thyroid function. For some patients, the doctor may recommend an eye examination to check for uveitis (inflammation of part of the eye). A blood test to look for the presence of antinuclear antibodies (a type of autoantibody) may also be done. This test helps determine if the patient has another autoimmune disease.

How Can People Cope With The Emotional And Psychological Aspects Of Vitiligo?

The change in appearance caused by vitiligo can affect a person's emotional and psychological well-being and may create difficulty in getting or keeping a job. People with this disorder can experience emotional stress, particularly if vitiligo develops on visible areas of the body, such as the face, hands, arms, and feet, or on the genitals. Adolescents, who are often particularly concerned about their appearance, can be devastated by widespread vitiligo. Some people who have vitiligo feel embarrassed, ashamed, depressed, or worried about how others will react.

Several strategies can help a person cope with vitiligo. First, it is important to find a doctor who is knowledgeable about vitiligo and takes the disorder seriously. The doctor should also be a good listener and be able to provide emotional support. Patients need to let their doctors know if they are feeling depressed because doctors and other mental health professionals can help people deal with depression. Patients should also learn as much as possible about the disorder and treatment choices so that they can participate in making important decisions about medical care.

Talking with other people who have vitiligo may also help a person cope. The National Vitiligo Foundation can provide information about vitiligo and refer people to local chapters that have support groups of patients, families, and physicians. Family and friends are another source of support.

Some people with vitiligo have found that cosmetics that cover the white patches improve their appearance and help them feel better about themselves. A person may need to experiment with several brands of concealing cosmetics before finding the product that works best.

What Treatment Options Are Available?

The goal of treating vitiligo is to restore the function of the skin and to improve the patient's appearance. Therapy for vitiligo takes a long time—it

Vitiligo

usually must be continued for 6 to 18 months. The choice of therapy depends on the number of white patches and how widespread they are and on the patient's preference for treatment. Each patient responds differently to therapy, and a particular treatment may not work for everyone. Current treatment options for vitiligo include medical, surgical, and adjunctive therapies (therapies that can be used along with surgical or medical treatments).

> **☞ Remember!!**
>
> In summary form, here are the treatment options for vitiligo:
>
> - Medical therapies
>   - ◊ Topical steroid therapy
>   - ◊ Topical psoralen photochemotherapy
>   - ◊ Oral psoralen photochemotherapy
>   - ◊ Depigmentation
> - Surgical therapies
>   - ◊ Skin grafts from a person's own tissues (autologous)
>   - ◊ Skin grafts using blisters
>   - ◊ Micropigmentation (tattooing)
>   - ◊ Autologous melanocyte transplants
> - Adjunctive therapies
>   - ◊ Sunscreens
>   - ◊ Cosmetics
>   - ◊ Counseling and support

Medical Therapies

Topical Steroid Therapy

Steroids may be helpful in repigmenting the skin (returning color to white patches), particularly if started early in the disease. Corticosteroids are a group of drugs similar to the hormones produced by the adrenal glands (such as cortisone). Doctors often prescribe a mild topical corticosteroid cream for children under 10 years old and a stronger one for adults. Patients must apply the cream to the white patches on their skin for at least three months before seeing any results. It is the simplest and safest treatment but not as effective as psoralen photochemotherapy. The doctor will closely monitor the patient for side effects such as skin shrinkage and skin striae (streaks or lines on the skin).

Psoralen Photochemotherapy

Psoralen photochemotherapy (psoralen plus ultraviolet A therapy, or PUVA) is probably the most beneficial treatment for vitiligo available in the United States. The goal of PUVA therapy is to repigment the white patches. However, it is time-consuming and care must be taken to avoid side effects, which can sometimes be severe. Psoralens are drugs that contain chemicals that react with ultraviolet light to cause darkening of the skin. The treatment involves taking psoralen by mouth (orally) or applying it to the skin (topically). This is followed by carefully timed exposure to ultraviolet A (UVA) light from a special lamp or to sunlight. Patients usually receive treatments in their doctors' offices so they can be carefully watched for any side effects. Patients must minimize exposure to sunlight at other times.

Topical Psoralen Photochemotherapy

Topical psoralen photochemotherapy often is used for people with a small number of depigmented patches (affecting less than 20 percent of the body). It is also used for children two years old and older who have localized patches of vitiligo. Treatments are done in a doctor's office under artificial UVA light once or twice a week. The doctor or nurse applies a thin coat of psoralen to the patient's depigmented patches about 30 minutes before UVA light exposure. The patient is then exposed to an amount of UVA light that turns the affected area pink. The doctor usually increases the dose of UVA light slowly over many weeks. Eventually, the pink areas fade and a more normal skin color appears. After each treatment, the patient washes his or her skin with soap and water and applies a sunscreen before leaving the doctor's office.

There are two major potential side effects of topical PUVA therapy: severe sunburn and blistering, and too much repigmentation or darkening of the treated patches or the normal skin surrounding the vitiligo (hyperpigmentation). Patients can minimize their chances of sunburn if they avoid exposure to direct sunlight after each treatment. Hyperpigmentation is usually a temporary problem and eventually disappears when treatment is stopped.

Oral Psoralen Photochemotherapy

Oral PUVA therapy is used for people with more extensive vitiligo (affecting greater than 20 percent of the body) or for people who do not respond to topical PUVA therapy. Oral psoralen is not recommended for children under 10 years of age because of an increased risk of damage to the eyes, such as cataracts. For oral PUVA therapy, the patient takes a prescribed dose of psoralen by mouth about two hours before exposure to artificial UVA light or sunlight. The doctor adjusts the dose of light until the skin areas being treated become pink. Treatments are usually given two or three times a week, but never two days in a row.

For patients who cannot go to a PUVA facility, the doctor may prescribe psoralen to be used with natural sunlight exposure. The doctor will give the patient careful instructions on carrying out treatment at home and monitor the patient during scheduled checkups.

Known side effects of oral psoralen include sunburn, nausea and vomiting, itching, abnormal hair growth, and hyperpigmentation. Oral psoralen photochemotherapy may increase the risk of skin cancer. To avoid sunburn and reduce the risk of skin cancer, patients undergoing oral PUVA therapy should apply sunscreen and avoid direct sunlight for 24 to 48 hours after each treatment. Patients should also wear protective UVA sunglasses for 18 to 24 hours after each treatment to avoid eye damage, particularly cataracts.

Depigmentation

Depigmentation involves fading the rest of the skin on the body to match the already white areas. For people who have vitiligo on more than 50 percent of their bodies, depigmentation may be the best treatment option. Patients apply the drug monobenzylether of hydroquinone (monobenzone or Benoquin®) twice a day to pigmented areas until they match the already depigmented areas. Patients must avoid direct skin-to-skin contact with other people for at least two hours after applying the drug.

The major side effect of depigmentation therapy is inflammation (redness and swelling) of the skin. Patients may experience itching, dry skin, or abnormal darkening of the membrane that covers the white of the eye. Depigmentation is permanent and cannot be reversed. In addition, a person who undergoes depigmentation will always be abnormally sensitive to sunlight.

Surgical Therapies

All surgical therapies must be viewed as experimental because their effectiveness and side effects remain to be fully defined.

Autologous Skin Grafts

In an autologous (use of a person's own tissues) skin graft, the doctor removes skin from one area of a patient's body and attaches it to another area. This type of skin grafting is sometimes used for patients with small patches of vitiligo. The doctor removes sections of the normal, pigmented skin (donor sites) and places them on the depigmented areas (recipient sites).

There are several possible complications of autologous skin grafting. Infections may occur at the donor or recipient sites. The recipient and donor sites may develop scarring, a cobblestone appearance, or a spotty pigmentation, or they may fail to repigment at all. Treatment with grafting takes time and is costly, and most people find it neither acceptable nor affordable.

Skin Grafts With Blisters

In this procedure, the doctor creates blisters on the patient's pigmented skin by using heat, suction, or freezing cold. The tops of the blisters are then cut out and transplanted to a depigmented skin area. The risks of blister grafting include the development of a cobblestone appearance, scarring, and lack of repigmentation. However, there is less risk of scarring with this procedure than with other types of grafting.

Micropigmentation (Tattooing)

Tattooing implants pigment into the skin with a special surgical instrument. This procedure works best for the lip area, particularly in people with dark skin; however, it is difficult for the doctor to match perfectly the color of the skin of the surrounding area. Tattooing tends to fade over time. In addition, tattooing of the lips may lead to episodes of blister outbreaks caused by the herpes simplex virus.

Autologous Melanocyte Transplants

In this procedure, the doctor takes a sample of the patient's normal pigmented skin and places it in a laboratory dish containing a special cell culture solution to grow melanocytes. When the melanocytes in the culture solution have multiplied, the doctor transplants them to the patient's depigmented skin patches. This procedure is currently experimental and is impractical for the routine care of people with vitiligo.

Additional Therapies

Sunscreens

People who have vitiligo, particularly those with fair skin, should use a sunscreen that provides protection from both the UVA and UVB forms of ultraviolet light. Sunscreen helps protect the skin from sunburn and long-term damage. Sunscreen also minimizes tanning, which makes the contrast between normal and depigmented skin less noticeable.

Cosmetics

Some patients with vitiligo cover depigmented patches with stains, makeup, or self-tanning lotions. These cosmetic products can be particularly effective for people whose vitiligo is limited to exposed areas of the body. Dermablend, Lydia O'Leary, Clinique, Fashion Flair, Vitadye, and Chromelin offer makeup or dyes that patients may find helpful for covering up depigmented patches.

Counseling And Support Groups

Many people with vitiligo find it helpful to get counseling from a mental health professional. People often find they can talk to their counselor about issues that are difficult to discuss with anyone else. A mental health counselor can also offer patients support and help in coping with vitiligo. In addition, it may be helpful to attend a vitiligo support group.

What Research Is Being Done On Vitiligo?

For more than a decade, research on how melanocytes play a role in vitiligo has greatly increased. This includes research on autologous melanocyte transplants. At the University of Colorado, the National Institute of Arthritis and Musculoskeletal and Skin Diseases supports a large collaborative project involving families with vitiligo in the United States and the United Kingdom. To date, over 2,400 patients are involved. It is hoped that genetic analysis of these families will uncover the location—and possibly the specific gene or genes—conferring susceptibility to the disease. Doctors and researchers continue to look for the causes of, and new treatments for, vitiligo.

Chapter 39

Sebaceous Cysts

Alternative Names

Epidermal cyst; keratin cyst; epidermoid cyst.

Definition

A closed sac found just under the skin containing "pasty" or "cheesy"-looking skin secretions.

Causes And Risks

Sebaceous cysts most often arise from swollen hair follicles. Skin trauma can also induce a cyst to form. A sac of cells is created into which a protein called keratin is secreted.

These cysts are usually found on the face, neck, and trunk. They are usually slow-growing, painless, freely movable lumps beneath the skin. Occasionally, however, a cyst will become inflamed and tender.

Symptoms

- Usually a nontender, small lump beneath the skin.

About This Chapter: © 2002 A.D.A.M., Inc. Reprinted with permission.

- Redness, tenderness, or increased temperature of the skin over the area may indicate infection.

- Grayish white, cheesy, foul-smelling material may drain from the cyst.

Signs And Tests

In most cases, your physician can diagnose a cyst based on its appearance. Occasionally, a biopsy may be needed to rule out other conditions with a similar appearance.

Treatment

Sebaceous cysts are not dangerous and can usually be ignored. At times, they may become inflamed and tender. Others may grow large and interfere with day-to-day life. In these cases, you can have them surgically removed in a physician's office. Alternatively, small inflamed cysts can be treated by injection of steroid medications.

> **Weird Words**
>
> Cyst: Any abnormal, saclike growth filled with gas, liquid, or semisolid material.
>
> Excision: Surgical removal by cutting out abnormal or diseased tissue.
>
> Source: Adapted from *Stedman's Medical Dictionary*, 27th Edition, © 2000. Lippincott Williams, and Wilkins. All rights reserved. Reprinted with permission.

Prognosis

Most cysts may be ignored or treated with simple surgery.

Complications

These cysts may occasionally become infected and form into painful abscesses. Recurrence after excision is also not unusual.

When To Call Your Health Care Provider

Call your health care provider if you notice any new growths on your body. Though cysts are not dangerous, your doctor should examine you to ensure that skin cancer is not present.

Chapter 40

Warts

What Causes Warts?

Warts are a type of infection caused by viruses in the human papillomavirus (HPV) family. Warts can grow on all parts of your body. They can grow on your skin, on the inside of your mouth, on your genitals, and on your rectal area. Some types of HPV tend to cause warts on the skin, while other HPV types tend to cause warts on the genitals and rectal area. Some people are more naturally resistant to the HPV viruses and don't seem to get warts as easily as other people.

Will Warts Go Away On Their Own?

Sometimes yes and sometimes no. Often warts disappear on their own, although it may take many months, or even years, for the warts to go away. Some warts won't go away on their own. It is not known why some warts disappear and others don't.

Do Warts Need To Be Treated?

Generally, yes. Warts are often bothersome. They can bleed and cause pain when they're bumped. They also can cause embarrassment, for example,

---

About This Chapter: Reprinted with permission from at http://familydoctor.org/handouts/209.html. Copyright © 2002 American Academy of Family Physicians. All rights reserved.

if they grow on your face. Treatment may also decrease the chance that the warts will be spread to other areas of your body or to other people.

How Are Warts On The Skin Removed?

First of all, it's important to know that warts on the skin (such as on the fingers, feet, and knees) and warts on the genitals are removed in different ways. Don't try any home remedies or over-the-counter drugs to remove warts on the genital area. You could damage your genital area by putting certain chemicals on it. You also shouldn't treat warts on your face without talking to your doctor first.

The following are some ways to remove warts from the skin:

> ♣ It's A Fact!!
> ### Can Warts Be Passed From One Person To Another Person?
> Yes. Warts on the skin may be passed to another person when that person touches the warts. It is also possible to get warts from using towels or other objects that were used by a person who has warts.
>
> Warts on the genitals can be passed to another person during sexual intercourse. It is important not to have unprotected sex if you or your partner has warts on the genital area. In a woman, warts can grow on the cervix (inside the vagina), and she may not know she has them. The woman may pass the infection to her sexual partner without even knowing it.

- *Applying salicylic acid.* For warts on places such as the hands, feet, or knees, one treatment method is to put salicylic acid (one brand name: Compound W®) on the warts. To get good results, you must apply the acid every day for many weeks. After you take a bath or shower, pat your skin dry lightly with a towel. Then put salicylic acid on your warts. The acid sinks in deeper and works better when it is applied to damp skin. Before you take a shower or a bath the next day, use an emery board or pumice stone to file away the dead surface of the warts.

- *Applying cantharidin.* Your doctor may use cantharidin on your warts. With this treatment, the doctor "paints" the chemical onto the wart. Most people don't feel any pain when the chemical is applied to the wart. You'll experience some pain and blistering of the wart in about three to eight hours. After treatment with cantharidin, a bandage is put over the wart. The bandage can be removed after 24 hours. When mixtures of cantharidin and other chemicals are used, the bandage is removed after two hours. When you see your doctor again, he or she will remove the dead skin of the wart. If the wart isn't gone after one treatment, your doctor may give you another treatment.

- *Applying liquid nitrogen.* Your doctor may use liquid nitrogen to freeze the wart. This treatment is called cryotherapy. Applying liquid nitrogen to the wart causes a little discomfort. To completely remove a wart, liquid nitrogen treatments may be needed every one to three weeks for a total of two to four times. If no improvement is noted, your doctor may recommend another type of treatment.

- *Other treatments for warts on the skin.* Other ways that your doctor can remove warts on the skin include burning the wart, cutting out the wart, and removing the wart with a laser. These treatments are stronger, but they may leave a scar. Ask your doctor about the risks and benefits of these treatments before you decide what kind of treatment to have for your warts.

How Are Warts In The Genital Area Treated?

Warts on the genital area aren't treated exactly like warts

> ### ✏ Weird Words
>
> Cryotherapy: The use of extreme cold to kill or remove abnormal or diseased tissue. Liquid nitrogen is commonly used in cryotherapy because its temperature is −320° F.
>
> Human papillomavirus (HPV): A group of over 70 closely related, easily transmitted viruses. Some HPVs cause warts; others cause cancer of the cervix.
>
> Interferon: A type of protein produced by cells in response to infection by viruses. Interferon acts as a natural antiviral agent to stop or reverse the infection.
>
> Podophyllin: A resinous extract of the North American mayapple plant (*Podophyllum peltatum*) used medicinally since precolonial times. Podophyllin's caustic properties make it useful in treating warts.
>
> Source: Adapted from *Stedman's Medical Dictionary, 27th Edition,* © 2000. Lippincott Williams, and Wilkins. All rights reserved. Reprinted with permission.

on other parts of the skin. The following are some ways to treat warts on the genitals:

- *Applying liquid nitrogen.* Warts on the genitals may be frozen with liquid nitrogen (cryotherapy). With liquid nitrogen treatment, the doctor applies the liquid nitrogen at a number of different office visits until the warts are completely gone.

- *Applying podophyllin.* Warts on the genitals may be treated weekly with podophyllin by your doctor. You may also put a medicine called podofilox (brand name: Condylox®) on the warts at home twice a day for three days, and then rest for four days. This process is repeated weekly until the warts are gone.

- *Loop electrosurgical excision procedure* (LEEP. With this method for removing genital warts, the doctor passes a sharp instrument shaped like a loop underneath the wart, cutting the wart out of the skin.

> ✔ **Quick Tip**
> **Do Warts Ever Come Back?**
>
> Most of the time, treatment of warts is successful and the warts are gone for good. Your body's immune system can usually get rid of any tiny bits of wart that may be left after a wart has been treated. If warts come back, though, see your doctor to talk about other ways to treat them.

- CO_2 *laser surgery.* For large warts in the genital area, laser surgery may be needed for complete removal.

- *Interferon injections.* If genital warts don't go away after they've been treated with different methods, your doctor may try an interferon injection into the warts. Interferon is a chemical that our bodies make. It helps our immune system fight infection. An injection of interferon into the wart may help your body's immune system fight the virus that is causing the wart. Generally, interferon is injected into warts twice a week for up to eight weeks, or until the warts are gone.

Chapter 41

Fever Blisters And Cold Sores

Cold sores and fever blisters are names for a common medical condition called herpes labialis. They are uncomfortable, annoying little blisters that form on the lips and around the mouth and nose. Up to 25 percent of all adults are troubled by this incurable condition, which can recur for many people time and time again.

What Causes Cold Sores And Fever Blisters?

Cold sores and fever blisters are caused primarily by the herpes simplex virus type 1 (HSV-1). Herpes simplex virus type 2 (HSV-2), which usually causes genital herpes infections, is also now known to infect the face and mouth and cause cold sores. HSV-1 and HSV-2 are very common viruses among humans and are easily spread from person to person.

Infection occurs when someone is exposed to the herpes virus by contact with fluids containing herpes virus from an infected person. Simple things like kissing, sharing utensils and drinks, and not washing hands after touching blisters can result in the spread of HSV to others and cause infection. Furthermore, it is suspected that oral-genital sexual contact with an infected person can also lead to HSV-1 or HSV-2 cold sores.

About This Chapter: Taken from "Cold Sores and Fever Blisters," University of Arizona, Campus Health Pharmacy, http://rx.health.arizona.edu/coldsores.htm, © 2001. Reprinted with permission; all rights reserved.

Once infected, the virus continues to live in nerve cells within the skin. The virus lies dormant in nerve roots until the time it might resurface and cause a cold sore outbreak. Recurrent cold sore outbreaks can be triggered by emotional or physical stress. Trauma, illness, menstruation, and sun exposure can all activate dormant herpes virus. It is not possible to predict the frequency or severity of recurrences; in fact, some people may never have a recurrence at all.

What Are The Symptoms?

There are two types of HSV infections: primary and recurrent. Primary infection after initial exposure is often associated with fever, headache, sore throat, and malaise, as well as the characteristic blisters. Sores of a primary infection appear 2 to 20 days after contact with an infected person and can last from 7 to 10 days.

Recurrent cold sores usually affect the same location as the initial outbreak. They are usually less severe than primary infections, and associated

---

✔ **Quick Tip**

Avoiding Cold Sores

Avoiding infection by HSV is the only sure way to avoid getting cold sores; unfortunately, this is no easy task. It requires careful avoidance of contact with virus-containing fluids from infected people. Kissing or sharing of foods, beverages, utensils, towels, toothbrushes, and so forth with someone with active cold sores is a sure way to get infected. Individuals infected with HSV-1 or HSV-2 should actively avoid exposing others to the virus. Sexual partners should be informed of herpes status prior to engaging in behaviors with a high risk of transmitting HSV.

Avoiding triggers, such as physical or emotional stress, can minimize recurrent cold sore outbreaks.

Fever Blisters And Cold Sores

symptoms are often absent. Sores tend to be smaller, less painful, and of shorter duration, resolving in an average of five days.

Both primary and recurrent cold sore outbreaks are often preceded by a sense of numbness, itching, tingling, or burning around the area where blisters will form. These "prodromal symptoms" may occur one to 48 hours prior to the appearance of blisters.

As the blisters emerge, they fill with virus-containing fluid and can be painful. Over the next two to three days the sores may ooze and then form a yellow crust. Eventually, the crusts fall off, leaving slightly red skin, which usually heals completely and rarely leaves a scar.

How Can I Treat Active Cold Sores?

Herpes labialis is often left untreated, and outbreaks usually resolve on their own without scarring. Good wound care is essential to avoid secondary bacterial infection of the involved tissue. The sores should be kept clean, and picking at sores or crusts should be avoided in order to promote quick healing and limit spreading of the virus containing blister fluids. Prescription and nonprescription medications may be used to effectively control symptoms and expedite healing.

Your physician may prescribe certain oral or topical antiviral medications in order to treat HSV infections. Topical antiviral medications such as 5 percent acyclovir ointment (Zovirax®) and 1 percent penciclovir cream (Denavir®) are frequently used for recurrent herpes labialis cold sores. Both products may shorten the duration of pain and time to healing of the sores. They must be applied soon after the first sign of a recurrence and every two or three hours while awake for four or more days. Antiviral drugs like acyclovir (Zovirax), famciclovir (Famvir®), and valacyclovir (Valtrex®) may also be taken orally to shorten the duration and severity of primary infections and severe recurrences.

Over-the-counter products are also effective in treating cold sore outbreaks. Analgesics such as acetaminophen (Tylenol®) or ibuprofen (Advil®, Motrin®) can help control, fever, aches, and pain associated with primary infection or recurrent outbreaks.

Topical anesthetics, such as tetracaine, benzocaine, lidocaine, or camphor, are effective for quick relief of pain and itching. Tetracaine cream has also been shown to reduce time to healing of cold sores in clinical trials compared with placebo. These agents are available as creams, ointments, gels, and lotions under a variety of brand names, such as Hurricaine®, Campho-Phenique®, Orabase®, Orajel®, Zilactin®, and others. All usually require frequent application and are suitable for use around the mouth.

Newly available is 10 percent docosanol cream (Abreva®), approved by the FDA for the over-the-counter treatment of herpes labialis. Docosanol appears to inhibit viral entry into cells, which is required for viral replication and infection, a mechanism different from prescription antiviral medications. In clinical studies docosanol showed a similar reduction in the average time to healing of sores as prescription penciclovir cream. Like the prescription topical antiviral medications, Abreva must be started early after the first sign of recurrence and applied five times daily.

Chapter 42

Lyme Disease

What Is Lyme Disease?

Lyme disease is a bacterial illness caused by a bacterium called a spirochete. The actual name of the bacterium is *Borrelia burgdorferi*. Lyme disease is spread by ticks when they bite the skin, permitting the bacterium to infect the body. Lyme disease can cause abnormalities in the skin, joints, heart, and nervous system.

Interestingly, the disease only became apparent in 1975 when mothers of a group of children who lived near each other in Lyme, Connecticut, made researchers aware that their children all were diagnosed with rheumatoid arthritis. This unusual grouping of illness that appeared "rheumatoid" eventually led researchers to the identification of the bacterial cause of Lyme disease in 1982.

The number of cases of the disease in an area depends on the amount of ticks in an area and how often the ticks are infected with the bacteria. In certain areas of New York, where Lyme disease is common, over half of the ticks are infected. Lyme disease appears most often in the northeastern United States, but has been reported in all 50 states as well as China, Europe, Japan,

About This Chapter: Source: MedicineNet, Inc. (wwwmedicinet.com). © 2002; reprinted with permission.

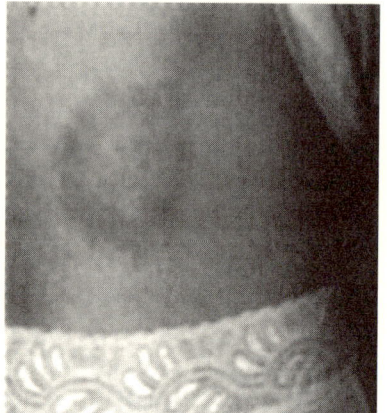

Figure 42.1. The characteristic bull's-eye rash—known technically as erythema migrans—of early-stage Lyme disease. Source: © California Department of Health Services, 2001; reprinted with permission.

Australia, and parts of the former Soviet Union. In the United States, it is primarily contracted in the Northeast from Maine to Maryland, in the Midwest in Minnesota and Wisconsin, and in the West in Oregon and northern California.

What Are Symptoms And Signs Of Lyme Disease?

Lyme disease affects different areas of the body in varying degrees as it progresses. The site where the tick attaches to the body is where the bacteria enter through the skin. Initially, the disease affects the skin and also causes "flulike" symptoms. Later, it produces abnormalities in the joints, heart, and nervous system.

Lyme disease is medically described in three phases as: (1) early localized disease with skin inflammation; (2) early disseminated disease with heart and nervous system involvement, including palsies and meningitis; (3) late disease featuring motor and sensory nerve damage, brain inflammation, and arthritis.

In the early phase of the illness, within hours to weeks of the tick bite, the local skin develops an expanding ring of unraised redness (see Figure 42.1). There may be an outer ring of brighter redness and a central area of clearing, leading to a bull's-eye appearance. This classic initial rash is called erythema migrans (formerly called erythema chronicum migrans). Patients often can't recall the tick bite (the ticks can be as small as the periods in this paragraph). Also, they may not have the identifying rash to signal the doctor. More than one in four patients never gets a rash. The redness of the skin is often accompanied by generalized fatigue, muscle and joint stiffness, swollen glands, and headache.

Weeks to months after the initial redness of the skin, the bacterium and its effects spread throughout the body. It is then that disease in the joints, heart, and nervous system occurs.

The later phases of Lyme disease can affect the heart, causing inflammation of the heart muscle. This can result in abnormal heart rhythm and heart failure. The nervous system can develop facial muscle paralysis (Bell's palsy), abnormal sensation due to disease of peripheral nerves (peripheral neuropathy), meningitis, and confusion. Arthritis, or inflammation in the joints, begins with swelling, stiffness, and pain. Usually, only one or a few joints become affected, most commonly the knees. The arthritis of Lyme disease can look like many other types of arthritis and can become chronic.

How Is Lyme Disease Diagnosed?

In early Lyme disease doctors can sometimes make a diagnosis simply by finding the classic red rash. The doctor might review the patient's history and examine the patient in order to exclude diseases with similar findings in the joints, heart, and nervous system. Blood testing for antibodies to Lyme bacteria also can help in diagnosis. (Antibodies are produced by the body to attack the bacteria and can be evidence of exposure to the bacteria. These antibodies can be detected with a laboratory method called an ELISA assay.) Antibodies, however, can be false indicators of disease, since they can remain for years after the disease is cured. Currently, the confirmatory test that is most reliable is the Western blot assay antibody test. More accurate tests are being developed.

How Is Lyme Disease Treated?

Most Lyme disease is curable with antibiotics. This is so true that some authors of Lyme disease research have stated that the most common cause of lack of response of Lyme disease to antibiotics is a lack of Lyme disease to begin with! The type of antibiotic depends on the stage of the disease (early or late) and what areas of the body are affected. Early illness is usually treated with oral medicines, for example, doxycycline (Vibramycin®). Therefore, if a person finds the typical bull's-eye skin rash developing in an area of a tick bite, he or she should seek medical attention as soon as possible. Later illness such as nervous system disease might require intravenous drugs, such as ceftriaxone (Rocephin®).

For the relief of symptoms, pain-relieving medicines might be added. Swollen joints can be reduced by the doctor removing fluid from them (arthrocentesis). An arthrocentesis is a procedure whereby fluid is removed from a joint using a needle and syringe under sterile conditions. It is usually performed in a doctor's office. Rarely, even with appropriate antibiotics, arthritis persists. The doctor also can inject cortisone into swollen joints or use oral medications, such as ibuprofen (Motrin®, Nuprin®), to reduce inflammation and improve function.

How Can Lyme Disease Be Prevented?

Because Lyme disease is transmitted by ticks attaching to the body, it is important to use tick-bite avoidance techniques when you are visiting known tick areas. Wearing long clothing can protect the skin. Clothing, children, and pets should be examined for ticks. Ticks can be removed gently with tweezers and saved in a jar for later identification. Bathing the skin and scalp and washing clothing upon returning home might prevent the bite and transmission of the disease.

Scientists have recently completed studies of vaccines against Lyme disease, and these vaccines are now available. These vaccines are particularly beneficial for persons living in areas where Lyme disease is known to be common and who have frequent exposure to the ticks that carry the Lyme disease bacterium. The vaccine is not recommended for persons who are not significantly exposed to such ticks. The vaccines require a series of three injections; the second injection is given one month after the first, and the third 12 months after the first. The full benefits of the vaccines are achieved only after the third booster dose (one year after the vaccination series is begun). After the second vaccination (the second month), there is only about 50 percent protection against Lyme disease. The complete series of vaccinations, however, confers about 80 percent to 90 percent protection.

—by William C. Shiel, Jr., M.D., F.A.C.P., F.A.C.R.

☞ Remember!!

- Lyme disease is a bacterial illness that is spread by tick bites.
- Lyme disease can affect the skin, joints, heart, and the nervous system.
- Lyme disease occurs in phases, the early phase beginning at the site of the tick bite with an expanding ring of redness.
- Lyme disease is diagnosed based on the patient's clinical signs of illness and the detection of Lyme antibodies in the blood.
- Lyme disease is treated with antibiotics.

Chapter 43

Cat Scratch Disease

Signs And Symptoms

Cat scratch disease is an infection that causes swelling of the lymph nodes (swollen glands) after an animal scratch—most often from a cat.

A blister or a small bump often develops 3 to 10 days after the scratch and may be mistaken for an insect bite. The blister or bump at the site of a cat scratch is called an inoculation lesion (injury site where germs enter the body), and it is most commonly found on the arms and hands, head, and scalp.

The first clue to diagnosing this illness is history of exposure to a cat or kitten. About 55 percent to 70 percent of people with the infection have a cat scratch somewhere on their bodies.

Usually within two weeks of a cat scratch, lymph nodes close to the area of the inoculation lesion will swell and become tender (lymph nodes are bean-shaped organs of the immune system that are often called glands).

These swollen lymph nodes or glands appear most often in the underarm area, neck, and above the collar bone. They range in size from about 1/2 inch

---

About This Chapter This information was provided by KidsHealth, one of the largest resources online for medically reviewed information written for parents, kids, and teens. For more articles like this one, visit www.KidsHealth.org or www.TeensHealth.org. © 2001 The Nemours Center for Children's Health Media, a division of the Nemours Foundation.

to 2 inches (1 to 5 centimeters) in diameter and may be surrounded by a larger area of swelling under the skin. The swollen lymph nodes may also be painful or tender, and the skin over them may be red. Swollen lymph nodes may persist for months.

In most children and adolescents, swollen lymph nodes are the main symptom of the disease. About one third of people with cat scratch disease have other, more generalized symptoms. These include fever (usually less than 101 degrees Fahrenheit or 38.3 degrees Celsius), fatigue, loss of appetite, headache, and a generally "ill" feeling.

Cat scratch disease does not appear in its usual form in about 9 percent to 14 percent of cases. Instead, it may appear in a form called Parinaud oculoglandular syndrome, with the following symptoms: an inoculation site that looks like a small sore on the conjunctiva (membrane lining the eye surface) of one eye; swollen lymph nodes in the area around the ears; and (sometimes) redness of the involved eye. Other unusual forms of cat scratch disease include osteomyelitis (bone infection), pneumonia (lung infection), liver and spleen abscesses, and prolonged fevers without any other findings.

Very rarely, people with cat scratch disease have symptoms that may include seizures. These symptoms usually begin one to six weeks after swollen lymph nodes appear and are severe for one to two weeks. People usually recover slowly, but completely.

Description

Bartonella henselae is the bacterium that causes cat scratch disease. It is found in all parts of the world, and over 80 percent of cases affect people under age 21. Most cases occur in fall and winter. In the United States, about 22,000 cases occur annually. Worldwide, the disease affects nine out of every 100,000 persons each year, and multiple cases within families are common, especially among those who have the same cat.

A cat with *Bartonella henselae* infection does not look sick. Experts believe that up to 44 percent of cats have a *Bartonella henselae* infection at some time in their lives.

Cat Scratch Disease

Incubation

It usually takes 3 to 10 days for a blister or small bump to appear at the site of a cat scratch. Lymph node swelling usually begins about 2 weeks after the cat scratch, with a range of 7 to 60 days.

Duration

Swollen lymph nodes usually disappear within two to six months in nearly all cases. Having one episode of cat scratch disease usually makes people immune for the rest of their lives.

Contagiousness

Cat scratch disease is not contagious from person to person. It is transmitted by the scratch of an infected animal, most often a kitten. Kittens or cats may carry these bacteria in their blood for months. Cats with these bacteria do not need to be put to sleep.

Prevention

Teaching children to avoid stray or unfamiliar cats can prevent cat scratch disease. If your child is scratched by a pet—even one of your own household pets—wash the injured area thoroughly with soap and water.

If you have a cat in your home, ask your veterinarian's advice about having the cat declawed. If you suspect that someone in your family has caught cat scratch disease from your family pet, you don't need to worry that the animal will need to be put to sleep. Talk with your veterinarian about the problem.

Professional Treatment

Diagnosis is usually based on the following (although not all of the following are necessary for diagnosis):

- Your child's history of being exposed to cats or kittens
- A physical examination for signs of a cat scratch and swollen lymph nodes

- Negative skin tests, blood tests, and cultures to rule out other causes of swollen lymph nodes

- A positive cat scratch blood test, available through your child's doctor or hospital

- A microscopic examination of a removed lymph node consistent with cat scratch disease

Rarely, a swollen lymph node becomes so large and painful that your child's doctor may recommend its removal. This is usually done in a very simple surgical procedure with a small incision.

Antibiotics are generally used to treat the disease, especially the unusual forms of cat scratch disease. If your child's doctor has prescribed antibiotics, give medication to your child on schedule for as many days as your child's doctor has advised. Use nonprescription medicines, like acetaminophen, to relieve pain of swollen lymph nodes and to lower fever.

In most cases, swollen lymph nodes usually subside within two to four months.

Home Treatment

A child with cat scratch disease doesn't need to be isolated from other family members. Bed rest is not necessary, but it may help a child with cat scratch disease who tires easily. If your child feels like playing, encourage quiet play, taking care to avoid injuring areas of swollen lymph nodes. For localized care of swollen lymph nodes, try moist compresses of salty water.

Chapter 44

Impetigo

What Is Impetigo?

Impetigo is an infection of the skin caused primarily by the bacterium *Streptococcus pyogenes*, also known as Group A beta-hemolytic streptococcus (GABS). Sometimes another bacterium, *Staphylococcus aureus*, can also be isolated from impetigo lesions.

What Are The Symptoms Of Impetigo?

Impetigo begins as a cluster of small blisters that expand and rupture within the first 24 hours. The thin yellow fluid that drains from the ruptured blisters quickly dries, forming a honey-colored crust. Impetigo develops most frequently on the legs, but may also be found on the arms, face, and trunk. There is usually no fever.

How Does A Person Get Impetigo?

Impetigo may develop after the skin is infected with GABS. The bacterium is usually acquired from skin-to-skin contact with another person with impetigo. Less commonly, impetigo may develop when open skin lesions

---

About This Chapter: Taken from "Impetigo," Wisconsin Department of Health and Family Services, available electronically at http://www.dhfs.state.wi.us/healthtips/BCD/Impetigo.htm, July 2001.

(such as insect bites or burns) are infected following exposure to a person with streptococcal pharyngitis ("strep throat").

Who Gets Impetigo?

The infection is most common in settings where there is crowding or activities leading to close person-to-person contact, such as schools and military installations. Impetigo occurs more commonly during the summer and early fall.

How Long Does It Take To Develop Impetigo Following Exposure?

Impetigo may develop up to 10 days after the skin becomes infected with GABS.

How Is Impetigo Treated?

Impetigo may be treated with an antibiotic taken by mouth or by application of an antibiotic ointment to the affected areas.

How Long Is A Person Considered Infectious?

A person with impetigo is probably no longer infectious after 24 hours of adequate antibiotic treatment. Without treatment, a person may be infectious for several weeks.

What Are The Complications Of Impetigo?

Rarely, GABS may invade beyond the skin of a person with impetigo and cause more serious illnesses. Persons with

> **Weird Words**
>
> Glomerulonephritis: A disease in which the glomeruli—tufts of very small blood vessels in the kidneys—become inflamed. The word "nephritis" is built from Greek roots meaning "kidney inflammation."
>
> Impetigo: An infectious skin disease characterized by blisters and a yellow crust. The word "impetigo" comes from Latin and means "a scabby eruption."
>
> Source: Adapted from *Stedman's Medical Dictionary, 27th Edition*, © 2000. Lippincott Williams, and Wilkins. All rights reserved. Reprinted with permission.

impetigo may also develop post-streptococcal scarlet fever, or glomerulonephritis, a condition that may result in temporary kidney failure. Post-streptococcal glomerulonephritis follows roughly 10 days after the onset of streptococcal infection. However, the long-term prognosis is excellent. Scarlet fever is caused by a toxin produced by certain strains of GABS and is characterized by high fever, chills, sore throat, headache, vomiting, and a fine red rash.

What Can Be Done To Prevent Impetigo?

Simple cleanliness and prompt attention to minor wounds will do much to prevent impetigo. Persons with impetigo or symptoms of GABS infections should seek medical care and, if necessary, begin antibiotic treatment as soon as possible to prevent spread of the disease to others. Individuals with impetigo should be excluded from school, day care, or other situations where close person-to-person contact is likely until at least 24 hours after appropriate antibiotic therapy is begun. Sharing of towels, clothing, and other personal articles should be discouraged.

Chapter 45

Poison Oak, Ivy, And Sumac

As you venture outdoors this summer, you may encounter these aggravating plants. Be wary of them! They are the most common plants that cause skin rashes. Don't let them ruin your summer vacation!

Poison ivy, poison oak, and poison sumac all belong to the same genus, *Toxicodendron*. All three plants produce an oil, urushiol, that can penetrate the skin very easily. This oil is not really "poisonous." However, if you come into contact with it, you can develop an allergic reaction. The allergic reaction usually takes the form of a bothersome skin rash.

How Do I Get Poison Ivy, Oak, Or Sumac?

You can get the skin rash simply by touching the plant and coming into direct contact with the chemical, urushiol, that is produced by the plant. The urushiol is found in all parts of the plant, not only the leaves.

Sometimes, you don't even have to touch a plant to get the rash. You can get it by indirect contact. You can get the skin rash if you touch inanimate objects (such as clothes, shoes, garden tools, golf clubs, or furniture) that have the urushiol on them. You can also get the rash after touching a pet with urushiol on its fur.

About This Chapter: Taken from "Poison Ivy, Poison Oak, and Poison Sumac," written by Joyce Chen, M.D., © 2002 The Johns Hopkins University Student Health & Wellness Center, http://www.jhu.edu/~shcenter/poisonivy.html; reprinted with permission.

The urushiol can remain active for a long time on objects if they are not cleaned. Did you know that you can get the skin rash after touching an object exposed to urushiol years ago? Therefore, it is important to clean all objects and pets that may have urushiol on them.

Rubber or latex gloves are not effective against poison ivy or poison oak. Heavy-duty vinyl gloves, however, are protective against the urushiol.

It is estimated that 50 to 70 percent of the general population is clinically susceptible to the urushiol. Only humans and higher primates react to urushiol. Dogs and cats are lucky. They do not get poison oak or poison ivy rashes.

Persons who are allergic to poison oak, ivy, and sumac may also be allergic to other members of the same family (Anacardiaceae). This family includes the cashew nut tree, mango tree, and the Japanese lacquer tree.

What Are The Symptoms?

Symptoms include a very itchy rash with red patches or linear streaks. Occasionally blisters can develop. New lesions can appear up to three weeks after exposure. The rash usually develops on exposed areas of skin. However, any part of the body that comes into contact with the urushiol can develop an allergic reaction. For example, if you have urushiol on your hands and then you touch your forehead, then it is possible that you may develop a rash on your forehead.

Despite popular belief, the fluid from the sores or blisters is not contagious.

Usually the rash doesn't develop immediately after exposure to the plant. Sometime, it may take days before the rash appears.

What Can I Do To Prevent The Rash?

- The best prevention is to stay away from poison ivy, oak, and sumac. Learn to recognize them.
- Wear long pants or socks when hiking.

> ✔ Quick Tip
> **Recognizing Poisonous Ivy, Oak, And Sumac**
>
> The majority of poison oak and poison ivy plants have leaves in groups of three. However, some may have more. To be safe, avoid all plants that have three large green leaves on each stem. Poison oak, poison ivy, and poison sumac tend to produce greenish white berries in the autumn. Another helpful tip is to avoid plants with black spots. The urushiol, after it leaks out of the plant, can turn black.
>
> Each of the three varieties tends to grow in different parts of the country:
>
> - Poison ivy can be found all over the country but it is most predominant on the East Coast. It often grows as a vine, but it can also be found as a shrub.
> - Poison oak is generally found on the west coast and Canada. It can appear as a shrub or a vine.
> - Poison sumac is more commonly found in the southeastern United States in woody, swampy areas. Poison sumac has 7 to 13 leaves per stem. One leaf is located at the terminal end of the stem. The other leaves are located opposite each other in two rows.

- Bathe pets who come into contact with poison oak, ivy, and sumac. Try not to let your cat or dog run through the woods, where it may play in patches of poison ivy or oak.
- Don't burn any plants that look like poison ivy, sumac, or oak. The smoke can contain urushiol, which can cause an allergic reaction or lung irritation.
- Ivy Block® cream, which contains bentoquatam, may be applied prior to potential contact. However, it must be applied every four hours.
- If you have had contact with any of these plants, wash the exposed areas of skin with water and soap as soon as possible. Try to remove the urushiol from your skin within 10 minutes of exposure. All contaminated clothes should be removed as soon as possible.

What Can I Do If I Develop A Rash From Poison Ivy, Oak, Or Sumac?

Make sure that you wash all clothes and other items that may have been exposed to the plant. Also make sure you wash under your fingernails in order to remove any remaining traces of urushiol.

The rash usually disappears within two to three weeks.

You can do several things to ease the discomfort associated with the rash:

- Cool soaks or wet compresses may provide relief.
- Topical steroid creams (such as hydrocortisone) may help with mild rashes.
- Oral antihistamines (such as Benadryl®) can help the itching. Be aware that they can also make you sleepy or drowsy.
- You may use calamine lotion to help ease the itching.
- Aveeno® oatmeal baths may be soothing and help dry up the blisters.

Seek medical attention if:

- The itching becomes severe.
- The rash is severe or painful.
- You have shortness of breath.
- You develop swelling of the tongue, lips, throat, or mouth.
- You develop fever.

Chapter 46

Hives

Urticaria, commonly known as hives, usually strikes suddenly. First the skin itches, then it erupts into red welts. The itching may be severe, keeping people from working or sleeping. It's a distressing disorder that affects an estimated 20 percent of the population at one time or another in their lives.

What Is Urticaria?

Most cases of urticaria are acute, lasting from a few hours to less than six weeks. Some cases are chronic, lasting more than six weeks. The welts may appear in one place, disappear after a short time, then erupt at another spot, then another. They are made worse by scratching. Each individual hive lasts no more than 24 hours.

What Kinds Of Things Can Trigger Attacks Of Urticaria?

Bouts of urticaria have been traced to such triggers as infections, drugs (including aspirin), certain foods and additives, cold, sun exposure, insect stings, alcohol, exercise, endocrine disorders, and emotional stress. In some people, pressure caused by belts and constricting clothing causes eruption. Urticaria may be a response to infection including the common cold, strep throat, and infectious mononucleosis.

About This Chapter: Taken from "Urticaria," updated March 8, 2002, © 2002 The American College of Allergy, Asthma, and Immunology; reprinted with permission. Available online at http://www.allergy.mcg.edu/advice/urtic.html.

In the urticaria-prone person, these triggers cause the body to release chemical mediators, including histamine, from cells. Histamine (which causes itchy, runny noses and watery eyes in hay fever sufferers) dilates the walls of blood vessels, allowing fluids to leak out into the surrounding tissues. Swelling and itching are the result.

How Are Urticaria "Triggers" Identified?

In some cases, the trigger is obvious—a person eats strawberries or shrimp, then develops urticaria within a short time. But because there are so many possible causes for urticaria, other cases require determined detective work on the part of the patient and physician. In some cases, the cause is never identified.

A single episode of uncomplicated acute urticaria probably does not need formal evaluation. In the cases of patients with recurrent episodes of acute urticaria, with chronic urticaria, or with urticaria complicated by swelling, trouble breathing, or other potentially serious problems, an evaluation is recommended. See your regular physician first, in order to evaluate for non-allergic causes of urticaria. If allergy is suspected, keep a diary of foods eaten, any unusual exposures, and when you have hives. Bring the diary with you to the allergist's office. To unravel the urticaria puzzle, your allergist-immunologist will take a detailed history, looking for clues in your lifestyle that will help pinpoint the cause of your symptoms. You'll be asked about the

---

❧ Weird Words

Urticaria: Medical term for hives. The word is derived from the Latin *urtica*, which means "stinging nettle." The name for a plant that causes hives became attached to the hives themselves as a formal name.

Dermographism: Hives that arise from stroking a firm object against the skin. The word comes from Greek roots meaning "skin writing." A person with dermographism can "write" on the skin by tracing letters and words with an object like an eating utensil or matchstick.

Source: Adapted from *Stedman's Medical Dictionary, 27th Edition*, © 2000. Lippincott Williams, and Wilkins. All rights reserved. Reprinted with permission.

frequency and severity of your symptoms, your family's medical history, medications you're taking, your work and home environment, and miscellaneous matters. The allergist will want to review your diary for further clues.

In some cases you may require tests to analyze blood and urine, and other procedures such as x-rays. Skin testing may provide useful information in some cases. Your allergist-immunologist will decide which tests to order based on the different types of urticaria and the suspected cause.

What Are The Different Types Of Urticaria?

They can be classified into two categories: allergic and nonallergic.

Allergic urticaria is the least common form, although it is somewhat more common in children than in adults. It is caused by the immune system's overreaction to foods, drugs, infection, insect stings, blood transfusions, or other substances. Foods, such as eggs, nuts and shellfish, and drugs, such as penicillin and sulfa, are common causes of allergic or immunologic urticaria. Recent studies also suggest that some cases of chronic urticaria are caused by autoimmune mechanisms, when the patient develops immune reactions to components of his or her skin.

Nonallergic urticaria are those types of urticaria where a clear-cut allergic basis cannot be proven. These take many forms:

- Dermographism is urticaria that develops when the skin is stroked with a firm object.
- Cold-induced urticaria appears after a person is exposed to low temperatures—for example, after a plunge into a swimming pool or when an ice cube is placed against the skin.
- Cholinergic urticaria, which is associated with exercise, hot showers, and anxiety, is a form of hives that is related to release of certain chemicals from parts of the nervous system that controls such body functions as blood pressure and heart rate.
- Pressure urticaria develops from the constant pressure of constricting clothing such as sock bands, bra straps, belts, or other tight clothing.

- Solar urticaria arises on parts of the body exposed to the sun; this may occur within a few minutes after exposure.

Some cases of nonallergic urticaria may be caused by reactions to aspirin and, possibly, certain food dyes, sulfites, and other food additives. In many cases, particularly in chronic urticaria, the trigger for the problem can't be found; in this instance it is called idiopathic urticaria.

Certain types of urticaria are more painful than itchy and may go away, leaving a bruise on the skin; individual hives may last more than 24 hours. In such cases and certain other situations, a biopsy of the skin may be necessary for diagnosis.

How Is Urticaria Treated?

Your allergist first will prescribe medications, such as antihistamines, to alleviate the discomfort. Severe, complicated attacks of urticaria can be temporarily relieved by injections of epinephrine; rarely, corticosteroids may be prescribed for a short period. Other drugs may be required for specific types of urticaria.

If the cause can be identified, the best course of treatment is avoidance of the substance that triggers urticaria. If a problem with a specific food is strongly suspected, then it should be avoided. This may require a careful reading of packaged food labels and inquiry about ingredients in restaurant meals. Persons with solar urticaria should wear protective clothing and apply sunscreen lotions when outdoors. Loose-fitting clothing will help relieve pressure urticaria. Avoid harsh soaps and frequent bathing to reduce the problem of dry skin, which can cause itching and scratching that can aggravate urticaria. Vigorous toweling after a bath may precipitate hives.

Although success in identifying the cause of chronic urticaria varies from clinic to clinic according to patient populations, it usually is no higher than 20 percent of cases. Chronic urticaria may last for months or for years and burn itself out, never to bother the sufferer again.

Chapter 47

Swimmer's Itch

What Is Swimmer's Itch?

Swimmer's itch, also called cercarial dermatitis, is a skin rash caused by an allergic reaction to infection with certain parasites of birds and mammals. These microscopic parasites are released from infected snails to swim in fresh and salt water, such as lakes, ponds, and oceans used for swimming and wading. Infection is found throughout the world. Swimmer's itch generally occurs during summer months.

What Are The Signs And Symptoms Of Swimmer's Itch?

Within minutes to days after swimming in contaminated water, you may experience tingling, burning, or itching of the skin. Small reddish pimples appear within 12 hours. Pimples may develop into small blisters. Itching may last up to a week or more, but will gradually go away.

Because swimmer's itch is caused by an allergic reaction to infection, the more often you swim or wade in contaminated water, the more likely you are to develop more serious symptoms. The greater the number of exposures to

---

About This Chapter: Taken from "Fact Sheet: Cercarial Dermatitis," Division of Infectious Diseases, Centers for Disease Control; available online at http://www.cdc.gov/ncidod/dpd/parasites/schistosomiasis/factsht_cardmermatitis.htm, March 2002.

contaminated water, the more intense and immediate symptoms of swimmer's itch will be.

Be aware that there are other causes of rash that may occur after swimming in fresh and salt water.

Do I Need To See My Health Care Provider For Treatment?

No. Most cases do not require medical attention.

If you have a rash, you may try the following for relief:

- Corticosteroid cream
- Cool compresses
- Bath with baking soda
- Baking soda paste
- Anti-itch lotion
- Calamine® lotion
- Colloidal oatmeal baths, such as Aveeno®

> **Weird Words**
> Cercarial dermatitis: A skin rash caused by an allergic reaction to infection with certain parasites of birds and mammals; also known as swimmer's itch.

Try not to scratch. Scratching may cause the rash to become infected. If itching is severe, your health care provider may prescribe lotion or creams to lessen your symptoms.

How Does Water Become Infested With The Parasite?

The adult parasite lives in the blood of infected birds, such as ducks, geese, gulls, and swans, as well as certain aquatic mammals, such as muskrats and beavers. The parasites produce eggs that are passed in the feces of infected birds or mammals.

If the eggs land in the water, the water becomes contaminated. Eggs hatch, releasing small, free-swimming larvae. These larvae swim in the water in search of a certain species of aquatic snail.

If the larvae find one of these snails, they infect the snail and undergo further development. Infected snails release a different type of larvae (cercariae, hence the name cercarial dermatitis) into the water. This larval form then searches for a suitable host (bird, muskrat) so it can start the lifecycle over again. Although humans are not a suitable host, the larvae burrow into the skin of swimmers, which may cause an allergic reaction or rash. The larvae cannot develop inside a human, and they soon die.

Can Swimmer's Itch Be Spread From Person To Person?

No.

Who Is At Risk For Swimmer's Itch?

Anyone who swims or wades in infested water may be at risk. Larvae are more likely to be swimming along shallow water by the shoreline. Children are most often affected because they swim, wade, and play in the shallow

---

✔ **Quick Tip**

What Can Be Done To Reduce The Risk Of Swimmer's Itch?

- Avoid swimming in areas where swimmer's itch is a known problem or where signs have been posted warning of unsafe water.
- Avoid swimming near or wading in marshy areas where snails are commonly found.
- Towel dry or shower immediately after leaving the water.
- Encourage health officials to post signs on shorelines where swimmer's itch is a current problem.
- Do not attract birds by feeding them to areas where people are swimming.

For further information on protecting yourself from recreational water illnesses, please visit www.healthyswimming.org.

water more than adults. Also, they do not towel dry themselves when leaving the water.

Once An Outbreak Of Swimmer's Itch Has Occurred In Water, Will The Water Always Be Unsafe?

No. Many factors must be present for swimmer's itch to become a problem in water. Since these factors change (sometimes within a swim season), swimmer's itch will not always be a problem. However, there is no way to know how long water may be unsafe. Larvae are generally infective for 24 hours once they are released from the snail. However, an infected snail will continue to produce cercariae throughout the remainder of its life. For future snails to become infected, migratory birds or mammals in the area must also be infected so the lifecycle can continue.

Is My Swimming Pool Safe To Swim In?

Yes. As long as your swimming pool is well maintained and chlorinated, there is no risk of swimmer's itch.

Chapter 48

Athlete's Foot, Jock Itch, And Ringworm

What Is Tinea?

Tinea is a fungus that can grow on your skin, hair, or nails. As it grows, it spreads out in a circle, leaving normal-looking skin in the middle. This makes it look like a ring. At the edge of the ring, the skin is lifted up by the irritation and looks red and scaly. To some people, the infection looks like a worm is under the skin. Because of the way it looks, tinea infection is often called "ringworm." However, there really isn't a worm under the skin.

How Did I Get A Fungal Infection?

You can get a fungal infection by touching a person who has one. Some kinds of fungi live on damp surfaces, like the floors in public showers or locker rooms. You can easily pick up a fungus there. You can even catch a fungal infection from your pets. Dogs and cats, as well as farm animals, can be infected with a fungus. Often this infection looks like a patch of skin where fur is missing.

What Areas Of The Body Are Affected By Tinea Infections?

Fungal infections are named for the part of the body they infect.

About This Chapter: Reprinted with permission from http://familydoctor.org/handouts/316.html. Copyright © 2002 American Academy of Family Physicians. All rights reserved.

Tinea corporis is a fungal infection of the skin on the body ("corporis" is the Latin word meaning "of the body"). If you have this infection, you may see small, red spots that grow into large rings almost anywhere on your arms, legs, or chest.

Tinea pedis is usually called athlete's foot ("pedis" is the Latin word for "of the foot"). The moist skin between your toes is a perfect place for a fungus to grow. The skin may become itchy and red, with a white, wet surface. The infection may spread to the toenails (tinea unguium; "unguium" comes

---

✔ **Quick Tip**

Preventing Tinea Infections

Skin that is kept clean and dry is your best defense. However, you're also less likely to get a tinea infection if you do the following things:

- When you're at home, take your shoes off and expose your feet to the air.
- Change your socks and underwear every day, especially in warm weather.
- Dry your feet carefully (especially between the toes) after using a locker room or public shower.
- Avoid walking barefoot in public areas. Instead, wear "flip-flops," sandals, or water shoes.
- Don't wear thick clothing for long periods of time in warm weather. It will make you sweat more.
- Throw away worn-out exercise shoes. Never borrow other people's shoes.
- Check your pets for areas of hair loss. Ask your veterinarian to check them too. It's important to check pets carefully, because if you don't find out whether they're causing your fungal infection, you may get it again from them, even after treatment.

Athlete's Foot, Jock Itch, And Ringworm

from the Latin word for nail). Here it causes the toenails to become thick and crumbly. It can also spread to your hands and fingernails.

When a fungus grows in the moist, warm area of the groin, the rash is called tinea cruris ("cruris" is the Latin word meaning "of the leg"). The common name for this infection is "jock itch." Tinea cruris generally occurs in men, especially if they often wear athletic equipment.

Tinea capitis, which is called "ringworm," causes itchy, red areas, usually on the head ("capitis" is the Latin word meaning "of the head"). The hair is destroyed, leaving bald patches. This tinea infection is most common in children.

How Do I Know If I Have A Fungal Infection?

The best way to know for sure is to ask your doctor. Other skin problems can look just like a fungal infection but have very different treatments. To find out what is causing your rash, your doctor may scrape a small amount of the irritated skin onto a glass slide (or clip off a piece of nail or hair). Then he or she will look at the skin, nail, or hair under a microscope. After doing this, your doctor will usually be able to tell if your skin problem is caused by a fungus.

Sometimes a piece of your skin, hair, or nail will be sent to a lab to grow the fungus in a test tube. This is another way the lab can tell if your skin problem is caused by a fungus. They can also find out the exact type of fungus. This process takes a while because fungus grows slowly.

How Do I Get Rid Of A Tinea Infection?

Once your doctor decides that you have a tinea infection, medicine can be used to get rid of it. You may only need to put a special cream on the rash for a few weeks. This is especially true for jock itch.

It can be harder to get rid of fungal infections on other parts of the body. Sometimes you have to take medicine by mouth. This medicine usually has to be taken for a long time, maybe even for months. Irritated skin takes time to heal. New hair or nails will have to grow back.

Some medicines can have unpleasant effects on the rest of your body, especially if you're also taking other medicines. There are some newer medicines that seem to work better with fewer side effects. You may need to have blood tests to make sure that your body is not having a bad reaction to the medicine.

Can Tinea Cause Serious Illness?

A fungus rarely spreads below the surface of the body to cause serious illness. Your body usually prevents this. However, people with weak immune systems, such as people with AIDS, may have a hard time getting well from a fungal infection.

Tinea infections usually don't leave scars after the fungus is gone. Sometimes, people don't even know they have a fungal infection and get better without any treatment.

Chapter 49

Nail Disorders And Treatments

In their protective role, nails bear the brunt of daily activities. Walking, running, wearing shoes, or participating in sports are just a few of the stresses and strains the feet must endure. All or a portion of the nail plate can be damaged when the feet are injured or abused.

Nail problems are commonly caused by improper trimming, minor injuries, or repeated trauma. Some nail disorders can also be congenital.

Proper trimming (along the contour) on a regular basis can help keep the toenails in the pink, as can wearing well-fitted, low to moderately heeled shoes.

Nail Problems And Their Care

Ingrown Nail

Painful ingrown nails may be congenital, caused by an overcurvature of the nail, or an imbalance between the width of the nail plate and the nail bed. Toe injuries that change the nail's contour also can lead to an ingrown toenail. Toe deformities (such as a bunion that forces the big toe to lean toward the second toe), high-heeled or narrow, pointed shoes can put pressure between the nail and soft tissues, eventually forcing the nail to grow into the skin.

About This Chapter: Taken from "Nail Disorders and Treatments," available on http://www.acfas.org/brnailds.html and as a printed brochure from The American College of Foot and Ankle Surgeons, © 2001. Reprinted with permission.

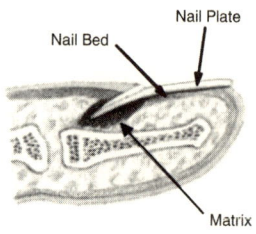

Figure 49.1. Resting on a bed of sensitive tissue, the nail plate is made up of several layers of keratin, a hard, horny protein material.

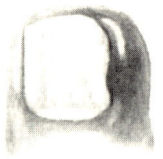

Figure 49.2. Most ingrown nails result from cutting the nail too deeply into the tissue.

> ✔ **Quick Tip**
>
> *Symptoms Of Ingrown Toenail*
>
> Redness, swelling, and infection make the toe very painful.

Ingrown nails can be accompanied by other toe disorders, such as excess surrounding tissue or an outgrowth of bone beneath the nail.

Treatments For The Ingrown Nail

Surgery is often necessary to ease the pain and remove the offending nail. Only a portion of the nail may be removed. If the entire nail is affected or there is a severe nail deformity, the nail plate and matrix (the cells that grow the nail) may be completely removed (see "Surgical Treatments for Nail Disorders" below).

Nail Disorders And Treatments

Fungal Infections

Various types of fungi are present everywhere in the environment. The dark, moist surroundings created by shoes and stockings make the feet especially susceptible to fungal infection.

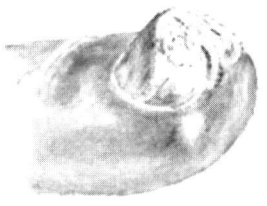

Figure 49.3. Fungus usually attacks a small portion of the nail and spreads slowly.

> ✔ **Quick Tip**
>
> *Symptoms Of Fungal Nails*
>
> Fungus may cause the nail to thicken and become yellow or brownish. As the fungus grows, foul-smelling, moist debris can be seen. Pressure from a thickened nail or the build-up of debris may make the toe painful.

Most fungi are harmless until they penetrate the skin. A fungus can invade through minor cuts; it may also appear after injury or repeated irritation to the toes has caused the nail to separate from the bed.

Fungal infections of the nail plate and nail matrix are quite common.

Treatments For Fungal Infections

Treatment is best begun at the early stages of infection. The accumulation of debris under the nail plate can lead to an ingrown nail, or to a more serious bacterial infection that can spread beyond the foot.

To reduce pain associated with a thickened, infected nail, the surgeon may reduce its thickness by filing the nail plate down with a surgical burr. Filing will not, however, prevent the infection from spreading.

Oral and topical medications may be prescribed when:

- Only a small portion of one nail is infected.
- Several nails are affected.
- Keeping the nail is desired.

Medication may or may not completely eliminate the fungus. Often, after medication is discontinued, the fungus recurs. Your podiatric surgeon will monitor the results of oral prescriptions carefully, and will explain any possible side effects.

While topical ointments usually do not eliminate the fungus, they may be effective when used directly on the nail bed, after the nail plate has been removed.

Eliminating the infection, in some cases, can only be achieved by permanent removal of the nail plate (see "Surgical Treatments for Nail Disorders" below).

Blood Beneath The Nail

A very common result of active lifestyles is blood, or a hematoma, beneath the toenail. Hematomas are especially common among people who jog or play tennis; they are caused by the toes repeatedly rubbing against the shoe.

A hematoma might indicate a fractured bone, especially after an injury (such as dropping a heavy object on the end of the toe). The toe should be examined by the podiatric surgeon, who may take an x-ray to determine the most appropriate treatment.

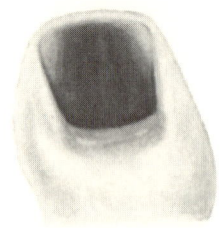

Figure 49.4. Sports injuries are common causes of hematomas under the toenail.

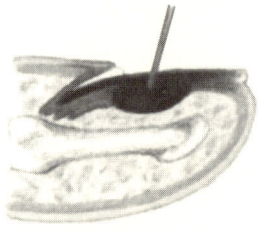

Figure 49.5. Treatment of a hematoma in the first few hours after injury consists of drilling a tiny hole into the nail to let the blood out.

Nail Disorders And Treatments

Hematoma Treatments

If the hematoma is treated within the first few hours of forming, the podiatric surgeon will create a tiny hole in the nail plate using a fine-point drill or scalpel. This releases the blood and relieves pain.

If several days have passed and the blood clot becomes painful, the nail plate may require removal so that the nail bed can be cleaned. Some podiatric surgeons prefer to remove the nail plate whenever blood forms beneath it, because the blood can attract fungi and lead to infection.

The nail may also be removed to treat a bone fracture beneath the hematoma. If the bone has fractured but has not moved out of its normal position, a splint may be used to keep the toe aligned during healing.

Nail plates that have been removed will grow again within three to six months.

Surgical Treatments For Nail Disorders

If the problem is severe or chronic, surgery to remove all or a portion of the nail may be recommended.

Most surgeries are performed very comfortably under local anesthesia, and require less than one hour at the podiatric surgeon's office. Laser surgery, because it requires special equipment, may be performed at a hospital.

Partial Nail Removal

For some cases of ingrown nails, only the portion of nail that is growing into the skin is removed. If both sides of the nail are ingrown, they may be removed during one procedure.

After the affected portion of nail (one-eighth to one-quarter inch) is taken, the nail bed is removed along with any enlarged tissue adjacent to the nail plate. The nail root and matrix are then destroyed by phenol, surgical removal, or laser heat (see "Permanent Nail Removal" below). Finally, the skin may be remodeled around the nail.

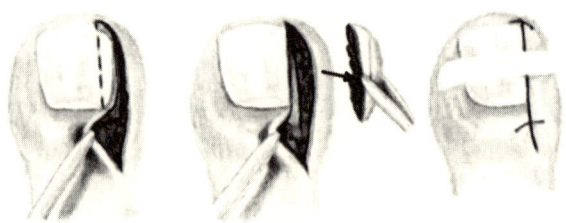

Figure 49.6. The surgical procedure for removing part of the toenail.

Permanent Nail Removal

Complete removal of the nail plate is a common remedy for fungal infections and ingrown nails.

During this procedure, the nail plate is removed and the nail matrix is destroyed by one of three methods:

- Phenol—an acidic chemical called phenol is applied only to the nail matrix. This destroys the growth cells of the nail.
- Surgical removal—the nail matrix and bed are cut away. Stitches are only occasionally necessary.
- Laser—a form of burning in which laser heat is focused on the matrix cells.

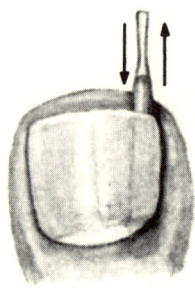

Figure 49.7. After the nail plate is cut away, the nail bed is destroyed to make the removal permanent.

Nail Disorders And Treatments

Removal Of Bone Overgrowth

Bone directly beneath the nail plate may become enlarged, developing a spur or outgrowth that can deform the nail plate or lead to an ingrown nail. Removal of excess bone may be performed concurrently with surgery to partially or permanently remove the nail plate.

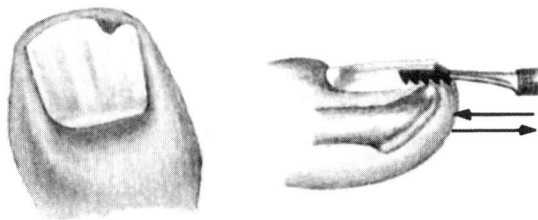

Figure 49.8. The surgical procedure for eliminating bone spurs under the nail.

Care After Surgery

Most people experience very little pain immediately following nail surgery and during the healing process, which lasts approximately two to three weeks. If bone has been removed during surgery, a longer healing process should be anticipated.

Total Nail Removal/Partial Nail Removal

The podiatric surgeon may prescribe medication for pain and may sometimes advise that the toe be soaked two or three times daily for one week. Some amount of drainage is normal when the nail has been removed chemically or by laser. If the nail has been partially removed and stitches were used to form a new nail fold, they are removed in approximately 10 days.

Ingrown Nail

Daily soaking in a saline solution may be recommended. If the toe is inflamed or infected, a topical antibiotic is applied for three to seven days; if the infection is severe, an oral antibiotic may be prescribed. In very few cases, the infection may invade the bone beneath the nail, requiring hospitalization and further treatment. The healing process generally does not interfere with daily activities.

Hematoma

Following simple drainage of a hematoma, the podiatric surgeon may advise that the toe be soaked and treated with topical antibiotics.

How Will The Toe Look After Surgery?

After surgery to permanently remove the nail plate, the body generates a hardened skin covering over the sensitive nail bed. When this covering has developed, normal activities can be resumed. Women can also use nail polish on this area.

Will The Nail Regrow After Removal?

Partial growth of the nail plate after permanent removal is rare, but possible. Because the nail matrix has been destroyed, the nail should not grow again.

Chapter 50

Dandruff

What Is Seborrheic Dermatitis?

Seborrheic dermatitis is a disease that causes flaking of the skin. It usually affects the scalp. In adolescents and adults, it is commonly called dandruff. In babies, it is known as cradle cap.

Seborrheic dermatitis can also affect the skin on other parts of the body, such as the face and chest, and the creases of the arms, legs, and groin. Seborrheic dermatitis usually causes the skin to look a little greasy and scaly or flaky.

How Common Is It?

Seborrheic dermatitis most often occurs in babies younger than three months of age and in adults from 30 to 60 years of age. In adults, it's more common in men than in women.

What Causes Seborrheic Dermatitis?

The exact cause isn't known. The cause may be different in infants and adults. Seborrheic dermatitis may be related to hormones, because the disorder often appears in infancy and disappears before puberty. Or the cause might

---

About This Chapter: Reprinted with permission http://familydoctor.org/handouts/157.html. Copyright © 2002 American Academy of Family Physicians. All rights reserved.

be a fungus called *Pityrosporum ovale*. This organism is normally present on the skin in small numbers, but sometimes its numbers increase, resulting in skin problems.

Seborrheic dermatitis has also been linked to neurologic disorders such as Parkinson's disease and epilepsy. The reason for this relationship isn't known.

How Is Seborrheic Dermatitis Treated?

The treatment of seborrheic dermatitis depends on its location on the body. Treatment also depends on the person's age.

Seborrheic Dermatitis Of The Scalp (Dandruff) In Adults And Adolescents

Dandruff is usually treated with a shampoo that contains salicylic acid (some brand names: X-Seb®, Scalpicin®), the prescription medicine selenium sulfide (brand names: Selsun®, Exsel®), or pyrithione zinc (some brand names: DHS Zinc®, Head & Shoulders®). These shampoos can be used two times a week. Shampoos with coal tar (some brand names: DHS Tar®, Neutrogena T/Gel®, Polytar®) may be used three times a week. If you have dandruff, you might start by using one of these shampoos daily until your dandruff is controlled, and then use it two or three times a week.

When you use a dandruff shampoo, rub the shampoo into your hair thoroughly and let it stay on your hair and scalp for at least five minutes before rinsing. This will give it time to work.

If the shampoo alone doesn't help, your doctor might want you to use a prescription steroid lotion once or twice daily in addition to the shampoo.

Seborrheic Dermatitis Of The Skin Creases In Adolescents And Adults

Steroid lotions may be used in adolescents and adults.

Seborrheic Dermatitis Of The Scalp (Cradle Cap) In Babies

Seborrheic dermatitis of the scalp in babies is treated with products that are not as strong as those used in adults. You might start with a mild,

Dandruff

nonmedicated baby shampoo. Brushing your baby's scalp with a soft brush, like a toothbrush, can help loosen scales or flakes. But be gentle when massaging or brushing your baby's scalp—a break in the skin makes it vulnerable to infection. If a nonmedicated shampoo doesn't work, talk to your doctor about switching to a shampoo that contains tar. Or your doctor may recommend a prescription shampoo that contains 2 percent ketoconazole (brand name: Nizoral®).

Seborrheic Dermatitis Of The Skin Creases In Babies

Gentle steroid lotions or creams may be used to treat seborrheic dermatitis in the skin creases of babies.

Chapter 51

Bald Too Soon: Alopecia Areata

What Is Alopecia Areata?

Alopecia areata is a common disease that results in the loss of hair on the scalp and elsewhere. It usually starts with one or more small, round, smooth patches. It occurs in males and females of all ages, but onset most often occurs in childhood. Over 4 million people in the United States are affected by alopecia areata.

In alopecia areata, the affected hair follicles become very small, drastically decrease production, and grow no hair visible above the surface for months or years. The scalp is the most commonly affected area, but the beard or any other hair-bearing site can be affected alone or together with the scalp.

Some people develop only a few bare patches that regrow hair within a year. In others, extensive patchy loss occurs, and in a few, all scalp hair is lost (this is referred to as alopecia totalis), or hair is lost from the entire scalp and body (this is referred to as alopecia universalis). No matter how widespread the hair loss, the hair follicles remain alive and are ready to resume normal

---

About This Chapter: The information in this chapter is reprinted with permission from the National Alopecia Areata Foundation (NAAF). © 2002 by the National Alopecia Areata Foundation. For additional information, contact NAAF, P.O. Box 150760, San Rafael, CA 94915; (415) 472-3780 (voice), (415) 472-5343 (fax), or info@naaf.org (e-mail); or visit the **NAAF** website at www.naaf.org.

hair production whenever they receive the appropriate signal. In all cases, hair regrowth may occur even without treatment and even after many years.

What Is The Signal That Triggers The Condition To Start Or Stop?

Current research suggests that something triggers the immune system to suppress the hair follicle. We do not yet know what this trigger is or whether it comes from outside the body, like a virus, or from inside. Recent research indicates that some persons have genetic markers that may increase their susceptibility to develop alopecia areata.

Is Alopecia Areata Hereditary?

Yes, heredity plays a role. In one out of five persons with alopecia areata, someone else in the family also has it. Those who develop alopecia areata for the first time after the age of 30 years are less likely to have another family member with it. Those who develop their first patch of alopecia areata before the age of 30 are more likely to have other family members with it.

Alopecia areata often occurs in families whose members have had asthma, hay fever, atopic eczema, or other autoimmune conditions such as thyroid disease, early-onset diabetes, rheumatoid arthritis, lupus erythematosus, vitiligo, pernicious anemia, or Addison's disease.

What Other Parts Of The Body Are Affected?

In some people, the nails develop stippling that looks as if a pin had made rows of tiny dents. In a few, the nails are severely distorted. However, other than the hair and occasionally the nails, no other part of the body is affected.

How Will Alopecia Areata Affect My Daily Life?

Alopecia areata is not medically disabling; persons with alopecia areata are usually in excellent health. But emotionally, this disease can be challenging, especially for those with extensive hair loss. One of the purposes of the National Alopecia Areata Foundation is to reach out to individuals and families with alopecia areata and help them live full, productive lives. There are thousands of successful, well-adjusted, contented people living with this condition. The emotional pain of alopecia areata can be overcome with one's own inner resources, sound medical facts, and the support of others. Sometimes professional counseling from a psychiatrist, psychologist, or social worker is needed to develop one's self-confidence and positive self-image.

Does The Hair Ever Grow Back?

Yes, the hair definitely can completely regrow even after years of extensive hair loss. It can also fall out again.

Is Alopecia Areata Due To Nerves?

No, it is not a nervous disorder. Those who have alopecia areata have not caused it and have no control over its course.

Is It Necessary To Change Plans Regarding School, Sports, Friends, Career, Dating, And Marriage?

No, not at all. People with alopecia areata do not need to limit their activities or expectations. They can do whatever they want to do.

Is There A Cure For Alopecia Areata?

At present, there is no cure for alopecia areata, although the hair may return by itself. There are various treatments, which are most effective in milder cases, but none are universally effective.

Are Treatments Available?

There are several available treatments; choice of treatment depends mainly on a person's age and the extent of hair loss.

Alopecia areata occurs in two forms: a mild patchy form where less than 50 percent of scalp hair is lost, and an extensive form where greater than 50 percent of scalp hair is lost. These two forms of alopecia areata behave quite differently, and the choice of treatment depends on which form is present.

Current treatments do not turn alopecia areata off; they stimulate the follicle to produce hair again, and treatments need to be continued until the condition turns itself off. Treatments are most effective in milder cases.

What Treatments Are Available For Mild, Patchy Alopecia Areata (Less Than 50 Percent Scalp Hair Loss)?

Cortisone Injections

The most common treatment is the injection of cortisone into the bare skin patches. The injections are usually given by a dermatologist who uses a tiny needle to give multiple injections into the skin in and around the bare patches. The injections are repeated once a month. Both the needle prick and the slight tingling are usually well tolerated, and there is no discomfort after leaving the doctor's office. If new hair growth occurs, it is usually visible within four weeks. Treatment, however, does not prevent new patches from developing. There are few side effects from local cortisone injections. Occasionally, temporary depressions in the skin result from the local injections, but these "dells" usually fill in by themselves.

Topical Minoxidil

Five percent topical minoxidil solution (Rogaine Extra Strength®) applied twice daily may grow hair in alopecia areata. Scalp, eyebrows, and beard hair may respond. If scalp hair regrows completely, treatment can be stopped. Two percent topical minoxidil solution (Rogaine Regular Strength®) alone is not effective in alopecia areata; response may improve if cortisone cream is applied 30 minutes after the minoxidil. Topical minoxidil is safe and easy to use, and it does not lower blood pressure in persons with normal blood pressure. Topical minoxidil solution is not effective in treating those with 100 percent scalp hair loss.

Anthralin Cream Or Ointment

Another treatment is the application of anthralin cream or ointment. Anthralin is a synthetic, tar-like substance that has been used widely for psoriasis. Anthralin is applied to the bare patches once daily and washed off after a short time, usually 30 to 60 minutes later. If new hair growth occurs, it is seen in 8 to 12 weeks. Anthralin can be irritating to the skin and can cause temporary, brownish discoloration of the treated skin. By using short treatment times, skin irritation and skin staining are reduced without decreasing effectiveness. Care must be taken not to get anthralin in the eyes. Hands must be washed after applying it.

What Treatments Are Available For Extensive Alopecia Areata (Greater Than 50 Percent Scalp Hair)?

Cortisone Pills

Cortisone pills are sometimes given for extensive scalp hair loss. Cortisone taken internally is much stronger than local injections of cortisone into the skin. It is necessary to discuss possible side effects of cortisone pills with your physician. Healthy young adults often tolerate cortisone pills with few side effects. In general, however, cortisone pills are used in relatively few patients with alopecia areata due to health risks from prolonged use. Also, regrown hair is likely to fall out when the cortisone pills are stopped.

Topical Minoxidil

See previous explanation under mild, patchy alopecia areata.

Topical Immunotherapy

Another method of treating extensive alopecia areata, alopecia totalis, or alopecia universalis is known as topical immunotherapy, which involves producing an allergic rash or allergic contact dermatitis. Chemicals such as diphencyprone (DPCP), dinitrochlorobenzene (DNCB), or squaric acid dibutyl ester (SADBE) are applied to the scalp to produce an allergic rash that resembles poison oak or ivy. Approximately 40 percent of patients treated with topical immunotherapy will regrow scalp hair after about six months of treatment. Those who do regrow scalp hair still need to continue the treatment to maintain the hair regrowth, at least until the condition turns itself off. An itchy rash may be uncomfortable in very hot weather, especially under a wig. These treatments are not available everywhere in the United States although they are used frequently in Canada and Europe.

♣ It's A Fact!!

The National Alopecia Areata Foundation

The National Alopecia Areata Foundation was founded in 1981 when a young Californian with the disease looked for others to share and understand her problems. It has grown into the world center of alopecia areata information, research, and service. Located in San Rafael, California, the foundation is governed by a volunteer board of directors and has a professional chief executive officer and staff. The foundation is represented in Washington, D.C., and the chief executive officer and others have testified before congressional committees.

The foundation engages in the following activities:

- Raises funds and awards research grants to study the cause of alopecia areata, to develop effective treatments, and to seek a cure

- Provides emotional support through personal contact and written materials to help those with alopecia areata and their families

- Acts as the international center for alopecia areata information

- Co-sponsors international research workshops on alopecia areata with the National Institute of Arthritis and Musculoskeletal and Skin Diseases of the National Institutes of Health every four years

- Conducts ongoing public awareness programs and nationwide campaigns

- Organizes an annual conference attended by people with alopecia areata and their families, doctors, researchers, and exhibitors

- Educates state and federal officials on the need for fair insurance laws and greater government-sponsored medical research

- Provides brochures for doctors to give to their patients

- Publishes a quarterly newsletter that provides a forum for people with alopecia areata and their friends and families to interact and receive the latest information on all aspects of the disease

- Sponsors volunteer support groups all over the world as well as telephone support contacts

Wigs

In general, treatments are much less effective for extensive alopecia areata (particularly alopecia totalis or alopecia universalis). For this reason, an attractive wig is an important option for some people. Proper attention will make a quality wig look completely natural; every wig has to be cut, thinned, and styled, often several times. To keep a net base wig from falling off, even during active sports, special double-sided tape can be purchased in beauty supply outlets and fastened to the inside of the wig.

For those with completely bare heads, there are suction caps to which any wig can be attached, and there are entire suction cap wig units. These state-of-the-art wigs, which make use of a silicon base to create a secure, vacuum fit, are comfortable and easily removed by the wearer. Proper fit of a vacuum wig requires that any existing scalp hair be shaved. These wigs are generally more expensive than other types of wigs.

What Research Is Being Done?

There is extensive worldwide research focusing on the cause and treatment of all forms of alopecia areata. The National Alopecia Areata Foundation (NAAF) is leading this research effort by raising private funds and awarding grants to university centers in the United States, Canada, and Europe, and by working closely with the government to increase federal funding for alopecia areata research. The NAAF has awarded millions of dollars to fund research at over 40 university centers throughout the world.

Part 6
Caring For Injuries To The Skin

Chapter 52

Cuts, Scrapes, And Puncture Wounds

What Is The Best Way To Care For A Cut Or Scrape?

The most important first step is to thoroughly clean the wound with soap and water and be careful to remove any foreign material, such as dirt or bits of grass, that might be in the wound and can lead to infection. The area should then be kept clean and dry.

Covering the area with a bandage (such as gauze or a Band-Aid) helps prevent infection and dirt from getting in the wound. A first aid ointment, such as Bacitracin®, can be applied to help prevent infection. Generally, however, these products are best avoided on the hands and feet beyond the first day because they can delay healing in these areas.

Continued care to the wound is also important. Washing the area gently with soap and water daily without scrubbing is best as the wound heals.

Avoid putting products such as hydrogen peroxide, alcohol, or iodine solutions in the wound. These only delay wound healing and do not do anything to prevent infection.

About This Chapter: Source: MedicineNet, Inc. (www.medicine.net). © 2002; reprinted with permission.

Who Should Seek Medical Care For A Cut?

People who have diabetes or other long-term illnesses such as cancer, or who are taking drugs that suppress the immune system such as steroids (cortisone medications like prednisone and prednisolone) or chemotherapy, are more likely to develop a wound infection and should be seen by a health care professional.

Any cut that goes beyond the top layer of skin and might need stitches (sutures) should be seen by a health care professional. Generally, the sooner sutures are put in, the lower the risk of infection. Therefore, any cut that might need suturing should be seen as soon as possible.

What Are The Signs Of A Wound Infection?

If the wound begins to drain greenish fluid (pus) or if the skin around the wound becomes red, warm, swollen, or increasingly painful, a wound infection may be present and medical care should be sought.

Any red streaking of the skin around the wound may indicate an infection in the system that drains fluid from the tissues, called the lymph system. This infection (lymphangitis) can be serious, especially if it is accompanied by a fever. Prompt medical care should be sought if streaking redness from a wound is noticed.

How Are Puncture Wounds Different?

There are two risks with puncture wounds. First, a wound infection can occur because of dirt pushed deep into the skin by the object (typically a nail) puncturing the tissue. As you can imagine, these wounds are very difficult to clean out. The second problem that can occur is an infection of the bone. If a nail penetrates deep into the foot, it can hit a bone and introduce bacteria into the bone. This risk is especially great if the nail has gone through a pair of tennis shoes. The foam in tennis shoes can harbor bacteria (*Pseudomonas*) that can lead to serious infection in the tissues.

First aid for puncture wounds includes cleaning the area well and keeping the foot elevated for several days (depending on the severity of the puncture

Cuts, Scrapes, And Puncture Wounds

> ✔ **Quick Tip**
>
> **Cuts, Scrapes, And Puncture Wounds At A Glance**
>
> - Washing a cut or scrape with soap and water and keeping it clean and dry is all that is required to care for most wounds.
>
> - Putting alcohol, hydrogen peroxide, and iodine into a wound can delay healing and should be avoided.
>
> - Seek medical care early if you think that you might need stitches. Any delay can increase the risk of wound infection.
>
> - Any puncture wound through tennis shoes has a high risk of infection and should be seen by your health care professional.
>
> - Any redness, swelling, increased pain, or pus draining from the wound may indicate an infection that requires professional care.

wound). Especially if the puncture wound occurred through tennis shoes, an evaluation by a health care professional should be sought. Additionally, diabetics, the elderly, those persons taking drugs that can suppress the immune system (such as cortisone-related medications), or any particularly deep puncture wound should be seen by a health care professional. This is particularly true if it was difficult to remove the nail, indicating that it may have penetrated the bone. Most puncture wounds do not become infected, but if redness and swelling persist, see your health care professional.

Puncture wounds commonly occur when someone steps on a nail. It is a good idea to wear shoes to minimize the risk of a puncture wound, especially if you have diabetes or loss of sensation in the feet for any reason.

Will I Need A Tetanus Shot?

Most people in the United States have been immunized against tetanus (lockjaw). If you have been immunized, you will need a booster shot if you have not had one in over five years. If you have never had a tetanus shot, or if your series is incomplete (fewer than three shots), you might need tetanus immunoglobulin, a medication that can prevent lockjaw.

Chapter 53

Those Big Scars: Keloids

What Is A Keloid?

A keloid is a scar that doesn't know when to stop. When the skin is injured, cells grow back to fill in the gap. Somehow, they "know" when the scar tissue is even with the contour of the skin, at which point they stop multiplying. When the cells keep on reproducing, the result is a what is called a overgrown (hypertrophic) scar or a keloid.

A hypertrophic scar is a thick, raised, smooth area that is confined to the site of injury. It diminishes over a period of one year or more.

A keloid, by contrast, may extend beyond the site of injury. Keloids do not subside.

What Does A Keloid Look And Feel Like?

A keloid looks shiny and is often dome-shaped. It can range in color from slightly pink to red. It feels hard and thick and is always raised above the surrounding skin.

Where On The Body Do Keloids Tend To Appear?

Keloids are most commonly located on the chest, upper back, and shoulders. However, they can appear almost anywhere, such as in surgical scars

---

About This Chapter: Source: MedicineNet, Inc. (www.medicinenet.com). © 2000; reprinted with permission.

any place on the body and in the earlobes or other areas that have been pierced for cosmetic purposes.

Do Keloids Cause Symptoms?

They may or may not. If they do, the symptoms may include itching, tenderness, and mild pain.

Who Is Particularly Prone To Develop Keloids?

People of African or Asian descent are more likely to get keloids than people with lighter skin. (In this respect, keloids are exactly the opposite of most skin cancers, which tend to occur in light-skinned people and spare people of color.)

How About High-Risk Areas Of The Body?

People of any skin type can get a keloid in a high-risk area of the body such as the mid-chest. A keloid can develop even when there has been no apparent injury to the skin.

How Do I Know If I Am Susceptible To Keloids?

This is an important question and one to which only a partial answer can be given. If you belong to a high-risk group, or if the surgery you plan or need to have involves a high-risk area of the body, your chances of forming a keloid are (by definition) greater. There are many exceptions, however, and these scars may form on a given person after some injuries, but not others, for no obvious reason.

The sensible preventive approach, therefore, is to avoid any elective surgery or body piercing if you have darker skin or have developed keloids in the past.

How Are Keloids Treated?

It is difficult, if not impossible, to remove keloids completely. Cutting them out, though tempting, is not a good idea. Doing so often results in another keloid and sometimes a larger one.

Those Big Scars: Keloids

> ### ✎ Weird Words
> ### Where Does "Keloid" Come From?
>
> The dense tumorlike scar was called a "keloid" (*chéloïde* in French) in 1835 by the dermatologist Jean-Louis Albert. However, the word "keloid" was already in use in France as early as 1817, according to the *Nouveau Petit Robert Dictionaire*. The origin of the term "keloid" is not entirely certain. The *Petit Robert* attributes it to the Greek word *chele* meaning in French *pince* and in English "a talon, claw, or hoof." Other authorities such as *Dorland's Illustrated Medical Dictionary* attribute "keloid" to the Greek *kelis*, "blemish," or to the Greek *kele*, "a rupture." And still other sources state that the word "keloid" comes from Greek roots *kel* (tumor) + *eidos* (form) = tumor form. A keloid is a tumor in the strict sense of being an abnormal mass of tissue. It is, of course, a benign tumor, not a malignant one.

Treatment methods include:

- *Injections of cortisone.* Safe and not very painful, injections of cortisone given once a month can significantly flatten keloids, especially small ones of recent onset.

- *Surgery.* Surgery, as we've said, can be counterproductive and accomplish little or nothing except to cause a second keloid to form.

- *Surgery plus injections of cortisone.* Some doctors cut keloids out and inject the healing site to help prevent recurrences.

- *Laser.* Other doctors may treat keloids with lasers. Lasers may lessen the redness but, unfortunately, they do little or nothing to the bulk of the keloid.

- *Laser plus injections of cortisone.* Still other doctors may zap the keloids with lasers and then inject the site.

- *Cryosurgery.* Freezing keloids with liquid nitrogen may flatten them, although sometimes this method produces discoloration of the skin.

- *Silicone sheeting.* For reasons that are not clear, applying a silicone sheet (which is available in pharmacies without a prescription) nightly for several months can gradually and safely minimize some keloids. Persevering with this routine can, however, be difficult.

- *Compression*. Long-term compression of keloids with pressure bandages can help soften them, too.

How Can Keloids Be Prevented?

Although preventing keloids is better than treating them, this is, obviously, not always possible. When injury or bad luck produces one, initiating therapy soon with cortisone injections can make the final outcome more satisfactory.

Chapter 54

Taking Care Of Burns

What Causes Burns?

You can get burned by heat and fire, radiation, sunlight, electricity, or chemicals. There are three degrees of burns:

- Thin or superficial burns (also called first-degree burns) are red and painful. They swell a little. They turn white when you press on them. The skin over the burn may peel off in one or two days.

- Thicker burns, called superficial partial-thickness and deep partial-thickness burns (also called second-degree burns), have blisters and are painful.

- Full-thickness burns (also called third-degree burns) cause damage to all layers of the skin. The burned skin looks white or charred. These burns may cause little or no pain if nerves are damaged.

How Long Does It Take For Burns To Heal?

- Superficial burns—three to six days
- Superficial partial-thickness burns—usually less than three weeks

---

About This Chapter: Reprinted with permission from http://familydoctor.org/handouts/638.html. Copyright © 2002 American Academy of Family Physicians. All rights reserved.

- Deep partial-thickness burns—usually more than three weeks
- Full-thickness burns—without skin grafts, heal only at the edges by scarring. A skin graft is a very thin layer of skin that is cut from an unburned area and put on a badly burned area.

How Are Burns Treated?

The treatment depends on what kind of burn you have.

Superficial Burn

Soak the burn in cool water. Then treat it with a skin care product like aloe vera cream or an antibiotic ointment. To protect the burned area, you can put a dry gauze bandage over the burn. Take acetaminophen (brand name: Tylenol®) to help with the pain.

> ✔ **Quick Tip**
> It is not good to put butter, oil, ice, or ice water on burns. This might cause more damage to the skin.

If a first- or second-degree burn covers a large area or is on your face, hands, feet, or genitals, you should see a doctor right away.

Superficial Partial-Thickness Or Deep Partial-Thickness Burn

Soak the burn in cool water for 15 minutes. If the burned area is small, put cool, clean, wet cloths on the burn for a few minutes every day. Then put on an antibiotic cream or other creams or ointments prescribed by your doctor. Cover the burn with a nonstick dressing (for example, Telfa®) and hold the dressing in place with gauze or tape.

Check the burn every day for signs of infection, such as increased pain, redness, swelling, or pus. If you see any of these signs, go to your doctor right away. To prevent infection, avoid breaking blisters.

Change the dressing every day. First, wash your hands with soap and water. Then gently wash the burn and put antibiotic ointment on it. If the burn area is small, a dressing may not be needed during the day. Make sure you are up-to-date on tetanus shots. If you aren't sure, check with your doctor's office.

Taking Care Of Burns

Burned skin itches as it heals. Keep your fingernails cut short, and don't scratch the burned skin. The burned area will be sensitive to sunlight for up to one year.

Full-Thickness Burns

If you get a bad burn, you should see your doctor or go to the hospital right away. Don't take off any clothing that is stuck to the burn. Don't soak the burn in water. Take off other clothing and jewelry near the burn area.

What Do I Need To Know About Electrical And Chemical Burns?

A person with an electrical burn (for example, from a power line) should go to the hospital right away. Electrical burns often cause serious injury inside the body. This injury may not show on the skin.

A chemical burn should be washed with large amounts of water. Take off any clothing that has the chemical on it. Don't put anything on the burn area. This might start a chemical reaction that could make the burn worse. If you don't know what to do, call your local poison control center or see your doctor right away.

Chapter 55
Over-The-Counter Medications For Skin Injuries

A half-inch scar on my left knee is a graphic reminder of a painful scrape at age seven. Also painful was the burn of Merthiolate® antiseptic applied as first aid to ward off infection.

Today's approved over-the-counter (OTC) topical (used on the skin) first-aid antimicrobials are less irritating and more effective than Merthiolate, which contains the mercury drug thimerosal. The Food and Drug Administration (FDA) has approved seven topical OTC antibiotics and is evaluating OTC topical antiseptics under a proposed rule. The proposal would ban numerous antiseptics, including mercurials, as ineffective and some, including thimerosal, as also unsafe.

Antibiotics are also available by prescription as injectable and oral medicines and medicines for the eye and ear. They are used to treat infections. While some can kill a limited number of bacterial species, other varieties affect many types of bacteria.

Antiseptics weaken microbes, but don't usually kill them. Health-care antiseptics in soaps and other products help prevent the spread of infection in medical facilities.

> About This Chapter: Adapted from "OTC Options: Help for Cuts, Scrapes, and Burns," *FDA Consumer Magazine*, May 1996; available at http://www.fda.gov/fdac/features/496_cuts.html. Reviewed by David A. Cooke, M.D., December 19, 2002.

OTC first-aid antibiotics and antiseptics are applied to the skin to help prevent infection in minor cuts, scrapes and burns.

"Used topically, OTC antimicrobials inhibit the growth of bacteria, but don't necessarily kill them all," says Audrey Love, a microbiologist with the division of OTC drug evaluation in FDA's Center for Drug Evaluation and Research. "If an injury is extensive," Love says, "it should be taken care of by a doctor. But consumers have to consider for themselves, based on reading the labeling, whether a product is something they should use."

FDA has published rules (monographs) establishing adequate labeling for OTC antimicrobials, and conditions under which products would be generally recognized as safe and effective for use without medical supervision. The final antibiotics rule (1987) and proposed antiseptics rule (1991) specify active ingredients and concentrations, as well as labeling information such as product identification, indications for use, warnings, and directions for use. All drugs must meet the agency's good manufacturing practice requirements for product identity, strength, quality, and purity.

Some Restrictions

OTC first-aid antimicrobials are to be used for only up to one week. If an injury persists or worsens after this time, the label warns consumers to stop use and consult a doctor.

The products are not for existing infections, animal bites, sunburn, punctures, or eye injuries. Nor should they be used for cuts, scrapes, or burns needing medical care, such as:

- Cuts that are deep, continue bleeding, or may require stitches
- Scrapes with imbedded particles that can't be flushed away

> ### ❧ Weird Words
>
> Antibiotic: A substance, usually derived from bacteria or molds, that inhibits the growth of disease-causing microorganisms.
>
> Antiseptic: A substance that weakens microorganisms and makes it more difficult for them to grow.
>
> Antimicrobial: A substance that tends to destroy microorganisms, keep them from multiplying, or prevent their disease-causing action.

- Large wounds
- Burns more serious than a small reddened area

Use of an antibiotic or antiseptic does not in itself constitute first-aid treatment of a minor wound.

A panel of experts convened by FDA defined first aid as "a process that includes initial adequate cleansing which may or may not be followed by application of a safe, nonirritating product which does not interfere with normal wound healing and which may reduce the bacterial numbers and help prevent infection."

FDA requires that labels for antibiotics advise users to first "clean the affected area." Antiseptics also would be labeled with the same advice.

Because topical antimicrobials are not totally effective in killing bacteria, FDA does not allow firms to place the claim "helps kill bacteria" in the same area as the required information. FDA believes the term "kill" implies the product will eliminate all bacteria and could be misleading if appearing with the required term "infection" (or alternate term "bacterial contamination") in the label's indications section. The claim may be used, though, as additional information elsewhere in the label.

More About Antibiotics

In its final rule, FDA listed these antibiotic active ingredients as safe and effective: bacitracin, bacitracin zinc, chlortetracycline hydrochloride, tetracycline hydrochloride, neomycin sulfate, oxytetracycline hydrochloride, and polymyxin B sulfate—the latter two only for combination products because of their limited effectiveness against certain microorganisms when used alone.

The rule does not allow the previously marketed antibiotic gramicidin, because it has the potential to break down red blood cells when absorbed through fresh wounds. The agency called for a well-designed, double-blind study (where neither patient nor doctor knows who gets the drug) to show gramicidin's effects.

✤ **It's A Fact!!**

OTC Antibiotics

The following antibiotic products have been approved by FDA for use without a prescription. They are ointments unless otherwise noted:

- Single-ingredient products

    ◊ bacitracin—Baciguent®

    ◊ bacitracin zinc—Bacitracin Zinc®

    ◊ chlortetracycline hydrochloride—Aureomycin®

    ◊ neomycin sulfate—Neomycin®, Myciguent Cream®

    ◊ tetracycline hydrochloride—Achromycin®

- Combination products

    ◊ bacitracin-neomycin—none currently marketed

    ◊ bacitracin-polymyxin B aerosol—none currently marketed

    ◊ bacitracin-neomycin-polymyxin B—Lanabiotic®, Medi-Quik Triple Antibiotic®, Clomycin Cream® (with lidocaine anesthetic), Mycitracin Plus Pain Reliever® (with lidocaine)

    ◊ bacitracin zinc-neomycin—none currently marketed

    ◊ bacitracin zinc-polymyxin B ointment, aerosol, or powder—Polysporin®, Polysporin Powder®

    ◊ bacitracin zinc-neomycin-polymyxin B—Neomixin®, Neosporin Original®

    ◊ neomycin-polymyxin B ointment or cream—Neosporin Plus Maximum Strength Cream® (with lidocaine)

    ◊ oxytetracycline-polymyxin B ointment or powder—none currently marketed

The data on which FDA based its approval of the other antibiotics included a well-controlled study of minor skin injuries or insect bites in 59 children. Streptococcal infection developed in 15 of the 32 receiving a topical placebo and in 3 of the 27 receiving a topical antibiotic. Twelve of the 15 eventually needed oral antibiotics, and one of the 3 did.

The agency agreed with comments that many such injuries are self-healing, but that some do not heal without treatment and it is impossible to make this distinction at the time of injury.

Also, says FDA's Love, there's always a chance someone can be allergic to a drug, prescription or OTC. "People who tend to be allergic," she says, "should talk to their doctor or pharmacist before trying any OTC medicine for the first time."

About one in 20 people is allergic to neomycin, according to an article in the August 1995 *Harvard Health Letter*. If a reaction such as redness, itching, or burning occurs, the article advises, "Stop using the preparation immediately, and consult a physician if symptoms worsen or persist for more than 48 hours."

Hypersensitivity reactions may also occur with bacitracin, according to the *Handbook of Nonprescription Drugs* (10th edition), published by the American Pharmaceutical Association and The National Professional Society of Pharmacists, Washington, D.C. The handbook also states that tetracycline products may trigger reactions in allergic patients, "some of whom may have severe reactions even if exposure is by topical application only."

With repeated use on large areas, neomycin also fosters development of neomycin-resistant strains of *Staphylococcus* bacteria. Neomycin products that include polymyxin B and bacitracin guard against this.

To prevent neomycin overuse, FDA limits the drug to ointments and creams, the most likely dosage forms for small wounds. Also, all OTC antimicrobials must be labeled for short-term use. The agency believes short-term use of neomycin ointments or creams on small wounds would not risk overuse. To reduce the risk even further, FDA requires labels for ointments and creams to identify a dose as "an amount equal to the surface area of the tip of a finger."

☞ **Remember!!**

What OTC Antibiotic Labels Should Tell You

- State the established name of the drug.

- Identify the drug as a "first-aid antibiotic."

- State the drug's approved use—for example: "First aid to help protect against infection in minor cuts, scrapes, and burns." (Allowed alternative wording includes "help prevent skin infection" or "help reduce the risk of bacterial contamination." Other descriptive statements may be added, provided they are truthful and not misleading.)

- Carry the warning: "For external use only. Do not use in the eyes or apply over large areas of the body. In case of deep or puncture wounds, animal bites, or serious burns, consult a doctor."

- Carry the warning: "Stop use and consult a doctor if the condition persists or gets worse. Do not use longer than one week unless directed by a doctor."

- Advise you to clean the area, use a small amount one to three times daily, and cover with a sterile bandage if desired.

- Specify on ointments and creams to use "an amount equal to the surface area of the tip of a finger."

- Combination products must give the established name of each active ingredient. Labels must identify any added anesthetic as such, include the directions and warnings in its monograph, and state: "First aid for the temporary relief of pain [or other approved alternative] in minor cuts, scrapes, and burns."

Another issue is the combination of a product with a local "-caine" anesthetic, such as benzocaine, as is allowed for bacitracin ointment or a combination ointment of bacitracin, neomycin, or polymyxin B. The review panel was concerned an anesthetic might mask symptoms of infection, delaying treatment by a doctor. But FDA believes the required warnings on the label adequately inform consumers when to consult a doctor.

More About Antiseptics

In its proposed rule, FDA listed these active antiseptic ingredients as tentatively safe and effective: ethyl alcohol (48 to 95 percent), isopropyl alcohol, benzalkonium chloride, benzethonium chloride, camphorated metacresol, camphorated phenol, phenol, hexylresorcinol, hydrogen peroxide solution, iodine tincture, iodine topical solution, povidone-iodine, and methylbenzethonium. Five ingredients listed as tentatively effective only in combination products are ethyl alcohol (26.9 percent), eucalyptol, menthol, methyl salicylate, and thymol.

The proposal would ban numerous mercury ingredients and cloflucarban, fluorosalan, and tribromsalan antiseptics as not generally recognized as safe and effective for OTC use.

FDA had requested study data on whether topical povidone-iodine affected thyroid function. In submitted data, iodine blood levels did increase after two weeks' use, but returned to normal when use was stopped. There was no effect on thyroid function.

Antiseptics would be labeled similarly to antibiotics, but with some differences.

Labels on camphorated metacresol, camphorated phenol, and phenol, for example, would warn, "Do not bandage."

"The drugs can be hard on the skin," says Debbie Lumpkins, a microbiologist in FDA's division of OTC drug evaluation. She explains that, "when bandaged, the skin gets damp, increasing absorption. Therefore, more drug enters the skin and may cause more damage than if you just left the wound uncovered."

Labels for ethyl alcohol (48 to 95 percent) and isopropyl alcohol (50 to 91.3 percent) would warn: "Flammable, keep away from fire or flame."

For liquid antiseptics, labels would direct users to let the product dry before bandaging.

Comments on the proposal were minimal, Lumpkins says, emphasizing that FDA's evaluation of the ingredients is still very much an evolving process.

"Frequently," she says, "we find that one study or one article says one thing, and there's another study or article on the other side. We have to determine the facts. Literature searches that we can now do so easily help, but we won't find everything. We rely on people to bring things to our attention."

Recent publications advise against two currently marketed antiseptics. The National Safety Council's 1996 *First Aid Pocket Guide* states: "DO NOT use hydrogen peroxide. It does not kill bacteria, and it adversely affects capillary blood flow and wound healing." And the *Handbook on Nonprescription Drugs* states ethyl alcohol "is not a desirable wound antiseptic because it irritates already damaged tissue. The coagulum [crust] formed may, in fact, protect the bacteria."

The final rule will reflect FDA's evaluation of all the data, Lumpkins says. Thus, antiseptic ingredients proposed as safe and effective could be found unsafe or ineffective, or new ingredients could be added, depending on new information.

Whether using an OTC antibiotic or antiseptic, consumers should realize "there are limits to what the products can do," Lumpkins says. "People should read the label, and use the product appropriately. If they notice a change in their condition, or if there's redness or swelling, they shouldn't continue to try to treat it. They should see a doctor."

—by Dixie Farley

Chapter 56

Bruises And Contusions

A football linebacker tackles another player using his shoulder. A soccer goalkeeper blocks the ball with her thigh. Athletes in all contact sports have many opportunities to get a muscle contusion (bruise). Contusions are second only to strains as a leading cause of sports injuries.

Contusions occur when a direct blow or repeated blows from a blunt object strike part of your body, crushing underlying muscle fibers and connective tissue without breaking the skin. You can also get a contusion by falling or jamming part of your body against a hard surface. Most contusions are minor and heal quickly without taking you out of the game. But severe contusions can cause deep tissue damage, lead to complications, and keep you out of sports for months.

First Aid

Contusions cause swelling and pain and limit joint range of motion near the injury. Torn blood vessels may cause bluish discoloration. The injured muscle may feel weak and stiff. To control pain, bleeding, and inflammation, keep the muscle in a gentle stretch position and use the RICE formula.

About This Chapter: © 2001 American Academy of Orthopaedic Surgeons. Reprinted with permission from Your Orthopaedic Connection, the patient education website of the American Academy of Orthopaedic Surgeons located at http://orthoinfo.aaos.org.

Severe Injuries

Sometimes a pool of blood collects within damaged tissue, forming a lump over the injury (hematoma). In severe cases swelling and bleeding beneath the skin may cause shock. If tissue damage is extensive, you may also have a fractured bone, dislocated joint, sprain, torn muscle, or other injuries. Contusions to the abdomen may damage internal organs.

See your doctor right away for complete diagnosis. A physical examination will determine the exact location and extent of injury. Diagnostic imaging tools may be used to better visualize inside the injured area of your body. These tools include ultrasound, MRI (magnetic resonance imaging), or CT (computed tomography) scans. For some injuries, your doctor may also need to check for nerve injury.

Treatment

Most athletes with contusions get better quickly without surgery. Your doctor may give you nonsteroidal anti-inflammatory drugs (NSAIDs) or other medications for pain relief. Do not massage the injured area. During the first 24 to 48 hours after injury (acute phase), you will probably need to continue using rest, ice, compression bandages, and elevation of the injured area to control bleeding, swelling, and pain. While the injured part heals, be

---

✔ **Quick Tip**

The RICE Formula For Treating Contusions

- *Rest*: Protect the injured area from further harm by stopping play. You may also use a protective device (i.e., crutches, sling).
- *Ice*: Apply ice wrapped in a clean cloth. (Remove ice after 20 minutes.)
- *Compression*: Lightly wrap the injured area in a soft bandage or ACE® wrap.
- *Elevation*: Raise the injury to a level above the heart.

sure to keep exercising the uninjured parts of your body to maintain your overall level of fitness. If you have a large hematoma that does not go away within several days, the doctor may drain it surgically to speed healing.

Rehabilitation

After a few days, inflammation should start to go down, and the injury may feel a little better. At this time, the doctor may tell you to apply gentle heat to the injury and start the rehabilitation process. Remember to increase your activity level gradually. Depending upon the extent of your injuries, returning to your normal sports activity may take several weeks or longer. If you put too much stress on the injured area before it has healed enough, excessive scar tissue may develop and cause more problems.

When you have normal, pain-free range of motion, the doctor may let you return to noncontact sports.

Return To Play

You may be able to return to contact sports when you get back your full strength, motion, and endurance. When the doctor says you are ready to return to play, he or she may want you to wear a customized protective device to prevent further injury to the area that suffered a contusion. Depending upon your sport, you may get special padding made of firm or semifirm materials. The padding spreads out the force of impact when direct blows from blunt objects strike your body.

Complications

Getting prompt medical treatment and following your doctor's advice about rehabilitation can help you avoid serious medical complications that occasionally result from deep muscle contusions.

Compartment Syndrome

In certain cases, rapid bleeding may cause extremely painful swelling within the muscle group of your arm, leg, foot, or buttock. Build-up of pressure from fluids several hours after a contusion injury can disrupt blood flow and prevent nourishment from reaching the muscle group. Compartment syndrome may require urgent surgery to drain the excess fluids.

Myositis Ossificans

Young athletes who try to rehabilitate a severe contusion too quickly sometimes develop myositis ossificans—a condition in which the bruised muscle grows bone instead of new muscle cells. Symptoms may include mild to severe pain that does not go away and swelling at the injury site. Abnormal bone formations can also reduce your flexibility. Vigorous stretching exercises may make the condition worse. Rest, ice, compression, and elevation to reduce inflammation will usually help. You may need to do gentle stretching exercises to improve flexibility. Surgery is rarely required.

☞ **Remember!!**

Two Phases Of Contusion Rehabilitation

- In the first phase, your doctor may prescribe gentle stretching exercises that begin to restore range of motion to the injured area.

- Later, when the doctor says range of motion has improved enough, he or she may prescribe weight-bearing and strengthening exercises.

Chapter 57
Animal Bites

Animal bites and scratches, even when they are minor, can become infected and spread bacteria to other parts of the body. Whether the bite is from a family pet or an animal in the wild, scratches and bites can carry disease. Cat scratches, for example, even from a kitten, can carry cat scratch disease, a bacterial infection. Other animals can transmit rabies and tetanus. Bites that break the skin are even more likely to become infected.

Care For Animal Bites

For superficial bites from a familiar household pet who is immunized and in good health:

- Wash the wound with soap and water under pressure from a faucet for at least five minutes, but do not scrub, as this may bruise the tissue. Apply an antiseptic lotion or cream.

- Watch for signs of infection at the site, such as increased redness or pain, swelling, drainage, or a fever. Call your physician or health care provider right away if any of these symptoms occur.

For deeper bites or puncture wounds from any animal, or for any bite from a strange animal:

About This Chapter: © 2001 University of Maryland Medical System. Reprinted with permission from the University of Maryland Medical Center, www.umm.edu.

- If the bite or scratch is bleeding, apply pressure to it with a clean bandage or towel to stop the bleeding.

- Wash the wound with soap and water under pressure from a faucet for at least five minutes, but do not scrub, as this may bruise the tissue.

- Dry the wound and cover it with a sterile dressing, but do not use tape or butterfly bandages to close the wound, as this could trap harmful bacteria in the wound.

- Call your physician or health care professional for guidance in reporting the attack and to determine whether additional treatment, such as antibiotics, a tetanus booster, or rabies vaccination is needed. This is especially important for bites on the face or for bites that cause deeper puncture wounds of the skin.

- If possible, locate the animal that inflicted the wound. Some animals need to be captured, confined, and observed for rabies. Do

---

✔ **Quick Tip**

Being safe around animals, even your own pets, can help reduce the risk of animal bites. Here are some general guidelines for avoiding animal bites and rabies:

- Do not try to separate fighting animals.

- Avoid strange and sick animals.

- Leave animals alone when they are eating.

- Keep pets on a leash when out in public.

- Select family pets carefully.

- Never leave a young child alone with a pet.

- All domestic dogs and cats should be immunized against rabies, and their shots kept current.

- Do not approach or play with wild animals of any kind, and be aware that domestic animals may also be infected with the rabies virus.

- Supervise pets so they do not come into contact with wild animals. Call your local animal control agency to remove any stray animals.

Animal Bites

- not try to capture the animal yourself; instead contact the nearest animal warden or animal control office in your area.
- If the animal cannot be found, or if the animal was a high-risk species (skunk or bat), or if the animal attack was unprovoked, the victim may need a series of rabies shots.
- Call your physician or health care provider for any flulike symptoms such as a fever, headache, malaise, decreased appetite, or swollen glands following an animal bite.

What Is Rabies?

Rabies is an infection of certain warm-blooded animals is caused by a virus in the Rhabdoviridae family. It attacks the nervous system and, once symptoms develop, it is 100 percent fatal in animals, if left untreated.

In North America, rabies occurs primarily in skunks, raccoons, foxes, and bats. In some areas, these wild animals infect domestic cats, dogs, and livestock. In the United States, cats are more likely than dogs to be rabid.

Generally, rabies is rare in small rodents such as beavers, chipmunks, squirrels, rats, mice, or hamsters. Rabies is also rare in rabbits. In the mid-Atlantic states, where rabies is increasing in raccoons, woodchucks can also be rabid.

How Does Rabies Occur?

The rabies virus enters the body through a cut or scratch or through mucous membranes (such as the lining of the mouth and eyes), then travels to the central nervous system. Once the infection is established in the brain, the virus travels down the nerves from the brain and multiplies in different organs.

The salivary glands and organs are most important in the spread of rabies from one animal to another. When an infected animal bites another animal, the rabies virus is transmitted through the infected animal's saliva. Scratches by claws of rabid animals are also dangerous because these animals lick their claws.

What Are The Symptoms Of Rabies?

The incubation in humans from the time of exposure to the onset of illness can range anywhere from five days to more than a year, although the average incubation period is about two months.

Table 57.1 details the most common symptoms of rabies. However, each individual may experience symptoms differently

The symptoms of rabies may resemble other conditions or medical problems. Always consult your physician for a diagnosis.

How Is Rabies Diagnosed?

In animals, the direct fluorescent antibody test (dFA) is most frequently used to detect rabies. Within a few hours, diagnostic laboratories can determine whether an animal is rabid and provide this information to medical professionals. These results may save a person from undergoing treatment if the animal is not rabid.

Table 57.1. Rabies Symptoms

Stage 1	Stage 2
Initial period of vague symptoms lasts 2 to 10 days.	Patients often develop difficulty in swallowing (sometimes referred to as "foaming at the mouth") due to the inability to swallow saliva; even the sight of water may terrify the patient.
Vague symptoms may include fever, headache, malaise, decreased appetite, vomiting.	Some patients become agitated and disoriented, while others become paralyzed.
Pain, itching or numbness and tingling at the site of the wound.	Immediate death, or coma resulting in death from other complications, may result.

Animal Bites

In humans, a number of tests are necessary to confirm or rule out rabies, as no single test can be used to rule out the disease with certainty. Tests are performed on samples of serum, saliva, and spinal fluid. Skin biopsies may also be taken from the nape of the neck.

Treatment For Rabies

Unfortunately, there is no known, effective treatment for rabies once symptoms of the disease occur. However, an effective new vaccine provides immunity to rabies when administered after an exposure. It may also be used for protection before an exposure occurs, for persons such as veterinarians and animal handlers.

> **☞ Remember!!**
>
> If you or someone you know is bitten by an animal, remember these facts to report to your health care provider:
>
> - Location of the accident
> - Type of animal involved (domestic pet or wild animal)
> - Type of exposure (cut, scratch, licking of open wound)
> - Part of the body involved
> - Number of exposures
> - Whether or not the animal has been immunized against rabies
> - Whether or not the animal is sick or well; if sick, what symptoms are present in the animal
> - Whether or not the animal is available for testing or quarantine

Chapter 58

Insect Bites And Stings

Alternative Names

Bedbug bite; bee sting; bites—insects; black widow bite; brown recluse bite; flea bite; honey bee sting; louse bite; mite bite; scorpion bite; spider bite; tick bite; yellow jacket sting.

Definition

This sting or bite is from an insect or spider.

Considerations

If bitten or stung by an insect, try to kill it and have it identified (if it can be done quickly and safely).

Most bites and stings do not require emergency medical care. However, possible complications to insect bites and stings include allergic reaction, shock, reaction to venom (see wasp and bee poison documents), toxic reaction, or infection.

Allergic reactions to insect bites or stings occur very quickly, usually within minutes, and severe reactions can be rapidly fatal if untreated. Approximately 0.5 percent of the population develops severe allergic reactions (anaphylaxis) to insect stings.

About This Chapter: © 2002 A.D.A.M., Inc. Reprinted with permission.

Ticks And Lyme Disease

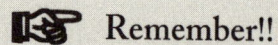 **Remember!!**

Lyme disease has become the leading tick-borne illness in the United States. In 1999, 16,273 cases of Lyme disease were reported to the Centers for Disease Control and Prevention (CDC). The deer tick, also known as the black-legged tick, is the species that most often transmits Lyme disease. With proper precautions, Lyme disease is preventable.

- Ticks are most active from April through October, so exercise additional caution when venturing into tick country during that time period.

- When in a tick-infested area, an insect repellent is good prevention is. However, consider a product designed to be applied to clothing rather than skin.

- Tuck pants cuffs into boots or socks, and wear long sleeves and light-colored clothing to make it easier to spot ticks.

- Stay to the center of hiking paths, and avoid grassy and marshy woodland areas.

- Inspect yourself for clinging ticks after leaving an infested area. Ticks are hard to see—nymphs are dot-sized; adults, smaller than a sesame seed.

- If you discover a tick feeding, do not panic. Studies indicate that an infected tick does not usually transmit the Lyme organism during the first 24 hours.

- If you suspect Lyme disease or its symptoms, contact your doctor immediately.

Ticks' mouthparts have reverse, harpoon-like barbs, designed to penetrate and attach to skin. Ticks secrete a cementlike substance that helps them adhere firmly to the host. If you find that you or your pet has been bitten by a tick, it is important to remove it properly. Figure 58.1 illustrates the correct procedure.

- Use fine-point tweezers to grasp the tick at the place of attachment, as close to the skin as possible.

- Gently pull the tick straight out.

Insect Bites And Stings

- Place the tick in a small vial labeled with the victim's name and address and the date.
- Wash your hands, disinfect the tweezers and bite site.
- Mark your calendar with the victim's name, place of tick attachment on the body, and general health at the time.
- Call your doctor to determine if treatment is warranted.
- Watch the tick-bite site and your general health for signs or symptoms of a tick-borne illness. Make sure you mark any changes in your health status on your calendar.
- If possible, have the tick identified or tested by a lab, your local health department, or veterinarian.

Source: "How To Use Insect Repellents Safely," Office of Pesticide Programs, Environmental Protection Agency, http://www.epa.gov/pesticides/citizens/insectrp.htm, April 17, 2002; and "Tick Removal," http://www.lyme.org/ticks/removal.html. Courtesy of the Lyme Disease Foundation, www.lyme.org.

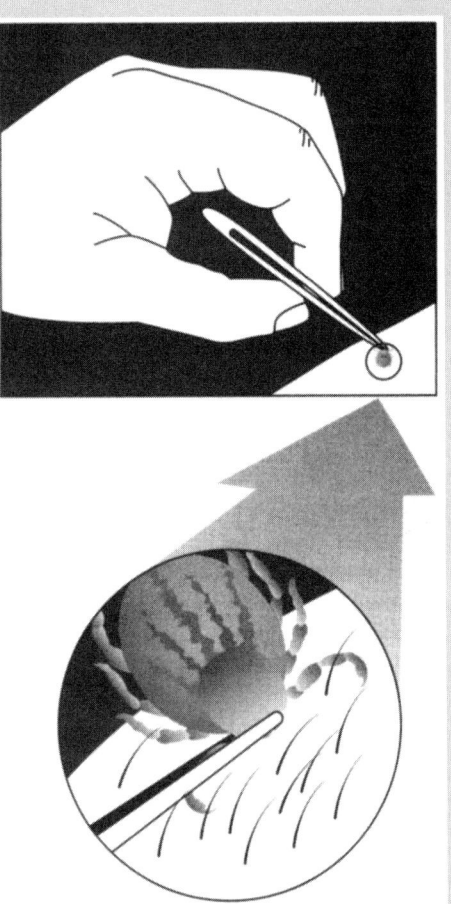

Figure 58.1. The right way to remove a tick. Source: FDA Consumer, July–August 2001, p. 7.

Causes

Common causes include:

- Black widow spider bite
- Brown recluse spider bite
- Bumblebee sting
- Fire-ant sting
- Honey bee sting
- Hornet sting
- Scorpion bite
- Tarantula bite
- Tick bite
- Wasp sting
- Yellow jacket sting

Choosing And Using Insect Repellents ✔ Quick Tip

Insect repellents are available in various forms and concentrations. Aerosol and pump-spray products are intended for skin applications as well as for treating clothing. Liquid, cream, lotion, spray, and stick products enable direct skin application. Products with a low concentration of active ingredient may be appropriate for situations where exposure to insects is minimal. Higher concentration of active ingredient may be useful in highly infested areas or with insect species that are more difficult to repel. And where appropriate, consider nonchemical ways to deter biting insects—screens, netting, long sleeves, and slacks.

The Environmental Protection Agency (EPA) recommends the following precautions when you are using insect repellents:

- Apply repellents only to exposed skin and or clothing (as directed on the product label). Do not use under clothing.
- Never use repellents over cuts, wounds, or irritated skin.
- Do not apply to eyes and mouth, and apply sparingly around ears. When using sprays, do not spray directly onto face; spray on hands first and then apply to face.
- Do not allow children to handle the products, and do not apply to children's hands. When using on children, apply to your own hands and then put it on the child.

Insect Bites And Stings

Symptoms

Symptoms vary according to insect and individual, but may include:

- Bite, sting, or wound
- Localized pain, redness, swelling, or itching
- Burning, numbness, or tingling
- Rash
- Difficulty breathing
- Coughing or wheezing
- Nausea or vomiting
- Headache

- Do not spray in enclosed areas. Avoid breathing a repellent spray, and do not use it near food.

- Use just enough repellent to cover exposed skin and clothing. Heavy application and saturation is generally unnecessary for effectiveness. If biting insects do not respond to a thin film of repellent, then apply a bit more.

- After returning indoors, wash treated skin with soap and water or bathe. This is particularly important when repellents are used repeatedly in a day or on consecutive days. Also, wash treated clothing before wearing it again. If you suspect that you are reacting to an insect repellent, discontinue use, wash treated skin, and then call your local poison control center. If you go to a doctor, take the repellent with you.

You can get specific medical information about the active ingredients in repellents and other pesticides by calling the National Pesticide Information Center (NPIC) at 800.858.7378. NPIC operates from 6:30 a.m. to 4:30 p.m. (Pacific Time), 9:30 a.m. to 7:30 p.m. (Eastern Time), seven days a week. The NPIC Web site is http://npic.orst.edu/.

Source: "How To Use Insect Repellents Safely," Office of Pesticide Programs, Environmental Protection Agency, http://www.epa.gov/pesticides/citizens/insectrp.htm, April 17, 2002.

Do Not

- Do *not* apply a tourniquet.

- Do *not* give the victim stimulants, aspirin, or other pain medication unless prescribed by the doctor.

- Do *not* allow the victim to exercise. If necessary, carry the victim to safety.

Call Your Health Care Provider If…

If the victim is having a severe reaction, or if the victim has been stung inside the mouth or throat, call immediately for emergency medical assistance.

First Aid

1. Check the victim's airway, breathing, and circulation. If necessary, begin rescue breathing and CPR.

2. Reassure the victim. Try to keep him or her calm, as anxiety will worsen the situation.

3. If the sting is from a honey bee, remove the stinger from the skin if it is still present. Carefully scrape the back of a knife or other thin straight-edged object across the stinger if the victim can remain still, and it is safe to do so. Otherwise, you can pull out the stinger with tweezers or your fingers, but avoid pinching the venom sac at the end of the stinger which will cause more venom to be released.

4. Wash the site thoroughly with soap and water.

5. Cover the site with a clean, cold compress or a clean, moist dressing to reduce swelling and discomfort.

6. Remove nearby rings and constricting items because the affected area may swell.

7. Give first aid for an allergic reaction, if necessary.

Insect Bites And Stings

8. If appropriate, treat the victim for signs of shock. Remain with the victim until medical help arrives.

9. Over the next 24 to 48 hours, observe the site for signs of infection (such as increasing redness, swelling, pain).

For Tick Bites

1. If a tick has bitten you and it is still attached, remove it. Grasp it close to its head or mouth with tweezers or with the fingernails, and pull it straight out with a slow and steady motion.

2. Clean the area thoroughly with soap and water.

3. Save the tick and watch carefully for the next week or two for signs of Lyme disease.

4. If all the parts of the tick cannot be removed, get medical help.

Prevention

- Avoid provoking insects, whenever possible.
- Avoid rapid, jerky movements around insect hives or nests.
- Wear light-colored clothing.
- Use appropriate insect repellents and/or protective clothing.
- Use caution when eating outdoors, especially with sweetened beverages or in areas around garbage cans which often attract bees.

Chapter 59

Itching

Alternative Names

Pruritus.

Definition

A peculiar tingling or uneasy irritation of the skin which causes a desire to scratch the affected part.

Considerations

Itching can be all over (generalized) or only in a particular location (localized).

There are many causes of itching, ranging from the simple to the complex. Some groupings would include:

- Localized itching
    - ◊ Skin irritation from insect bites and stings
- Localized or generalized
    - ◊ Chemical irritation, such as from poison ivy or stinging nettle

About This Chapter: © 2002 A.D.A.M., Inc. Reprinted with permission.

- ◊ Environmental causes (drying, sunburn)
- ◊ Hives (localized to general)
- ◊ Parasites (body lice, head lice, pubic lice)
- Generalized
  - ◊ Infectious diseases (chickenpox)
  - ◊ Allergic reactions
  - ◊ Kidney disease
  - ◊ Liver disease with jaundice
  - ◊ Medication reactions

Common Causes

- Insect bites
- Dry skin
- Contact dermatitis (poison ivy or poison oak)
- Contact irritants (such as soaps, chemicals, or wool)
- Atopic dermatitis
- Rashes (may or may not itch)
- Childhood infections (such as chickenpox or measles)
- Aging skin
- Allergy caused by food or drugs (antibiotics)
- Superficial skin infections, such as folliculitis and impetigo
- Pregnancy
- Hepatitis
- Iron deficiency anemia
- Parasites such as pinworm
- Pityriasis rosea
- Psoriasis
- Seborrheic dermatitis

> **Weird Words**
>
> Folliculitis: Inflammation of the hair follicles.
>
> Pityriasis rosea: A widespread, usually mild, itchy rash, most common in individuals between the ages of 10 and 35, that has no known cause and goes away on its own.
>
> Urticaria: The medical term for hives.
>
> Source: Adapted from *Stedman's Medical Dictionary, 27th Edition*, © 2000. Lippincott Williams, and Wilkins. All rights reserved. Reprinted with permission.

Itching

- Urticaria
- Drugs such as antibiotics (penicillin, sulfonamides), gold, griseofulvin, isoniazid, opiates, phenothiazines, or vitamin A

Home Care

For persistent or severe itching, have the dermatologist (a specialist in skin disorders) make the precise diagnosis and prescribe specific treatment. In the meantime, there are some steps you can take to help deal with the itch:

- Avoid scratching or rubbing the itchy areas. Keep fingernails short to avoid skin damage from any unconscious scratching. Family members or friends may help call attention to subconscious scratching.
- Wear cool, light, loose bedclothes. Avoid wearing rough clothing, particularly wool, over an itchy area.
- Take lukewarm baths, using little soap and rinsing thoroughly. Try a skin-soothing oatmeal or cornstarch bath.
- Apply a soothing lotion after bathing to soften and cool the skin.
- Apply cold compresses to an itchy area.
- Avoid prolonged exposure to excessive heat and humidity.
- Take up an enjoyable hobby that distracts from the itching during the day and makes you tired enough to sleep at night.
- Try over-the-counter oral antihistamines such as diphenhydramine (Benadryl®).
- Try over-the-counter hydrocortisone cream.

When To Call Your Health Care Provider

- If itching is associated with other unexplained symptoms
- If itching is severe, prolonged, or cannot be easily explained

The medical history will be obtained and a physical examination performed. Medical history questions documenting itching in detail may include:

- Time pattern
    - How long have you had this itch?
    - Does it itch all the time?
    - Does it seem to get worse?
    - Has it spread?
- Aggravating or triggering factors
    - What do you think caused this itch?
    - Have you ever had this kind of itch before? What caused it then?
    - Do you recall any irritant that you recently came in contact with?
    - Do you have any allergies or sensitivities?
    - What medications are you taking?
    - Have you started using any new products recently? What was it? Have you used any new soaps, fabric softeners, perfumes, deodorants, fabrics (wool), chemicals?
    - Have you been around animals?
    - Have you eaten shellfish or nuts recently?
    - Have you had insect bites recently?
    - Do you use lotions on your skin?
    - Have you been in the sun recently?
- Location
    - What part of your body itches?
    - Is it all over your body (generalized itch)?
    - Is the itch limited to a specific area? What area?
- Quality
    - What does the skin that itches look like?
    - Is there a rash?

Itching

◊ Are there blisters?

◊ Are there scales?

- Other

    ◊ Are you being treated for other medical conditions?

    ◊ What other symptoms do you have?

If there is no localized infection or skin lesion, then diagnostic studies such as blood tests, skin biopsies, or x-rays will focus on finding a systemic (whole body) cause.

Prescribed medications may include topical corticosteroids, antihistamines, or tranquilizers.

> ♣ **It's A Fact!!**
>
> Most itching does not require medical evaluation. Attempts should be made to rule out the obvious causes of itching. It is sometimes easy for a parent to discern the cause of a child's itching. Usually a simple visual examination will demonstrate the presence of bites, stings, rashes, dry skin, or irritation. Often the cause of itching is fairly obvious, such as a mosquito bite.
>
> Recurrent itching without obvious cause, total body itching, and recurrent hives are all indications that the itching should be evaluated as soon as possible. It may be a symptom of an underlying disease or condition.

Part 7
Additional Help And Information

Chapter 60
Directory of Skin-Related Resources

American Academy of Allergy, Asthma, and Immunology
611 East Wells Street
Milwaukee, WI 53202
Phone: (414) 272-6071
Website: http://www.aaaai.org

American Academy of Dermatology
P.O. Box 4014
Schaumburg, IL 60168
Phone: (847) 330-0230
Toll Free: (888) 462-DERM (3376)
Fax: (847) 330-0050
Website: http://www.aad.org

American Academy of Family Physicians
11400 Tomahawk Creek Parkway
Leawood, KS 66211-2672
Website: http://familydoctor.org
E-Mail: mail@familydoctor.org

American College of Allergy, Asthma, and Immunology
85 Algonquin Road, Suite 550
Arlington Heights, IL 60005
Website: http://www.allergy.mcg.edu/home.html
E-Mail: mail@acaai.org

About This Chapter: Information in this chapter was compiled from many sources deemed accurate; inclusion does not constitute endorsement. All contact information verified in December 2002.

American College of Foot and Ankle Surgeons
515 Busse Highway
Park Ridge, IL 60068
Phone: (847) 292-2237
Toll Free: (800) 421-2237
Website: http://www.acfas.org/index.shtml
E-Mail: mail@acfas.org

American Lyme Disease Foundation, Inc.
Mill Pond Offices
293 Route 100, Suite 204
Somers, NY 10589
Toll Free: 800-876-LYME
Phone: (914) 277-6970
Fax: (914) 277-6974
Website: http://www.aldf.com
E-Mail: inquire@aldf.com

American Podiatric Medical Association
9312 Old Georgetown Road
Bethesda MD 20814
Phone: (301) 571-9200
Toll Free: (800) ASK-APMA
Fax: (301) 530-2752
Website: http://www.apma.org

American Society for Dermatologic Surgery
5550 Meadowbrook Drive, Suite 120
Rolling Meadows, IL 60008
Phone: (847) 956-0900
Toll Free: (800) 441-2737
Fax: (847) 956-0999
Website: http://www.asds-net.org
E-Mail: info@aboutskinsurgery.com

Center for Young Women's Health
Children's Hospital Boston
333 Longwood Avenue
Boston, MA 02115
Phone: (617) 355-2994
Fax: (617) 232-3136
Website: http://www.youngwomenshealth.org
E-Mail: cywh@tch.harvard.edu

Centers for Disease Control
1600 Clifton Road
Atlanta, GA 30333
Toll Free: (800) 311-3435
Phone: (404) 639-3311
Website: http://www.cdc.gov

Federal Trade Commission
CRC-240
Washington, DC 20580
Phone: (202) 326-2222
Website: http://www.ftc.gov

Directory of Skin-Related Resources 405

Food and Drug Administration
5600 Fishers Lane
Rockville, MD 20857-0001
Toll Free: (888) INFO-FDA (463-6332)
Website: http://www.fda.gov

Healthlink
Office of Clinical Informatics
Medical College of Wisconsin
9200 West Wisconsin Avenue, Suite 2997
Milwaukee, WI 53226
Phone: (414) 805-6337
Fax: (414) 805-6337
Website: http://healthlink.mcw.edu
E-Mail: healthlink@mcw.edu

Lyme Disease Foundation
One Financial Plaza, 18th Floor
Hartford, CT 06103
Toll Free: (800) 886-LYME
Phone: (860) 525-2000
Fax: (860) 525-TICK
Website: http://www.lyme.org
E-Mail: lymefnd@aol.com

National Alopecia Areata Foundation
P.O. Box 150760
San Rafael, CA 94915-0760
Phone: (415) 472.3780
Fax: (415) 472.5343
Website: http://www.naaf.org/default2.asp
E-Mail: info@naaf.org

National Arthritis and Musculoskeletal and Skin Diseases Information Clearinghouse
National Institutes of Health
1 AMS Circle
Bethesda, MD 20892-3675
Toll Free: (877) 22-NIAMS (226-4267)
Phone: (301) 495-4484
TTY: (301) 565-2966
Fax: (301) 718-6366
Website: http://www.niams.nih.gov/hi/index.htm

National Cancer Institute
6116 Executive Boulevard, MSC8322
Suite 3036A
Bethesda, MD 20892-8322
Toll Free:(800) 4-CANCER or (800) 422-6237
Website: http://www.cancer.gov

National Eczema Association
6600 SW 92nd Ave
Suite 230
Portland, OR 97223-0704
Toll Free: (800) 818.7546
Phone: (503) 228-4430
Fax: (503) 224.3363
Website: http://www.nationaleczema.org
E-Mail: info@nationaleczema.org

National Vitiligo Foundation
611 South Fleishel Avenue
Tyler, TX 75701
Phone: (903) 531-0074
Fax: (903) 525-1234
Website: http://www.nvfi.org
E-Mail: vitiligo@trimofran.org

National Vulvodynia Association
P.O. Box 4491
Silver Spring, MD 20914-4491
Phone: (301) 299-0775
Fax: (301) 299-3999
Website: http://www.nva.org

Nemours Foundation
12735 West Gran Bay Parkway
Jacksonville, FL 32258
Phone and Fax: (904) 288-5750
Website: http://www.nemours.org

Skin Cancer Foundation
245 Fifth Avenue, Suite #1403
New York, NY 10016
Toll Free: (800) SKIN-490
Fax: (212) 725-5751
Website: http://www.skincancer.org
E-Mail: info@skincancer.org

Virtual Hospital
University of Iowa Health Care
200 Hawkins Drive
Iowa City, IA 52242
Toll Free: (800) 777-8442
Website: http://www.vh.org

Chapter 61

Suggested Reading For Skin-Related Concerns

Balin, Arthur K., Loretta Pratt-Balin, and Marietta Whittlesey. *The Life of the Skin*. New York: Bantam Books, 1997.

Barbour, Alan G., M.D. *Lyme Disease: The Cause, the Cure, the Controversy*. Baltimore: Johns Hopkins University Press, 1996.

Bark, Joseph P. *Skin Secrets: A Complete Guide to Skin Care for the Entire Family*. New York: McGraw-Hill, 1987.

Bark, Joseph P. *Your Skin: An Owner's Guide*. Englewood Cliffs, N.J.: Prentice-Hall, 1995.

Begoun, Paula. *The Beauty Bible: From Acne to Wrinkles and Everything in Between: Every Woman's Skin-Care and Make-up Application Guide*. Seattle: Beginning Press, 1997.

Boyd, Alan S. *The Skin Sourcebook*. Los Angeles: Lowell House, 1998.

Brumberg, Elaine. *Save Your Money, Save Your Face: What Every Cosmetics Buyer Needs to Know*. New York: Facts on File, 1986.

Brumberg, Elaine. *Take Care of Your Skin*. New York: Harper & Row, 1989.

Callan, Annette. *Skin Wise: A Guide to Healthy Skin for Women*. Melbourne, New York: Oxford University Press, 1995.

Camphausen, Rufus C. *Return of the Tribal: A Celebration of Body Adornment: Piercing, Tattooing, Scarification, Body Painting.* Rochester, Vt.: Park Street Press, 1997.

Cram, David L. *Coping with Psoriasis: A Patient's Guide to Treatment.* Omaha, Neb.: Addicus Books, 2000.

Delio, Michelle. *Tattoo: The Exotic Art of Skin Decorations.* New York: St. Martin's Press, 1994.

Fornay, Alfred. *The African American Woman's Guide to Successful Make-Up and Skin Care.* Los Angeles: Amber Books, 1998.

Gelman, Amy. *The Buzz on Beauty: A Girl's Guide to Looking and Feeling Your Best.* New York: Rosen Publishing Group, 1999.

Goldstein, Beth G., and Adam O. Goldstein. *Practical Dermatology.* Second edition. St. Louis: Mosby, 1997.

Goodman, Thomas, and Stephanie Young. *Smart Face: A Dermatologist's Guide to Saving Your Money and Saving Your Skin.* New York: Prentice Hall, 1988.

Hauser, Susan. *Nature's Revenge: The Secrets of Poison Ivy, Poison Oak, and Poison Sumac and Their Remedies.* New York: Lyons & Burford, 1996.

Inlander, Charles B., and Janet Worsley Norwood. *Skin: Head-to-Toe Tips for Health and Beauty.* New York: Walker, 1998.

Kent, Barney. *Saving Your Skin: Early Detection, Treatment, and Prevention of Melanoma and Other Skin Cancers.* New York: Four Walls Eight Windows, 1994.

Lane, I. William, and Linda Comac. *The Skin Cancer Answer.* Garden City, N.Y., 1999.

Lang, Denise V., with Joseph Territo. *Coping with Lyme Disease: A Practical Guide to Dealing with Diagnosis and Treatment.* New York: Henry Holt, 1997.

Leffell, David J. *Total Skin: The Definitive Guide to Whole Skin Care for Life.* New York: Hyperion, 2000.

Suggested Reading For Skin-Related Concerns

Litt, Jerome Z. *Your Skin: From Acne to Zits.* New York: Dembner Books, 1989.

Mackie, Rona M. *Clinical Dermatology: An Illustrated Textbook.* Third edition. Oxford and New York: Oxford University Press, 1991.

Mifflin, Margot. *Bodies of Subversion: A Secret History of Women and Tattoo.* New York: Juno Books, and St. Paul, Minn.: Consortium, 1997.

Miller, Jean-Chris. *The Body Art Book: A Complete Illustrated Guide to Tattoos, Piercings, and Other Body Modifications.* New York: Berkley Books, 1997.

Mindell, Earl, with Virginia L. Hopkins. *Dr. Earl Mindell's What You Should Know About Beautiful Hair, Skin, and Nails.* New Canaan, Conn.: Keats Publishing, 1996.

Montagna, William, Albert M. Kligman, and Kay S. Carlisle. *Atlas of Normal Human Skin.* New York: Springer-Verlag, 1992.

Peiss, Kathy Lee. *Hope in a Jar: The Making of America's Beauty Culture.* New York: Metropolitan Books, 1998.

Reybold, Laura. *Everything You Need to Know About the Dangers of Tattooing and Body Piercing.* New York: Rosen Publishing Group, 1998.

Robins, Perry, and Maritza Perez. *Understanding Melanoma: What You Need to Know.* New York: Skin Cancer Foundation, 1996.

Sacks, Stephen L. *The Truth About Herpes.* West Vancouver and Seattle: G. Soules Book Publishers, 1988.

Sadick, Neil S., Donald Charles Richardson, and the editors of Consumer Reports Books. *Your Hair: Helping to Keep It: Treatment and Prevention of Hair Loss for Men and Women.* Yonkers, N.Y.: Consumer Reports Books, 1991.

Siegel, Mary-Ellen. *Safe in the Sun.* New York: Walker, 1990.

Silverstein, Alvin, Virginia, and Robert. *Overcoming Acne: The How and Why of Healthy Skin Care.* New York: Morrow Junior Books, 1990.

Stoll, David, M.D. *A Woman's Skin.* New Brunswick, N.J.: Rutgers University Press, 1994.

Thompson, Wendy J. A., and Jerry Shapiro. *Alopecia Areata: Understanding and Coping with Hair Loss.* Baltimore: Johns Hopkins University Press, 1996

Turkington, Carol, and Jeffrey S. Dover. *Skin Deep: An A–Z of Skin Disorders, Treatments, and Health.* Updated edition. New York: Facts On File, 1998.

Vanderhoof-Forschner, Karen. *Everything You Need to Know About Lyme Disease and Other Tick-Borne Disorders.* New York: John Wiley, 1997.

Walzer, Richard A., and the editors of Consumer Reports Book. *Treating Acne.* Yonkers, N.Y.: Consumer Reports Books, 1992.

Winter, Ruth. *A Consumer's Dictionary of Cosmetic Ingredients.* New York: Three Rivers Press, 1999.

Index

Index

Page numbers that appear in *Italics* refer to illustrations. Page numbers that have a small 'n' after the page number refer to information shown as Notes at the beginning of each chapter. Page numbers that appear in **Bold** refer to information contained in boxes on that page (except Notes information at the beginning of each chapter).

A

Abreva (docosanol) 304
Accutane (isotretinoin) 141–42, **170**, 175–84, **176**
acetone 164–65
acetonitrile 106
Achromycin (tetracycline hydrochloride) 372
acitretin 274
acne (acne vulgaris)
   causes 138–39, **176**
   described 11
   over the counter medications 163–65
   overview 135–45
   prescription medications 167–74
   psychological effects 147–50
   research 144–45
   scars 143, 151–58, 185–87
   skin care 143–44
"Acne Scarring" (American Academy of Dermatology) 151n
acral lentiginous melanoma
   described 239
   see also melanoma
actinic keratosis 206
active ingredient, described 27
acyclovir 303
A.D.A.M., Inc., skin publications 15n

adapalene 140, 170
adrenocortical insufficiency, vitiligo 286
aeroallergens, described 256–57
age spots *see* benign solar lentigo
Agin, Patricia 218
alcohol
   acne 164–65
   blushing 20
   cosmetics 35
alcohol-free, described 31
Aldactone (spironolactone) 143
allergens
   atopic dermatitis 254–57
   defined **248**
allergic contact dermatitis
   described 34
allergic contact eczema
   described **250**
allergic urticaria 325
allergies
   body piercings 68
   cercarial dermatitis 327
   cosmetics 28–30
   hair dye 111–12
   nail products 99, 105–6
   tattoos 76–77
   urushiol 320

alopecia
  defined **118**
  described 12
  tattoos 76
  see also hair loss
alopecia areata
  defined **118**
  described 119
  overview 347–53
  vitiligo 286
alopecia totalis, described 347
alopecia universalis, described 347
alpha hydroxy acids 40
American Academy of Allergy, Asthma, and Immunology, contact information 403
American Academy of Dermatology
  contact information 403
  publications
    acne causes 151n
    acne medications 167n
    acne scars 151n
    acne treatments 163n
    birthmarks 47n
    hair concerns 113n
    skin care problems 33n
American Academy of Family Physicians, contact information 403
American College of Allergy, Asthma, and Immunology
  contact information 403
  urticaria publication 323n
American College of Foot and Ankle Surgeons
  contact information 404
  nail disorders publication 335n
American Lyme Disease Foundation, Inc., contact information 404
American Podiatric Medical Association, contact information 404
American Society for Dermatological Surgery (ASDS), publications
  chemical peels 185n
  skin cancer 227n
American Society for Dermatologic Surgery, contact information 404
anabolic steroids, acne 159–60
androgen
  acne 142
  defined **137**

androgenetic alopecia, described 119
angel's kisses *see* birthmarks; macular stains
angioedema, defined **160**
animal bites, described 381–85
anorexia, defined **118**
anthralin 270–71, 350–51
antiandrogen medications, acne 173
antibiotic medications
  acne 140, 141, 167–68
  atopic dermatitis 259
  burns 366
  cat scratch disease 314
  defined **370**
  described 369–75
  impetigo 316
  Lyme disease 307–8
  psoriasis 274
antibodies, defined **286**
antiepileptic medications, acne 161
antihistamines
  atopic dermatitis 259
  urushiol 322
antimicrobial medications
  defined **370**
  described 369–3707
antiperspirants 37
antiseptic medications
  defined **370**
  described 369–70, 375–76
antituberculosis medications, acne 161
antiviral medications 303
apocrine glands
  defined **8**
  described 7
apoptosis, described 271
Armstrong, Myrna L. **82**
Arnonette, Rex 217
Aropax (paroxetine) **150**
arthritis, Lyme disease 307
arthrocentesis, described 308
artificial nails
  infections 103–4
  precautions **105**
artificial tanning 204–5
ASDS *see* American Society for Dermatological Surgery
asteatosis, defined **16**
astringents, described 35
ateatosis *see* dry skin

Index

athlete's foot *see* tinea pedis
atopic
  defined **248**
  described 247
atopic dermatitis
  described 10, 247–49, **250**
  quality of life 261–62
  research 263–66
  skin features 251
  stages 251–52
  symptoms 249–51
  treatment 257–61
  see also eczema
atrophic macules, described 155
atypical nevi 44
  see also moles
Aureomycin (chlortetracycline hydrochloride) **372**
Aurorix (moclobemide) **150**
autoimmune disease
  alopecia areata 119
  defined **268**
  psoriasis 268
autoimmune diseases
  alopecia areata 348
  vitiligo 286
autologous fat transfer, described 156
autologous melanocyte transplants, vitiligo 293
autologous skin grafts, vitiligo 292
Aveeno 322
avobenzone 35
azelaic acid **42**, 140, 168

B

baciguent (bacitracin) **372**
Bacitracin 357
bacitracin 371, **372**, 373
Bailey, John E., Jr. 25–26, 32, **100,** 106, 124–25, 205
baldness *see* alopecia
Barrett, Stephen 65
Barsky, S. 78
Bartonella henselae 312
basal cell carcinoma
  described 191, 222, 227
  sunscreen 211

Begoun, Paula 29–30
Beitz, Julie 183
Bell's palsy 307
Benadryl 322
benign solar lentigo, described 41–42
Benoquin (monobenzone) 292
bentoquatam 321
benzalkonium chloride 375
benzethonium chloride 375
benzocaine 304
benzoyl peroxide
  acne 140, 144
  described 163, **164**
beta blockers
  hair loss 120
  psoriasis 268
beta hydroxy acid 40
betamethasone dipropionate **282**
bioflavinoids 58
biopsy
  atopic dermatitis 252
  described 235
  psoriasis 268
  sebaceous cysts 296
birthmarks, overview 47–52
blue nevi 43
  see also moles
blushing, described 19–21
bodybuilding, stretch marks 53
body piercing
  complications 92
  described 86–87
  healing process 95–98
  healing times **69, 87**
  history 81–83
  overview 67–74
  risks 83
  site care 89–97
"Body Piercing: Cleaning and Healing" (University of California at Berkeley) 95n
body wrap shops 57–58
Borrelia burgdorferi 305
bromine 162
Bronson, D. M. 78
bronzers, described 205, **215**
Brooks, Traci 74
Brown, Trudy 128–29
"Brown Spots and Freckles" (New Zealand Dermatological Society) 41n

bruises, descibed 377–80
bulimia, defined **118**
burns, overview 365–67

C

calamine lotion 322
calcipotriene 270
calcium hydroxide 110
camouflage, tattoos 80
CamphoPhenique 304
camphor 304
camphorated metacresol 375
cancer
   hair dye **108**
   hair loss 121
   lichen sclerosis 283
   see also skin cancer
candidal dermatitis, described 11
cantharidin 298–99
canthaxanthin **214–15**
canthaxanthin retinopathy, described **215**
capillary hemangioma *see* port wine stains
carbolic acid 187
carcinoid syndrome, defined **20**
cataracts
   atopic dermatitis 252
   sun exposure 222
cat scratch disease, overview 311–14
cavernous hemangiomas, described 48
ceftriaxone 308
Ceilley, Roger 217
Cellanese 58–61
CelluLean 61–62
cellulite
   described **56**
   overview 55–65
"'Cellulite' Removers" (Quackwatch, Inc.) 55n
cellulitis
   described 10
   overview 275–77
Centers for Disease Control and Prevention (CDC)
   contact information 404
   publications
      cercarial dermatitis 327n
      skin cancer 191n

cercarial dermatitis (swimmer's itch)
   defined **328**
   overview 327–30
cheilitis, atopic dermatitis **254**
chemical burns 367
"Chemical Peeling" (ASDS) 185n
chemical peels
   acne 165, 185–87
   brown spots **42**
chemotherapy
   hair loss 120
   skin cancer treatment 228
   see also photochemotherapy
Chen, Joyce 319n
Chiang, J. K. 78
Children's Hospital of Boston, Center for Young Women's Health, contact information 67n, 404
chlortetracycline hydrochloride 371, **372**
cholinergic urticaria 325
"Choose Your Cover Skin Cancer Prevention Campaign: Questions and Answers" (CDC) 191n
Cibis, Gerhard 203
cinnamates 35
Cipramil (citalopram) **150**
citalopram **150**
"Clearing up Cosmetic Confusion" (FDA) 25n
clindamycin 140, 168
clobetasol propionate **282**
cloflucarban 375
Clomycin Cream (bacitracin-neomycin-polymyxin B) **372**
coal tar
   hair dye 111, **112**
   psoriasis 270–71, 272
   shampoos 344
cold-induced urticaria 325
cold sores, overview 301–4
"Cold Sores and Fever Blisters" (University of Arizona) 301n
collagen
   acne treatment 156
   defined **8**
   described 7
   stretch marks 53
   sun damage 219–20
colored cosmetics, skin problems 37–38

Index

comedo
  defined **137**
  depicted *136*
  described 137
compartment syndrome, described 379–80
compound nevi 43
  see also moles
compression, keloids 364
conditioners 37, 113–16
  see also hair
congenital, defined **43**
congenital pigmented nevi 43
  see also moles
contact dermatitis
  cosmetics 34
  described 10
  nail products 106
contact eczema, described **250**
contusions, described 377–80
Cooke, David A. 81n, **90**, 99n, 167n, **169**, 199n, 221n
cortex
  defined **114**
  described 6
corticosteroid medications
  acne 143, 160, 173
  atopic dermatitis 259–60
  hair loss 122
  hemangiomas 50
  lichen sclerosis **282**, 282–83
  psoriasis 269, 270
  urticaria 326
cortisone 308, 350, 351, 363
cosmeceuticals, described 40
cosmetics
  acne 144
  nail products 101–2
  overview 25–32
  port wine stains 51
  skin problems 33–40
  sunscreens **214**
  vitiligo 288, 293–94
cosmetic surgery, tattoos 78
Cosmetic Voluntary Registration Program 102
counseling
  atopic dermatitis 262
  depression **150**
  vitiligo 294
cruelty-free, described 31

cryosurgery, keloids 363
cryotherapy
  brown spots **42**
  defined **43**, **299**
  skin cancer treatment 228
cuticle
  defined **114**
  described 6
cuts, treatments 357–59
cyclosporine
  acne 161
  defined **160**
  eczema 260
  psoriasis 273
Cyr, Howard 204
cysts
  defined **296**
  described 138

D

dandruff *see* seborrheic dermatitis
Daniel, Ralph **100**
Denavir (penciclovir) 303
Dennie-Morgan fold, described 250
deodorants 37
depigmentation
  defined **286**
  vitiligo 286–87, 292
depilatories, described 124–25
depressed fibrotic scars, described 154
depression
  Accutane 181–82
  acne 149–50
  atopic dermatitis 262
  psoriasis 268
  vitiligo 288
dermabrasion, described 79, 92, 143, 156–57
dermatitis
  defined **36**, **248**
  described 10, 247, **250**
dermatologists
  acne 139
  atopic dermatitis 248, 253
  chemical peels 185
  cosmeceuticals 40
  cosmetics 33
  defined **230**

dermatologists, continued
  hemangiomas 49–50
  lichen sclerosis 284
  melanoma 235
  stretch marks 54
dermis
  defined **8**
  depicted *5*
  described 6
dermographism
  defined **324**
  described 325
dFA *see* fluorescent antibody test
DHA *see* dihydroxyacetone
Diabinese 20
diet and nutrition
  atopic dermatitis 255–56
  hair loss 120–21, 122
  oily skin 15
diflorasone diacetate **282**
dihydroxyacetone (DHA) 205, **215**
dinitrochlorobenzene (DNCB) 351
diphencyprone (DPCP) 351
Diprolene 270
DMDM hydantoin 35
DNCB *see* dinitrochlorobenzene
docosanol 304
Dopress (dothiepin) **150**
dothiepin **150**
double-blind study, described **61**
Dovonex (calcipotriene) 270
doxycycline 140, 171
DPCP *see* diphencyprone
Draelos, Zoe Diana 113–16
Drake, Lynn 119
dry skin
  described 15–17
  home remedies **17**
  see also skin
D-TAG program **90**
dust mites, atopic dermatitis 257
  see also scabies
dyshidrotic eczema, described **250**
dysmorphic acne, described 150
dysplastic nevi
  characteristics **232**
  defined **230**
  described 229–30
  see also moles

E

eccrine glands
  defined **8**
  described 7
eczema
  defined **248**
  described **250**
  overview 247–66
  see also atopic dermatitis
eflorintine cream 125–26
eicosapentaenoic acid 265
elastin
  defined **8**
  described 7
electrical burns 367
electrical muscle stimulators (EMS) 56–57
electric epilators 127–30
electrolysis
  hair removal 127
  moles **44**
Endermologie 62–63
Environmental Protection Agency (EPA), insect repellent safety publication 391n
eosinophils 254
ephilides 41–42
epidermal cells, described 7
epidermal cyst *see* sebaceous cysts
epidermis
  defined **8**
  depicted *5*
  described 5, 250
epidermoid cyst *see* sebaceous cysts
epilatory waxes 126–27
epinephrine 326
Erysipelothrix rhusiopathiae 276
erythema migrans
  depicted *306*
  described 306–7
erythrodermic psoriasis, described 269
erythromycin 140, 168, 171
estrogen 172
ethyl alcohol 375–76
ethyl methacrylate 106
eucalyptol 375
evening primrose oil 59
excision, defined **296**

Index 419

excision biopsy
 defined **230**
 described 45
expiration date, described 31
extenders 205
eye cosmetics 37
eye damage
 cat scratch disease 312
 sun exposure 222–23
 vitiligo 285, 291

F

facial cosmetics 36
"Fact Sheet: Cercarial Dermatitis" (CDC) 327n
Fair Packaging and Labeling Act 26
famciclovir 303
Famvir (famciclovir) 303
Farley, Dixie 376
FDA *see* US Food and Drug Administration
Federal Trade Commission (FTC)
 cellulite-reducing products 63–64
 contact information 404
 indoor tanning publication 221n
Felten, Richard 130–31
fever blisters, overview 301–4
fibroblast, described 219
financial considerations
 body piercings 71–72
 tattoo removal 93
fingernails *see* nails
"Fingernails: Looking Good While Playing Safe" (FDA) 99n
fish oil 59
FK506 265
fluorescent antibody test (dFA) 384
fluorosalan 375
fluoxetine **150**
flushing, described 19–21
flutamine 173
follicles
 acne 135
 alopecia areata 347
 baldness 8
 defined **8**
 depicted *5*
 described 6, 117–18

follicles, continued
 hair removal 127
 sebaceous glands 7
follicular macular atrophy, described 155
folliculitis, defined **396**
Food, Drug, and Cosmetic (FD&C) Act 26
formaldehyde 35, 105
fragrance-free, described 31, 34
freckles 41–42
Freier, Pearl 111–12
FTC *see* Federal Trade Commission
Fucus vesiculosus 58
fungal infections
 nails 13, 103, 337–38
 skin 10–11
 tinea 331–34

G

GABS *see* group A beta-hemolytic streptococcus
genital warts 299–300
Ginko biloba 58
glaucoma, port wine stains 51
glomerulonephritis
 defined **316**
 described 317
glycerin 35
glycolic acid 40, 187
Goldstein, Norman 77
gonadotropin
 defined **160**
 described 159
Grace, Esterann 74
gramicidin 371
granulomas, tattoos 77
group A beta-hemolytic streptococcus (GABS) 315–17
guanidine carbonate 110
guttate psoriasis, described 269

H

Haemophilus influenzae 276
hair
 described 3–4, 6
 dyes 107–12

hair, continued
  maintenance 113–16
  melanin 8
  relaxing techniques 107–12
  see also conditioners
hair cosmetics 38–39
hair growth, described 8
"Hair Loss" (KidsHealth) 117n
hair loss, overview 117–22
  see also alopecia
hair removal, overview 123–31
"Hair Today, Gone Tomorrow" (FDA) 123n
Halber, Allen 80
halobetasol propionate **282**
halogenated, defined **160**
halogenated medications, acne 162
halo nevi 44
  see also moles
Halper, Allen 109, 112
Hamilton, Scott 204
"Handout on Health: Atopic Dermatitis" (NIAMS) 247n
Hauslaib, Lara 74
"Heading Off Hair-Care Disasters: Use Caution With Relaxers and Dyes" (FDA) 107n
Healthlink (Wisconsin), contact information 405
hemangiomas
  defined **50**
  described 48–51
hematoma
  described 378
  nails 338–39
  treatment 379
herbal products
  acne 165
  atopic dermatitis research 265
heredity
  acne 138
  alopecia areata 348
  atopic dermatitis 247, 249, 263
  body fat distribution **64**
  hair loss 119
  psoriasis 268
  vitiligo 286
herpes labialis, described 301–4
herpes simplex, described 11, 301

hexylresorcinol 375
Hill, Suzette 101
hirsutism, described 142, 173
histamine, urticaria 324
hives *see* urticaria
Honig, Peter 179, 182
hormones
  acne 159–60, 171–74
  androgen **137**, 142
  estrogen 172
  hair loss 119
  moles 234
  testosterone 159
"How To Use Insect Repellents Safely" (EPA) 391n
HPV *see* human papillomavirus
human papillomavirus (HPV)
  defined **299**
  warts **299**297
Hurricaine 304
Hydrea (hydroxyurea) 273
hydrocortisone 322
hydrogen peroxide 375
hydroquinone 292
hydroxy acids **42**
hydroxyurea 273
hyperlinear palms, atopic dermatitis **254**
hyperpigmented eyelids, described 250
hypersensitive reactions, antibiotics 373
hyperthyroidism, vitiligo 286
hypertrophic scars, described 153–54
  see also keloids
hypoallergenic
  defined **36**
  described 31

I

ice-pick scars, described 154
ichthyosis, atopic dermatitis **254**
IgE *see* immunoglobulin E
imidazolidinyl urea 35
immune system
  alopecia areata 348
  atopic dermatitis 264–65
  cellulitis 275
  cosmetics 33
  psoriasis 268, 272

Index

immunizations, tetanus 359, 366
immunoglobulin E (IgE)
  atopic dermatitis **254**, 264
  defined **248**
immunosuppresive drugs
  atopic dermatitis 260
  defined **248**
immunotherapy, described 351
impetigo
  versus cellulitis 275–77
  defined **316**
  described 10
  overview 315–17
"Impetigo" (Wisconsin Department of Health and Family Services) 315n
indoor tanning 204–5, 221–26
"Indoor Tanning" (FTC) 221n
infections
  atopic dermatitis 249, 251, 257, 258–59
  body piercing 67–69, **70**, 72–74, 83
  cellulitis 276–77
  fungus 332–33
  hair removal 128
  nail products 99, 103–4
  psoriasis 274
  skin 10–11
  tattoos 75, 76, 83, 86
  wounds 358–59
infestations, described 11
Ingram regime, described 272
ingrown nails
  described 12, 335–36
  treatment 341–42
inoculation lesion, described 311
insect bites, described 387–93
insect repellents **390–91**
in situ, described 237–38
interferon
  atopic dermatitis 264
  defined **299**
  wart removal 300
inverse psoriasis, described 269
iodine 58, 162, 375
iontophoresis devices 56–57
iron deficiency anemia, hair loss 121
irritant contact dermatitis, described 34
irritants, atopic dermatitis 254–55
isopropyl alcohol 375
isotretinoin 141–42, **149, 170,** 174

itching *see* pruritus
itch-scratch cycle, described 249, 254
Ivy Block 321

J

Jan, George 204
jock itch *see* tinea cruris
junctional nevi 43
  see also moles

K

Katz, Stephen 202
Kechijian, Paul **100**
"Keeping the Luster in Your Locks: The Four Most Common Hair Concerns" (American Academy of Dermatology) 113n
keloids
  acne 153, *154*, 158
  defined **363**
  overview 361–64
  tattoos 77
keratin
  defined **8**
  described 6, 8, 117–18
keratin cyst *see* sebaceous cysts
keratinization, described 8
keratinocytes
  defined **8**
  described 5, 137
keratosis, defined **186**
keratosis pilaris, atopic dermatitis 254
KidsHealth, publications
  hair loss 117n
  stretch marks 53n
Kurtzweil, Paula 106

L

labels
  Accutane 178–79, 181
  antibiotic medications **374**
  antimicrobial medications 370
  antiseptic medications 375–76

labels, continued
  cosmetics 25–27
  epilatory waxes 127
  hair relaxers 110
  sun protection factor 217–18
  tanning booths 223–24
lactic acid 187
Lambert, Lark 110–12
Lanabiotic (bacitracin-neomycin-polymyxin B) **372**
Langerhans cells, described 5
lanolin 35
lasers
  acne scars 143, 157
  brown spots **42**
  defined **130**
  hair removal 123, 130–31
  hemangiomas 51
  keloids 363
  nail removal 340
  port wine stains 52
  skin cancer treatment 228
  tattoo removal 79, 92–93
LEEP *see* loop electrosurgical excision procedure
lentigines, described 41–42
lentigo maligna, described 42, 238
  see also melanoma
lesions, psoriasis 269
Lewis, Carol 32
Ley, Ronald D. 210
lice, described 11
lichen sclerosis
  causes 281
  described 279–80, 283–84
  diagnosis 281
  symptoms 280
  treatment 281–83
lidocaine 304
lip cosmetics 38
Lipnicki, John 210, 213, 216
liquid nitrogen, wart removal 299, 300
lithium 161, 268
liver spots *see* benign solar lentigo
loop electrosurgical excision procedure (LEEP) 300
Love, Audrey 370, 373
Lucas, Lee 121
Lumpkins, Debbie 375–76

lunula
  defined **9**
  described 6
lupus, defined **118**
lye relaxers 110
Lyme disease
  described **388–89**
  overview 305–9
Lyme Disease Foundation, contact information 405

M

macular stains
  defined **50**
  described 48
macules, described **157**
magnetic resonance imaging (MRI), tattoos 77
makeup *see* cosmetics
malignant melanoma *see* melanoma
Marks, Robin 211, 213
matrix, described 6
Meadows, Michelle 112, 184
MED *see* minimal erythemal dose
"Medications That Cause Acne" (American Academy of Dermatology) 159n
Medi-Quick Triple Antibiotic (bacitracin-neomycin-polymyxin B) **372**
medulla
  defined **114**
  described 6
melanin
  brown spots **42**
  defined **9, 286**
  described 7, 237
melanocytes
  defined **9, 230**
  described 5, 7, 44, 235, 237
  vitiligo 285
melanocytic nevi 43
  see also moles
melanoma
  ABCDs, described 240
  causes 210
  characteristics 236
  defined **43, 230**
  depicted *241–42*

Index

melanoma, continued
  described 42, 222, 227, **228**, 230–31
  dysplastic nevi 230
  early detection 234–36
  overview 237–43
  prevention 233
  risk factors 231–33
  statistics 210, 213
  warning signs **243**
  see also skin cancer
meningitis 307
menthol 375
Merizzi, Gianfranco 58
Merthiolate 369
metastasis, defined **230**
meta tags, described 62–63
methotrexate 273
methylbenzethonium 375
methylchloroisothiazolinone 35
methyl methacrylate 105
methyl salicylate 375
microcomedo, depicted *136*
microdermabrasion, described 54, 143, 157
micropigmentation, vitiligo 293
  see also tattoos
Miller, Sharon 204, 213
Milstein, Stanley R. 124
mineral oil 35
minimal erythemal dose (MED), described 224–25
minocycline 140, 171
minoxidil 122, 350, 351
moclobemide **150**
MOHS micrographic surgery, described 228
moisturizers
  described 35
  psoriasis 271
"Moles" (New Zealand Dermatological Society) 41n
moles (nevi)
  ABCDs, described 240
  characteristics **232**
  depicted *241–42*
  overview 43–45, 229–36
  treatment **42**
monobenzone 292
monobenzylether 292
monocytes, atopic dermatitis 263

Moshell, Alan N. 184
MRI *see* magnetic resonance imaging
muscle stimulators 56–57
Myciguent Cream (neomycin sulfate) **372**
Mycitracin (bacitracin-neomycin-polymyxin B) **372**
myositis ossificans, described 380

N

NAAF *see* National Alopecia Areata Foundation
nail biting, described 12
nail cosmetics 39–40
"Nail Disorders and Treatments" (American College of Foot and Ankle Surgeons) 335n
nail growth, described 9
nail pitting, described 12
nail plate, defined **9**
nails
  described 4, 6
  disorders 12–13, 335–42
  safety concerns 99–106
Nash, Jay 218
National Alopecia Areata Foundation (NAAF)
  contact information 347n, 405
  described **352**
National Cancer Institute, contact information 405
National Eczema Foundation, contact information 406
National Institute of Arthritis and Musculoskeletal and Skin Diseases (NIAMS)
  contact information 405
  publications
    acne 135n
    atopic dermatitis 247n
    lichen sclerosis 279n
    psoriasis 267n
    vilitigo 285n
National Institutes of Health (NIH), moles publication 229n
National Pesticide Information Center (NPIC), contact information **391**
National Psoriasis Foundation Tissue Bank, contact information 274

National Vitiligo Foundation, contact information 406
National Vulvodynia Association, contact information 406
National Weather Service, Climate Prediction Center, Web site address **200**
natural, described 30–31
needle epilators 129–30
Nemours Foundation, contact information 406
Neomycin (neomycin sulfate) **372**
neomycin sulfate 371, **372**, 373
Neosporin (neomycin-polymixin B) **372**
nerves, depicted 5
neurodermatitis, described **250**
nevi *see* moles
nevus (nevi), defined **230**
nevus flammeus *see* port wine stains
New Zealand Dermatological Society, publications
  freckles 41n
  moles 41n
niacin 20
NIAMS *see* National Institute of Arthritis and Musculoskeletal and Skin Diseases
nipple eczema 252, **254**
nodular melanoma, described 239–40
  see also melanoma
nodules, described 138
nonacnegenic, defined **36**
nonallergic urticaria 325–26
noncomedogenic
  defined **36**, **137**
  described 144
noncomedogenic, described 31
NPIC *see* National Pesticide Information Center
nummular eczema, described **250**
nutrition *see* diet and nutrition

O

obesity, stretch marks 53
O'Connell, Kathy 177
oil glands, depicted 5
  see also sebaceous glands
"Oily Skin" (A.D.A.M., Inc.) 15n
oily skin, described 15
  see also skin
Orabase 304
Orajel 304
organic products, acne 165
"OTC Options: Help for Cuts, Scrapes, and Burns" (FDA) 369n
overgrown scar *see* keloids
"Over-the-Counter Products" (American Academy of Dermatology) 163n
oxytetracycline hydrochloride 371
ozone layer, ultraviolet rays 200

P

PABA esters 35
papilla, described 6
papillomavirus, described 11
papules, described 137
paraben 35
Parinaud oculoglandular syndrome 312
paronchia, described 13
paroxetine **150**
Pasteurella multocida 276
penciclovir 303
perifollicular elastolysis 155
peripheral neuropathy 307
permanent makeup *see* tattoos
permanent waving 39
pernicious anemia, vitiligo 286
personal care products, skin problems 36–37
petrolatum 35
phenol 187, 340, 375
phenoxyethanol 35
photoaging
  described 209–10
  sun exposure 220
photochemotherapy
  atopic dermatitis 260
  vitiligo 290–91
  see also chemotherapy
phototherapy
  atopic dermatitis 260
  defined **248**
  psoriasis 271–73
piercings *see* body piercing
pigmentation, defined **286**

Index

pigmented nevi 43
 see also moles
pilosebaceous units
 defined **137**
 depicted *136*
 described 135
pimples *see* acne
pityriasis rosea, defined **396**
Pityrosporum ovale 344
plaque psoriasis, described 268
plaques
 defined **268**
 described 267
podophyllin
 defined **299**
 described 300
poison ivy 319–22
"Poison Ivy, Poison Oak, and Poison Sumac" (Chen) 319n
poison oak 319–22
poison sumac 319–22
polymyxin B sulfate 371, 373
Polysporin (bacitracin zinc-polymixin B) **372**
pores, described 137
port wine stains
 defined **50**
 overview 51–52
postinflammatory pigmentation, described **157**
povidone-iodine 375
"The Power of Accutane: The Benefits and Risks of a Breakthrough Acne Drug" (FDA) 170n, 175n
"Prescription Medications" (American Academy of Dermatology) 167n
preservatives, cosmetics 34
pressure urticaria 325
prodromal symptoms, described 303
Propionibacterium acnes 137, 168
propylene glycol 35
Prothiaden (dothiepin) **150**
Prozac (fluoxetine) **150**
pruritus (itching)
 defined **16**
 overview 395–99
Pseudomonas 358
pseudoscars, described **157**
psoralen 260, 272, 290–91
Psorcon 270

psoriasis
 described 267
 diagnosis 268–69
 research 274
 treatment 269–74
psoriasis vulgaris 268
psoriatic arthritis, described 267
puncture wounds, treatment 357–59
pustular psoriasis, described 269
pustules, described 138
PUVA treatment
 described 272–73
 vitiligo 291
pyogenic granulomas, described 51
pyritione zinc 344

Q

Quackwatch, Inc., cellulite removers publication 55n
quaternium-15 35
"Questions and Answers About Acne" (NIAMS) 135n
"Questions and Answers About Lichen Sclerosis" (NIAMS) 279n
"Questions and Answers About Psoriasis" (NIAMS) 267n
"Questions and Answers About Vitiligo" (NIAMS) 285n

R

rabies, described 382–85
red face *see* blushing; flushing
remission, described 252
Reniers, Lynn 25
resorcinol 140, 164
retinal (vitamin A) 40
retinal damage, sun exposure 222
retinoic acid receptors, described 169
retinoids **42**, 140–41, 169–71, 270–71, 274
RICE formula, described **378**
ringworm *see* tinea capitis; tinea corporis; tinea unguium
Rocephin (ceftriaxone) 308
Ronsard, Nicole 55
root, defined **9**

rosacea, defined **20**
Ruffner, Brenda 126

S

SADBE *see* squaric acid dibutyl ester (SADBE)
Safer, Leslie F. 111
salabrasion, described 79, 92
salicylic acid 35, 40, 140, 164, 187, 271, 298, 344
scabies (dust mites), described 11
scarification, described 79
scarlet fever 317
scars, acne 143, 151–58, 185–87
 see also keloids
scrapes, treatments 357–59
scratches, animals 381
sebaceous cysts, overview 295–96
sebaceous glands
 defined **9**
 described 7, 135
seborrheic dermatitis (dandruff)
 described 10
 overview 343–45
seborrheic eczema, described **250**
sebum
 defined **9, 114**
 described 7, 135
Segal, Marian 131
selenium sulfide 344
shaft (hair)
 defined **9**
 described 8
shampoos 36, 344–45
 see also hair
shave biopsy
 defined **230**
 described 45
shelf life, described 31
Shiel, William C., Jr. 309
silicone 35
silicone sheeting, keloids 363
skin
 depicted 5
 disorders, described 10–13
 overview 3–13
 see also dry skin; oily skin

"Skin Blushing/Flushing" (A.D.A.M., Inc.) 19n
skin cancer
 described 11
 lichen sclerosis 283
 malignant melanoma 42
 self examination 234–35, **239**
 sun exposure 191–98
 symptoms **239**
 treatment 227–28
 see also cancer; melanoma
"Skin Cancer" (ASDS) 227n
Skin Cancer Foundation, contact information 406
"Skin Cancer: Preventing America's Most Common Cancer" (CDC) 191n
skin care products
 atopic dermatitis 258, 262
 described 33–40
 see also cosmetics
skin cleaners 36
"Skin-Dry" (A.D.A.M., Inc.) 15n
skin examinations, precancerous conditions 206
skin exfoliation, described 40
skin grafting, acne scars 158
skin grafts, vitiligo 292–93
skin type, sunburn **194**
social phobia, defined **149**
sodium hydroxide 110
sodium sulfonamide 168
soft scars, described 154
solar keratoses, described 42
solar urticaria 326
Solomon, Neil 55
"Solving Problems Related to the Use of Cosmetics and Skin Care Products" (American Academy of Dermatology) 33n
Soriatane (acitretin) 274
soya lecithin 59
SPF *see* sun protection factor
spironolactone 143, 173
squamous cell carcinoma
 described 191, 222, 227
 sunscreen 210
squaric acid dibutyl ester (SADBE) 351
staphylococcal infections
 cellulitis 275, 276
 described 10

Index

Staphylococcus aureus 315
stasis dermatitis, described **250**
static electricity 115
steroids
  erythrodermic psoriasis 269
  psoriasis 270
  seborrheic dermatitis 344
  stretch marks 53
  vitiligo 290
stork bites *see* birthmarks; macular stains
strawberry hemangiomas, described 48
streptococcal infections
  antibiotics 373
  cellulitis 276
  described 10
  psoriasis 274
Streptococcus pyogenes 315
stretch marks
  defined **54**
  described 53–54
striae cutis distensae, defined **54**
subcutaneous tissue
  defined **9**
  described 6
subungual hematoma, described 12
sulfonamide 168
sulfur 140, 164
sulfurated lime 164
sunburn 194–95, 209–10
sunglasses, ultraviolet rays 197–98, 203
sunless tanners, described **215**
sunlight
  brown spots **42**
  psoriasis 270
sun protection factor (SPF)
  described 193, 195–98, 202, **214**
  melanoma 233
  overview 216–17
sunscreens
  described 35–36, **214**
  overview 209–20
  statistics **212**
  tattoos 88–89
  ultraviolet rays 201–2
  vitiligo 293
"Sunscreens, Tanning Products, and Sun Safety" (USDA) 209n
suntan 194–95

superficial spreading melanoma, described 238
  see also melanoma
support groups, vitiligo 294
surgical procedures
  acne scars 156–58, 185–87
  autologous fat transfer 156
  keloids 363
  mole removal 44–45
  nail disorders 339–42
  port wine stains 52
  skin cancer treatment 228
  tattoo removal 79
  vitiligo 292
sweat glands
  depicted 5
  described 7
sweet clover extract 58
swimmer's itch *see* cercarial dermatitis

T

tanning *see* suntan
tanning accelerators, described **214**
tanning booths 204–5, 221–26
tanning pills, described 205, **214–15**
"Tattooing and Body Piercing: Decision Making for Teens" (University of Iowa) 81n, **90**
tattoos
  complications 91–92
  described 85–86
  history 81–83
  overview 75–80
  removal 83, 92–93
  risks 83
  site care 88–89
  vitiligo 293
"Tattoos and Permanent Makeup" (FDA) 75n
tazarotene 140, 171, 271
Tazorac (tazarotene) 271
T-cells
  described 268
  psoriasis 271
Telfa dressing 366
Temovate 270
temporary tattoos 80

testosterone 159
tests
    atopic dermatitis 252
    contusions 378
    cosmetic allergies **38**
    fungal infections 333
    Lyme disease 307
    rabies 384
    vitiligo 287–88
tetanus (lockjaw) 359, 366
tetracycline 140, 171, 304, 373
tetracycline hydrochloride 371, **372**
thimerisol 369
Thomas, Phaedra 74
Thompson, Larry 220
thymol 375
thymopentin 265
tinea, overview 331–34
tinea capitis (ringworm), described 12, 333
tinea corporis (ringworm), described 11, 332
tinea cruris (jock itch), described 333
tinea pedis (athlete's foot), described 11, 332
tinea unguium (ringworm), described 13, 332–33
titanium dioxide 36
toenails *see* nails
Toombs, Ella 77
toxic, defined **268**
Toxicodendron 319
traction alopecia, described 120
tretinoin 140, 144, 169
tribromsalan 375
trichloroacetic acid 187
trichoptilosis, defined **114**
trichotillomania
    defined **118**
    described 120
"Trying to Look SUNsational? Complexity Persists in Using Sunscreens" (FDA) 209n
tweezers epilators 129–30
tweezing, hair removal 126–27
tyrosine 205, **214**

U

ultrasound, cellulite 56
Ultravate 270
ultraviolet rays (UV)
    acne 165
    described 192–94
    hair 115–16
    overview 211–13
    psoriasis 271–73
    skin 4
    skin cancer 191–92
    sun protection factor 196
    suntans 199–200
    tanning booths 221–22
University of Arizona, cold sores publication 301n
University of California - Berkeley, body piercing publication 95n
University of Iowa, tattoos publication 81n, **90**
University of Iowa, Virtual Hospital, contact information 406
"Urticaria" (American College of Allergy, Asthma, and Immunology) 323n
urticaria (hives)
    defined **324**
    overview 323–26
urushiol 319–20
US Food and Drug Administration (FDA)
    Accutane information **180**
    contact information 405
    Office of Cosmetics and Colors, contact information **78**
    publications
        Accutane 170n, 175n
        cosmetics 25n
        fingernails 99n
        hair dyes 107n
        hair removal 123n
        skin injury medications 369n
        sun safety 209n
        tattoos 75n
UV *see* ultraviolet rays
UVB phototherapy 272
UV index, described 193–94, 200

V

vaccines, Lyme disease 308–9
valacyclovir 303
Valtrex (valacyclovir) 303

Index

varicella, described 11
vascular birthmarks *see* birthmarks
"Vascular Birthmarks" (American Academy of Dermatology) 47n
Vega, Amarilys 180
Vibramycin (doxycyline) 308
Virtual Hospital (Iowa), contact information 406
vitamin A (retinal; tretinoin) 40, 140, 169
vitamin C, brown spots **42**
vitamin D3 270
vitiligo
    coping strategies 288
    described 285–86
    diagnosis 287–88
    research 294
    symptoms 286–87
    tattoos 76
    treatment 288–94
Voorhees, John J. 219–20

W

Walker, Annette 77
warts, overview 297–300
Watson, Anthony 127, 129–30
waxing, hair removal 126–27
Wexler, Mona 127–28
"What Are Stretch Marks?" (KidsHealth) 53n
"What You Need To Know About Moles and Dysplastic Nevi" (NIH) 229n
"Why Acne Forms, and How Accutane Knocks It Out" (FDA) 175n
wigs, alopecia areata 353
Wilkin, Jonathan 181
winter itch *see* dry skin
Wisconsin Department of Health and Family Services, impetigo publication 315n
Wiskur, Lois 102
witch hazel 35
wounds, treatments 357–59
wrinkles 219–20

Z

Zilactin 304
zinc acetate 168
zinc oxide 36
zits *see* acne
Zovirax (acyclovir) 303
Zwerling, Charles 77

DATE DUE			

3 3396 02575396 6

616.5
SKI

Skin health
information for
teens : health tips
about dermatological

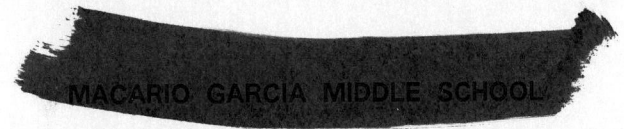

538655 07020   61783A   005